The Washington
Manual™ General
Internal Medicine
Consult

The Washington Manual™ General Internal Medicine Consult

Faculty Advisor
Thomas M. DeFer, M.D.
Assistant Professor of Medicine
Department of Internal Medicine
Washington University School of Medicine
Barnes-Jewish Hospital
St. Louis, Missouri

The Washington Manual™ General Internal Medicine Consult

Editors

Christopher H. Kwoh, M.D.
Nephrology Fellow
Former Internal Medicine Resident
Washington University School of Medicine
Barnes-Jewish Hospital
St. Louis, Missouri

Eric F. Buch, M.D.
Clinical Instructor
Department of Internal Medicine
Division of Hospital Medicine
Former Internal Medicine Resident
Washington University School of Medicine
Barnes-Jewish Hospital
St. Louis, Missouri

Jennifer M. Quartarolo, M.D.
Clinical Instructor
Department of Internal Medicine
Division of Hospital Medicine
Former Internal Medicine Resident
Washington University School of Medicine
Barnes-Jewish Hospital
St. Louis, Missouri

Series Editor

Tammy L. Lin, M.D.
Adjunct Assistant Professor of Medicine
Washington University School of Medicine
St. Louis, Missouri

Series Advisor

Daniel M. Goodenberger, M.D.
Professor of Medicine
Washington University School of Medicine
Chief, Division of Medical Education
Director, Internal Medicine Residency
Program
Barnes-Jewish Hospital
St. Louis, Missouri

 LIPPINCOTT WILLIAMS & WILKINS
A **Wolters Kluwer** Company
Philadelphia · Baltimore · New York · London
Buenos Aires · Hong Kong · Sydney · Tokyo

Acquisitions Editors: Danette Somers and James Ryan
Developmental Editors: Scott Marinaro and Keith Donnellan
Supervising Editor: Mary Ann McLaughlin
Production Editor: Brooke Begin, Silverchair Science + Communications
Manufacturing Manager: Colin Warnock
Cover Designer: QT Design
Compositor: Silverchair Science + Communications
Printer: RR Donnelley

© 2004 by Department of Medicine, Washington University School of Medicine

Printed in the USA

Library of Congress Cataloging-in-Publication Data

The Washington manual general internal medicine consult / editors, Christopher Kwoh, Eric
    Buch, Jennifer Quartarolo.
    p. ; cm. -- (The Washington manual subspecialty consult series)
    Includes bibliographical references and index.
    ISBN 0-7817-4369-9
    1. Internal medicine--Handbooks, manuals, etc. I. Kwoh, Christopher. II. Buch, Eric.
III. Quartarolo, Jennifer. IV. Title: General internal medicine consult. V. Series.
    [DNLM: 1. Internal Medicine--methods--Handbooks. WB 39 W3168 2003]
RC55.W367 2003
616--dc21

2003051677

10 9 8 7 6 5 4 3 2 1

Contents

*Denotes a "Top 25 consult."

Contributing Authors

Douglas R. Bree, M.D.

Cardiology Fellow
Former Internal Medicine Resident
Washington University School of
Medicine
St. Louis, Missouri

Eric F. Buch, M.D.

Clinical Instructor
Department of Internal Medicine
Division of Hospital Medicine
Former Internal Medicine Resident
Washington University School of
Medicine
Barnes-Jewish Hospital
St. Louis, Missouri

Michelle Cabellon, M.D.

Neurology Fellow
Former Internal Medicine Resident
Washington University School of
Medicine
St. Louis, Missouri

Rebecca Chandler, M.D.

Attending Physician
Internal Medicine
Washington University School of
Medicine
St. Louis, Missouri

Peter A. Crawford, M.D., Ph.D.

Cardiology Fellow
Former Internal Medicine Resident
Washington University School of
Medicine
St. Louis, Missouri

Thomas M. DeFer, M.D.

Assistant Professor of Medicine
Department of Internal Medicine
Washington University School of
Medicine
Barnes-Jewish Hospital
St. Louis, Missouri

Erik R. Dubberke, M.D.

Infectious Diseases Fellow
Former Internal Medicine Resident
Washington University School of
Medicine
Barnes-Jewish Hospital
St. Louis, Missouri

Elizabeth Friedman, M.D.

Fellow
Department of Internal Medicine
Division of Allergy and Immunology
Washington University School of
Medicine
St. Louis, Missouri

Evan D. Gross, M.D., M.S.

Nephrology Fellow
Former Internal Medicine Resident
Washington University School of
Medicine
Barnes-Jewish Hospital
St. Louis, Missouri

Barbara C. Jost, M.D.

Fellow
Department of Internal Medicine
Division of Allergy and Immunology
Washington University School of
Medicine
St. Louis, Missouri

Matthew J. Koch, M.D.

Instructor of Medicine
Division of Nephrology
Washington University School of
Medicine
Barnes-Jewish Hospital
St. Louis, Missouri

Christopher H. Kwoh, M.D.

Nephrology Fellow
Former Internal Medicine Resident
Washington University School of
Medicine
Barnes-Jewish Hospital
St. Louis, Missouri

Michael E. Lazarus, M.D.

Instructor of Medicine
Department of Internal Medicine
Division of Hospital Medicine
Washington University School of
Medicine
Barnes-Jewish Hospital
St. Louis, Missouri

Chris Leach, M.D.

Cardiology Fellow
Former Internal Medicine Resident
Washington University School of
Medicine
St. Louis, Missouri

Steven L. Leh, M.D.

Fellow
Department of Internal Medicine
Division of Pulmonary and Critical
Care
Former Internal Medicine Resident
Washington University School of
Medicine
Barnes-Jewish Hospital
St. Louis, Missouri

Ron Lubelchek, M.D.

Attending Physician
Former Internal Medicine Resident
Department of Internal Medicine
Washington University School of
Medicine
Barnes-Jewish Hospital
St. Louis, Missouri

Kyle C. Moylan, M.D.

Geriatrics Fellow
Division of Geriatrics and Nutrition
Science
Washington University School of
Medicine
Barnes-Jewish Hospital
St. Louis, Missouri

Jeanie Park, M.D.

Resident Physician
Department of Internal Medicine
Washington University School of
Medicine
Barnes-Jewish Hospital
St. Louis, Missouri

Jennifer M. Quartarolo, M.D.

Clinical Instructor
Department of Internal Medicine
Division of Hospital Medicine
Former Internal Medicine Resident
Washington University School of
Medicine
Barnes-Jewish Hospital
St. Louis, Missouri

Erin K. Quirk, M.D.

Clinical Fellow
Department of Internal Medicine
Division of Infectious Disease
Washington University School of
Medicine
Barnes-Jewish Hospital
St. Louis, Missouri

David Anand Rengachary, M.D.

Resident Physician in Neurology
Washington University School of
Medicine
Barnes-Jewish Hospital
St. Louis, Missouri

Michael J. Riley, M.D.

Resident Physician
Department of Internal Medicine
Washington University School of
Medicine
Barnes-Jewish Hospital
St. Louis, Missouri

Georges Saab, M.D.

Nephrology Fellow
Former Internal Medicine Resident
Department of Internal Medicine
Washington University School of
Medicine
Barnes-Jewish Hospital
St. Louis, Missouri

Rajesh Shah, M.D.

Gastroenterology Fellow
Former Internal Medicine Resident
Department of Medicine
Washington University School of
Medicine
St. Louis, Missouri

Aaron Shiels, M.D.

Gastroenterology Fellow
Former Internal Medicine Resident
Washington University School of
Medicine
St. Louis, Missouri

Rick Starlin, M.D.

Infectious Disease Attending
Former Infectious Disease Fellow
Former Chief Resident, Department
of Internal Medicine
Washington University School of
Medicine
Barnes-Jewish Hospital
St. Louis, Missouri

Stephen J. Wen, M.D.

Internal Medicine Hospitalist
St. John's Mercy Medical Center
Former Internal Medicine Resident
Barnes-Jewish Hospital
St. Louis, Missouri

Alan Zajarias, M.D.

Cardiology Fellow
Former Internal Medicine Resident
Washington University School of
Medicine
St. Louis, Missouri

Chairman's Note

Medical knowledge is increasing at an exponential rate, and physicians are being bombarded with new facts at a pace that many find overwhelming. The Washington Manual™ Subspecialty Consult Series was developed in this context for interns, residents, medical students, and other practitioners in need of readily accessible practical clinical information. They therefore meet an important unmet need in an era of information overload.

I would like to acknowledge the authors who have contributed to these books. In particular, Tammy L. Lin, M.D., Series Editor, provided energetic and inspired leadership, and Daniel M. Goodenberger, M.D., Series Advisor, Chief of the Division of Medical Education in the Department of Medicine at Washington University, is a continual source of sage advice. The efforts and outstanding skill of the lead authors are evident in the quality of the final product. I am confident that this series will meet its desired goal of providing practical knowledge that can be directly applied to improving patient care.

Kenneth S. Polonsky, M.D.
Adolphus Busch Professor
Chairman, Department of Medicine
Washington University
School of Medicine
St. Louis, Missouri

Series Preface

The Washington Manual™ Subspecialty Consult Series is designed to provide quick access to the essential information needed to evaluate a patient on a subspecialty consult service. Each manual includes the most updated and useful information on commonly encountered symptoms or diseases and highlights the practical information you need to gather before formulating a plan. Special efforts have been made to organize the information so that these guides will be valuable and trusted companions for medical students, residents, and fellows. They cover everything from questions to ask during the initial consult to issues in subsequent management.

One of the strengths of this series is that it is written by residents and fellows who know how busy a consult service can be, who know what information will be most helpful, and can detail a practical approach to patient care. Each volume is written to provide enough information for you to evaluate a patient until more in-depth reading can be done on a particular topic. Throughout the series, key references are noted, difficult management situations are addressed, and appropriate practice guidelines are included. Another strength of this series is that it was written in concert. All of the guides were designed to work together.

The most important strength of this series is the collection of authors, faculty advisors, and especially lead authors assembled to write this series. In addition, we received incredible commitment and support from our chairman, Kenneth S. Polonsky, M.D. As a result, the extraordinary depth of talent and genuine interest in teaching others at Washington University is showcased in this series. Although there has always been house staff involvement in editing The Washington Manual™ series, it came to our attention that many of them also wanted to be involved in writing and making decisions about what to convey to fellow colleagues. Remarkably, many of the lead authors became junior subspecialty fellows while writing their guides. Their desire to pass on what they were learning, while trying to balance multiple responsibilities, is a testament to their dedication and skills as clinicians, teachers, and leaders.

We hope this series fulfills the need for essential and practical knowledge for those learning the art of consultation in a particular subspecialty and for those just passing through it.

Tammy L. Lin, M.D., Series Editor
Daniel M. Goodenberger, M.D., Series Advisor

Preface

This book is a guide for the general internal medicine consult. It is intended to be used primarily by residents who are called on to do an inpatient consult, for students who work on an inpatient medicine service, and for specialists who seek information on general internal medicine management. We are hopeful that this is the first of many editions of the general internal medicine consult manual. As with other texts produced by our institution, we anticipate further improvement and maturation in subsequent editions of this manual. Comments from our readers on content selection and errata are, as always, greatly appreciated.

The manual is not meant to be an exhaustive or lengthy review of hospital medicine. The breadth of problems faced by today's hospitalist is enormous. It is therefore not possible to discuss all of the pertinent issues in a manual of this size. The topical content was chosen based on the 25 most common general internal medicine consults, as requested of the hospitalist service at the Barnes-Jewish Hospital of Washington University School of Medicine. These "Top 25" topics are indicated by asterisks in the Contents. This approach allows us to focus our content within the provided space. It has been a great challenge to provide adequate amounts of data and information, while still producing an efficient and readable clinical text of manageable size. We believe that we have accomplished this.

This manual is part of a series of subspecialty manuals published by Washington University and Lippincott Williams & Wilkins. The chapters are written primarily by residents, fellows, and attendings. Much of the material contained herein is adapted from chapters from other subspecialty manuals. The adaptations focus mainly on management issues, with additional material on the perioperative care of the patient with medical conditions. The chapters from the subspecialty manuals have also been made more concise for smooth review. There are also several specific chapters on certain common consult issues presented in this text that are not contained in the other manuals. In addition, we have included a section on the appropriate conduct and approach of a medical consultant. Further details on pathophysiology and more esoteric information on many of our topics may therefore be found in our companion texts.

Medical management is overflowing with discussion and debate; this is what allows our field to be both progressive and exciting. This also means that not all physicians agree on appropriate management in even the most commonly encountered clinical situations. The guidelines proposed here are either those followed by our own services or the most accepted approaches to management based on the available evidence. On topics of great debate, we have often chosen instead to present the appropriate clinical evidence and, when available, official guidelines advocated by major medical organizations. It is the role of the clinician to decide which evaluations and interventions are most appropriate.

Of great use to the reader is an appendix containing reviews of some of the most influential and most cited clinical trials, complete with details on trial design, results, and interpretation. In this age of evidence-based medicine, it is our aim to provide this detailed evidence at your fingertips for personal review and interpretation. In medical consultation, it is also valuable to include findings from clinical trials in consult notes and recommendations.

We would like to offer our thanks to all the contributing authors and editors for all of their hard work and diligence.

C.H.K.
E.F.B.
J.M.Q.

Key to Abbreviations

ABG	arterial blood gas
ACE	angiotensin converting enzyme
ACTH	adrenocorticotropic hormone
AIDS	acquired immune deficiency syndrome
ALT	alanine aminotransferase
ANA	antinuclear antibody
ANCA	antineutrophil cytoplasmic antibody
ASA	aspirin
AST	aspartate aminotransferase
BP	blood pressure
BUN	blood urea nitrogen
CBC	complete blood count
CK-MB	myocardial muscle creatine kinase isoenzyme
CMV	cytomegalovirus
CNS	central nervous system
COPD	chronic obstructive pulmonary disease
CPR	cardiopulmonary resuscitation
CSF	cerebrospinal fluid
CT	computed tomograph, -graphy
CVA	cardiovascular accident
DDAVP	desmopressin (deamino-8-D-arginine vasopressin)
DI	diabetes insipidus
DSM	*Diagnostic and Statistical Manual*
ECG	electrocardiogram, –graphic, –graphy
ER	emergency room
ESR	erythrocyte sedimentation rate
FEV_1	forced expiratory volume in 1 second
GERD	gastroesophageal reflux disease
GFR	glomerular filtration rate
GI	gastrointestinal
hCG	human chorionic gonadotropin
HEENT	head, ears, eyes, nose, and throat
HIV	human immunodeficiency virus
HSV	herpes simplex virus
HTN	hypertension
ICU	intensive care unit
INH	isoniazid
INR	international normalized ratio
ITP	idiopathic thrombocytopenic purpura
LMWH	low-molecular-weight heparin
LV	left ventricle
LVEF	left ventricular ejection fraction
LVH	left ventricular hypertrophy
MI	myocardial infarction
MRI	magnetic resonance imaging
NPO	nothing by mouth

NSAIDs	nonsteroidal antiinflammatory drugs
PCN	penicillin
PCR	polymerase chain reaction
PET	positron emission tomography
PT	prothrombin time
PTT	partial thromboplastin time
RBC	red blood cell
SBP	systolic blood pressure
SIADH	syndrome of inappropriate antidiuretic hormone secretion
SLE	systemic lupus erythematosus
SSRI	selective serotonin reuptake inhibitor
TB	tuberculosis
TCA	tricyclic antidepressant
TIA	transient ischemic attack
TMP-SMX	trimethoprim-sulfamethoxazole
TSH	thyroid-stimulating hormone
U/S	ultrasound
UNa	urinary sodium
UTI	urinary tract infection
$\dot{V}/\dot{Q}$	ventilation/perfusion
VDRL	Venereal Disease Research Laboratory
VZV	varicella-zoster virus
WBC	white blood cell

General Consultative Principles

Thomas M. DeFer

The inpatient general internal medicine consultation is essentially a service provided by internists (attending physicians, fellows, house officers, and students) to other noninternist physicians. Some of the strategies and politics of providing effective consultative services are unique. The physicians on other services are obviously not internists, and we should not expect them to behave as such. Their request for a consultation is a call for assistance with a problem(s) that they do not feel qualified to deal with on their own. Whereas an additional ill-formed consultative question on an already busy day may feel like a nuisance and more work to be done, it is better seen as an opportunity to assist a colleague in the care of a patient. Adhering to the "Ten Commandments for Effective Consultations" is especially good advice [1] (Table 1).

General surgery, subspecialty surgery, psychiatry, obstetrics and gynecology, neurology, and rehabilitation are common sources of consultations. The types of questions asked by these other services are often dictated by the characteristics of the patients on those services (Table 2)—for example, preoperative cardiovascular risk assessment of the general surgical patient, atrial fibrillation in the postoperative patient, routine management of diabetes in the psychiatric patient, and more comprehensive medical management of the rehabilitation patient. The expectations and needs of the requesting service also vary by service. Whereas surgeons tend to be single-problem oriented and want to maintain primary control, psychiatrists and rehabilitation doctors are often more inclined to yield the control of purely medical issues to the internist. Of course, individual physicians have individual habits and expectations. Being particularly knowledgeable and skillful regarding recurring questions and mindful of the needs and expectations of individual physicians are integral to providing successful and appreciated consultative services.

Discerning the specific clinical question being asked and its urgency is the first and most important task. Whenever possible, the consultant should speak directly to the requestor. This also serves as an excellent opportunity to discuss the requestor's expectations regarding your level of involvement. Not uncommonly, the clinical question is initially somewhat vague. A series of diplomatically delivered questions may be useful:

What are your major concerns?
Is there a problem you would like us to focus on?
What is the patient's medical history, and are any of those problems out of control?
Is the patient having a new problem?
Is there an abnormal lab/x-ray/ECG that we should focus on?
Is the patient going to have surgery in the near future?
How can we serve you the best?

On occasion, the requestor is unable to articulate a precise question, even with careful prompting. Accepting that the physician requesting the consultation is in need of your expertise, whatever the question, rather than making more work for you is important in this circumstance. An initial thoughtful evaluation of the patient usually reveals issues for which the internist can be of assistance. A follow-up conversation with the requestor can then take place to narrow the focus of the consultation.

On the other hand, there are times after an introductory conversation regarding a potential consult when it is clear that your particular skills as a general internist are

1

TABLE 1. TEN COMMANDMENTS FOR EFFECTIVE CONSULTATIONS

Determine the question	Provide contingency plans
Establish the urgency	Honor thy turf
Look for yourself	Teach with tact
Be as brief as appropriate	Talk is cheap and effective
Be specific	Follow up

Adapted from Goldman L, Lee T, Rudd P. Ten commandments for effective consultations. *Arch Intern Med* 1983;143:1753.

TABLE 2. COMMON CONSULTATIONS BY SERVICE

Service	Common consults
Psychiatry	BP control
	Blood sugar control
	Fever
	Any lab abnormality
	Pre-electroconvulsive therapy evaluation
	Evaluate for medical causes of altered mental status
OB/Gyn	BP control
	Blood sugar control
	Fever
	Any lab abnormality
	Preoperative assessment
Surgery	Preoperative assessment
	Postoperative atrial fibrillation or any other arrhythmia
	Postoperative chest pain and rule out myocardial infarction
	Postoperative hypotension
	Postoperative shortness of breath and rule out deep venous thrombosis/pulmonary embolism
	Postoperative delirium
	Postoperative reduced urine output and renal dysfunction
	Postoperative fever and infection of any kind
Neurology	BP control
	Blood sugar control
	Any lab abnormality
Rehabilitation	BP control
	Blood sugar control
	Fever
	Any lab abnormality
	Follow and manage all medical problems

not needed or that a full consultation is not warranted. If the patient is better served by a subspecialty consultation, offering to facilitate arranging this is much appreciated. If there is something else you can do, such as scheduling a follow-up medicine clinic appointment, contacting the patient's private physician, or arranging a diagnostic test, then offer to do this. When there is any uncertainty about the need for a full consult, you should err on the side of caution and at least briefly evaluate the patient. The last thing you want to do is leave the requestor with the impression that the general medicine consultation service just is not interested in business and/or that you personally are being difficult or lazy ("blocking a consult"). You could be on the requesting end of this situation at any time.

Calls for after-hours consultations (often in the middle of the night) are common. Discerning the nature and urgency of the question is particularly important in this instance. At least some of these calls are truly urgent or emergent, regarding acute decompensation of a patient (e.g., chest pain, shortness of breath, hypotension, acute mental status changes, etc.). Obviously, these patients must be attended to immediately. This is definitely not the time to worry about a specific question! For these types of patients it may be easier for you and better for the patient to arrange a rapid transfer to the medical service or intensive care unit after your initial evaluation. Consults are sometimes requested for patients about to undergo emergent surgery. There is often little that can be done preoperatively in the setting of emergent surgery. Nonetheless, the patient should be at least briefly evaluated and the willingness to follow the patient postoperatively should be clearly stated. Less-than-urgent requests can usually be dealt with the next morning—just be sure to pass the information on. For all of these late-night consults, do not forget to call your attending. They may be cranky, but you will not be faulted for keeping them informed.

When approaching any new consultation, it is, in general, prudent to provide answers only for the question(s) asked. Otherwise, the critical points can get lost in what may be perceived as an avalanche of unwanted recommendations. When the evaluation of the patient uncovers a new clinical problem that is not directly relevant to the question initially asked and it requires immediate attention, it should be discussed directly with the requestor. Again, emergent and urgent consultations should be handled accordingly. When in doubt, seeing the patient as soon as possible is the best strategy. Regardless, same-day service will be greatly appreciated.

Even when the clinical question is highly specific, in most instances the requestor has a reasonable expectation that a thorough evaluation of the patient is performed by the general internist. Never rely on the findings of others. The consultant should obtain as much information from the primary sources (e.g., the patient, lab data, old records, and family members) as is necessary.

The formulation of the written consultation is very important. From legal and billing standpoints, it is important to document everything that was asked, examined, and interpreted, as well as the assessment and recommendations. A useful and common strategy is to reiterate the specific question asked and by whom, the assessment, and the most important recommendations in a concise and very specific manner on the first page of the consultation report. A detailed history and physical exam follow. The requesting service is then able to easily get "the answer" without having to slog through "the details" (after all, that is what we are there for). In most instances, directly discussing your initial assessment and recommendations with the requesting service is highly desirable and provides an excellent opportunity for education. When new drugs are recommended, specifically stating the dose, route, and frequency may lead to more effective consultations [2]. It is also helpful to be as precise as possible about diagnostic tests. If what you really think the patient needs is a dobutamine stress echocardiogram today, say so, as opposed to just recommending a "stress test." It might seem trivial, but if your recommendations cannot be read, they cannot be followed. Neatness does count. Do leave your pager number.

Follow-up notes should be likewise brief, with clear subsequent recommendations. In almost all cases it is appropriate, if not mandatory, to follow the patient for at least 1–2 days. Knowing when to gracefully bow out can be a difficult decision. When in doubt, there is no harm in hanging on another day. It may be appropriate to follow some patients "at a distance" from time to time. When you do ultimately sign off, be sure to state your availability for any further questions that develop and how you can be easily reached. If appropriate, you should also leave specific instructions regarding follow-up after discharge (e.g., a private physician, the general medicine clinic, or a medical subspecialty clinic). If possible, setting up these appointments yourself is the best way to ensure that it gets done.

In the end, your recommendations are just that; the requesting service does not have to follow all of your suggestions to the letter. In fact, they probably have perfectly legitimate reasons for not doing so. Do not get hung up on your way being the only way. Be open to alternate but equivalent ways of getting things done. If you feel a crucial recommendation must be followed, then be sure to discuss this with the requesting service and document having done so. Expressing your willingness to assist in carrying out your recommendations is also important. It is often much easier for the internist to arrange a test specific to our specialty. You, rather than the surgery intern, are much more likely to be successful speaking directly to the cardiology fellow about getting a transesophageal echocardiogram done as quickly as possible. Some requesting services are happy to have you write orders, but definitely do not do this without asking. If you do accept this responsibility, you must also be prepared to accept the responsibility for this aspect of the patient's care. There must be no confusion in this regard. "I thought you were going to order that," is an unacceptable excuse and could leave a consultant open to serious liability issues. If you have written an order, you must follow up on it.

The written consultation can also be an effective educational vehicle, particularly for house officers. Again, brevity is crucial. Leaving one recent and directly relevant journal article in the chart is a nice touch. Anything more may be perceived as an annoyance or over-stepping bounds. Of note, the chart is not the appropriate place for open disagreements regarding the patient's management. Using journal articles as ammunition in this type of battle is unlikely to be educational or well received. Such disagreements are best dealt with verbally, most often between attendings.

Unfortunately, politics often come into play in the consultation business, particularly at busy, major teaching hospitals. Turf wars are never any fun and generally do not serve the patient well, so observe your boundaries closely. It should fall to the attending consultant to be the voice of reason. Following the above strategies often prevents such turf wars. If any of your recommendations are particularly critical and/or complicated, make sure that you specifically address these with the requestor directly. Attending-to-attending communication almost always resolves any disputes satisfactorily. Questions of patient safety should be referred to the appropriate chief residents or chiefs of service. If a transfer is requested and you feel that it is at least reasonably appropriate, do what you can to facilitate it as quickly as possible. As with any other transfer, you should consider speaking directly to the accepting physician (e.g., the house officer on the general or subspecialty medical service or the attending accepting the patient on the hospitalist service). You will probably do a much better job describing the situation to your internist colleague than a house officer from a different service will. Professionalism and collegiality are key components to successful consultations. Being "nice" pays, not only in more requests for consults but also in reciprocity.

Consultations for preoperative risk assessment are very common and deserve special mention. Most important, no one is ever "cleared for surgery." A patient may be low risk for surgery but not at no risk. Multiple factors influence the assessment of risk, and a structured approach is very desirable. Both the American Heart Association/American College of Cardiology Task Force [3] and American College of Cardiology [4] Guidelines are very practical tools for cardiovascular risk assessment. For the other aspects of risk assessment available, "guidelines" are not as directive and therefore less straightforward to use. Table 3 provides a sensible, although not necessarily complete, checklist for preoperative assessments.

General internal medicine consultations can be very challenging and rewarding. Developing a reputation as an outstanding consultant is a difficult but worthwhile goal. The authors are hopeful that readers find this manual to be an informative and effective resource to accomplish this goal.

TABLE 3. PREOPERATIVE RISK ASSESSMENT CHECKLIST

1. Is the surgery truly urgent/emergent or could it be delayed or canceled?
2. If the patient is older than 40 yrs and undergoing more than minor surgery, has a preoperative ECG been done?
3. What is the modality of anesthesia (e.g., general, regional, local ± IV sedation ± nitrous oxide)?
4. Is the patient at risk for postoperative delirium?
5. If the patient is elderly, has a preoperative mental status exam been done?
6. Does the patient abuse alcohol, sedatives, or illicit drugs?
7. Perform a preoperative cardiovascular risk assessment using the American Heart Association/American College of Cardiology or American College of Physicians guidelines.
8. Consider a beta blocker for all patients with cardiovascular risk factors.
9. If the patient has significant pulmonary symptoms or disease, has a preoperative chest x-ray and ABG been done?
10. If the patient is at risk for pulmonary complications, has the patient been taught deep-breathing exercises and incentive spirometry preoperatively?
11. What is the patient's risk of deep venous thrombosis/pulmonary embolism, and what is the appropriate prophylactic regimen?
12. Does the patient require endocarditis prophylaxis?
13. Is surgical wound antibiotic prophylaxis necessary?
14. If the patient is diabetic, what is the most appropriate way to alter the patient's therapy?
15. If the patient is taking a medication that increases the risk of bleeding, how and when will it be stopped before surgery and resumed after surgery?
16. What are the patient's current medications (including herbals and over-the-counters), and do any of them need to be altered in the perioperative period?
17. Is it possible that the patient may need to go to an extended care facility postoperatively?
18. Have you talked directly with the surgical team?

REFERENCES

1. Goldman L, Lee T, Rudd P. Ten commandments for effective consultations. *Arch Intern Med* 1983;143:1753.
2. Horwitz RI, Henes CG, Horwitz SM. Developing strategies for improving the diagnostic and management efficacy of medical consultations. *J Chronic Dis* 1983;36:213.
3. Eagle KA, Brundage BH, Chaitman BR, et al. Guidelines for perioperative cardiovascular evaluation for noncardiac surgery. *J Am Coll Cardiol* 1996;27:910.
4. Palda VA, Detsky AS. Guidelines for assessing and managing the perioperative risk from coronary artery disease associated with major noncardiac surgery. *Ann Intern Med* 1997;127:309.

General Issues

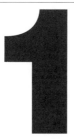

Approach to Perioperative Care

Michael E. Lazarus

INTRODUCTION

The most common reason to consult medicine at Barnes-Jewish Hospital is to "clear" a patient for surgery. However, your main objective should be to **stratify** patients according to their risk, as you can never say a patient has **no** risk.

Discussions of perioperative diabetes management (see Chap. 39, Inpatient Diabetes Management), anticoagulation and surgery (see Chap. 8, Anticoagulation and Surgical Procedures), and perioperative cancer considerations (see Chap. 37, Perioperative Cancer Issues) are included elsewhere in this manual.

PERIOPERATIVE CARDIAC EVALUATION

Preoperative testing should be limited to circumstances in which the results will affect patient treatment and outcomes.

Coronary artery disease (CAD) is the most frequent cause of perioperative cardiac mortality and morbidity after noncardiac surgery.

History

Functional status is critical in assessing a patient's preoperative risk. A cutoff of 4 metabolic equivalents (mets) has been used to indicate whether a patient has an adequate functional status to allow more accurate determination of cardiac risk [1]. Table 1-1 lists some activities, compiled from several sources, for 4 mets of exercise.

Comorbid conditions must be identified, especially diabetes, lung disease, heart disease, renal failure, immune status, hematologic diseases, and malignancy.

The most widely used algorithm for the preoperative assessment of cardiac risk for noncardiac surgery was published in 1996 and updated in 2002 by the American Heart Association (AHA) and uses the following 8 steps:

- **Step 1: What is the urgency of the surgery?** If the surgery is emergent, your time would best be spent concentrating on perioperative medical management and surveillance.
- **Step 2: Has the patient undergone coronary revascularization within the past 5 yrs?** If so and the patient is asymptomatic, then no further workup is needed. However, consider delaying in patients who have had intracoronary stents within the last 6 wks (see Angioplasty).
- **Step 3: Has the patient undergone an evaluation for coronary artery disease within the last 2 yrs?** If so and the patient is asymptomatic, then repeat testing may be redundant.
- **Step 4: Does the patient have an unstable coronary syndrome or major clinical predictors?** In the setting of unstable coronary disease, decompensated congestive heart failure (CHF), symptomatic arrhythmias, high-grade atrioventricular block, or severe valvular heart disease, patients will most often benefit from cardiac catheterization. Surgery may need to be delayed while medical therapy is optimized.
- **Step 5: Does the patient have intermediate predictors of risk?** These include a history of MI, stable angina pectoris (Canadian class I or II), compensated CHF, and diabetes

TABLE 1-1. METABOLIC EQUIVALENTS (METS) FOR CERTAIN ACTIVITIES

METS	Representative activities
≥ 4	Walking at 4 mph on level ground, climbing stairs, climbing hills, riding a bicycle at 8 mph, golfing, bowling, throwing a baseball/football, carrying 25 lbs (groceries from the store to the car), scrubbing the floor, raking leaves, mowing the lawn.
> 7	Jogging at 5 mph on level ground, carrying 60-lb objects.

mellitus. The most recent AHA recommendations have also included renal insufficiency in this list. Those with intermediate predictors are then further considered through step 6. If they have no intermediate predictors, then they may be evaluated through step 7. Consideration of the functional capacity (Table 1-1) and the level of surgery-specific risk will help identify those patients most likely to benefit from noninvasive cardiac testing:

- Surgery-specific cardiac risk:
  - The type of procedure (e.g., vascular procedures are more likely to be associated with underlying CAD than nonvascular surgery). The AHA has stratified surgical procedures into high, intermediate, or low in terms of cardiac risk:
    - High: emergent major operations, major vascular surgery, peripheral vascular surgery, anticipated prolonged procedures with large fluid shifts or blood loss.
    - Intermediate: carotid endarterectomy, head and neck, orthopedic, prostate, intraperitoneal surgery. (Cardiac event risk <5%.)
    - Low: endoscopic or superficial procedures, cataract, breast. (Cardiac event risk <1%.)
  - The degree of hemodynamic stress associated with specific procedures is important to consider. Certain procedures are more likely than others to result in prolonged perioperative alterations in heart rate and BP, fluid shifts, pain, bleeding, clotting tendencies, oxygenation, and neurohumoral activation.
- **Step 6: Patients with intermediate clinical predictors of risk who have moderate to excellent functional capacity (>4 mets) can generally undergo an intermediate risk operation with little likelihood of perioperative cardiac complications.** These patients should also tolerate low-risk procedures well. Further testing is often required for patients who have a poor functional capacity or are undergoing high-risk surgery, or both.
- **Step 7: Noncardiac surgery is generally safe in patients in whom no high or intermediate risk factors exist and in patients with moderate functional capacity >4 mets** (Table 1-1). If the patient has poor functional capacity and is going for a high-risk procedure, then the patient would likely benefit from noninvasive testing before surgery.
- **Step 8: Results of noninvasive testing guide further cardiac management, be it medical or invasive.** If the noninvasive cardiac test is positive, then strongly consider coronary angiography and maximize medical management.

Physical Exam

Vital signs are critical, with severe HTN being a treatable but potentially dangerous preoperative condition. Check the BP in both arms, and use the arm with the higher BP to guide management. A thorough head-to-toe physical exam is also necessary.

Focus on cardiac auscultation. The presence of a murmur may provide critical information on valvular disease or the need for endocarditis prophylaxis.

Look for signs of volume overload or heart failure, with an elevated jugular venous pressure, positive hepatojugular reflex, or S_3 being most reliable. Pulmonary auscultation may reveal pulmonary edema.

Look for evidence of peripheral vascular disease, including carotid bruits, which may be the only clue to underlying atherosclerosis.

Lab Evaluation

Adults age >50 yrs should have a 12-lead ECG to evaluate for rhythms other than normal sinus and any evidence of old infarcts or ischemia. Any additional evaluation should be based on symptoms, comorbid conditions, and physical exam findings.

Imaging Evaluation: Methods of Assessing Cardiac Risk

Resting Left Ventricular Function
Left ventricular (LV) ejection fraction <35% increases risk in noncardiac surgery, as does severe diastolic dysfunction. Knowledge of LV function provides valuable information when managing postoperative fluids.

Exercise Stress Testing
Evidence of myocardial ischemia on stress testing identifies patients with a sevenfold increased risk of untoward outcomes during noncardiac surgery. A gradient of increasing ischemic risk is seen in association with the degree of functional incapacity, symptoms of ischemia, and severity of ischemia (depth and rapidity of onset and the duration of ST-segment depression and evidence of hemodynamic or electrical instability during or after stress). This gradient also correlates with an increasing likelihood of severe and multivessel CAD.

In patients with left bundle branch block, exercise stress testing, even with nuclear imaging, has been found to be much less sensitive and specific than in those without left bundle branch block. Vasodilator (dipyridamole and adenosine)-based stress testing has maintained a high sensitivity and specificity in this situation, however.

Pharmacologic Stress Testing
Dipyridamole or adenosine thallium stress testing has a high sensitivity and specificity for perioperative events when used in patients with preexisting clinical predictors of risk such as angina, diabetes, and prior MI. Perioperative ischemic events correlate with the magnitude of ischemia (the presence of both ECG evidence of ischemia and thallium or technetium redistribution after pharmacologic stress testing). The long-term risk of death or MI may be better predicted by the presence of reversible or fixed defects.

Dobutamine Stress Echo
Dobutamine stress echo provides comparable information to thallium studies; however, it also provides the opportunity to evaluate the LV function and heart valves.

Ambulatory ECG Monitoring
Detection of ischemia by preoperative 24- to 48-hr monitoring correlates with an increased risk of perioperative ischemic events. Higher-risk patients may have baseline ECG abnormalities that preclude analysis.

Coronary Angiography
Indications for preoperative angiography are the same as those in the nonoperative setting. Before sending a patient for cardiac catheterization, make sure that percutaneous transluminal coronary angioplasty (PTCA) or coronary artery bypass graft (CABG) are options for the patient.

Specific Preoperative Cardiovascular Conditions

Hypertension
Continuation of preoperative antihypertensive treatment throughout the perioperative period is critical, especially when the patient is on beta blockers or clonidine (Catapres).

Severe HTN, as defined by the AHA as BP >180/11 mm Hg, preoperatively often results in wider fluctuations in intraoperative BP and has been associated with an increased rate of perioperative cardiac events. BP below this does not appear to confer a significant increased risk perioperatively. Long-term benefits of controlling

HTN are clear, however, and the consultant should take the opportunity to initiate appropriate management perioperatively. Certain beta blockers have been shown to have a dramatic effect in reducing perioperative cardiovascular events (see Medical Management).

Valvular Heart Disease
Symptomatic stenotic lesions, such as mitral stenosis and atrial stenosis, are associated with perioperative CHF and shock, and preoperative valvotomy or replacement is often needed. Symptomatic regurgitant lesions are generally better tolerated perioperatively and may be managed medically. If surgery is emergent, the patient should proceed with surgery and have elective valvular surgery at a later time. Exceptions to this are regurgitant lesions with LV dysfunction, because these patients have reduced hemodynamic reserve.

Myocardial Heart Disease
Dilated cardiomyopathy and hypertrophic obstructive cardiomyopathy are both associated with a higher incidence of perioperative CHF. These patients should be managed by maximizing preoperative hemodynamic status and providing intensive postoperative medical treatment and surveillance.

Arrhythmias and Conduction Anomalies
When an arrhythmia is detected preoperatively, then a thorough assessment for an underlying cause should be sought. The indications for preoperative arrhythmia management and pacemaker insertion are the same as in the nonoperative setting.

Coronary Artery Bypass Grafting
Several observational studies have shown that patients with CAD who have undergone CABG are at lower cardiac risk when they undergo subsequent noncardiac surgery.

Angioplasty
No large randomized trials have compared perioperative cardiac outcome after noncardiac surgery for patients who had PTCA vs. medical therapy. However, smaller observational studies have revealed that cardiac death is infrequent in patients who have PTCA before noncardiac surgery.

Medical Management
Surgical stress can lead to the release of large amounts of catecholamines, which can mediate arrhythmias and may predispose to coronary plaque rupture. Accordingly, a recent randomized controlled trial documented that perioperative beta blockade may reduce perioperative clinical events. Included were high-risk patients (defined as having ≥ 2 of the following risk factors: age >65 yrs, HTN, current smoking, cholesterol level >240 mg/dL, and diabetes) undergoing noncardiac surgery. Atenolol (Tenormin) produced a 15% absolute reduction compared to placebo in the combined end point of MI, unstable angina, CHF requiring hospital admission, myocardial revascularization, or death at 6 mos and reduced the mortality rate at 6 mos and 2 yrs. The dosing of atenolol used in the study was 5 mg administered IV 1 hr before surgery, immediately after surgery, and an oral dose of 50–100 mg daily throughout their hospital stay (up to 7 days). The use of bisoprolol (Zebeta, Ziac) has produced dramatic results as well; however, this trial selected those patients at highest risk. See Appendix A, Review of Selected Clinical Trials, for detailed summaries of both of these trials.

Intraoperative and Postoperative Period

Pulmonary Artery Catheters
Current evidence suggests that patients most likely to benefit from the use of pulmonary artery catheters are those with recent MI with associated CHF; patients with severe CAD undergoing procedures routinely associated with hemodynamic stress; and patients with LV dysfunction, cardiomyopathy, or valvular disease undergoing high-risk operations.

ECG Monitoring
Intraoperative and postoperative ST-segment changes are strong predictors of perioperative MI in patients at high clinical risk who undergo noncardiac surgery. Postoperative ischemia is a strong predictor of the risk of long-term MI and cardiac death.

Cardiac Enzymes
Routine postoperative assessments should be discouraged. They should be obtained in patients who have clinical, ECG, or hemodynamic evidence of cardiovascular dysfunction.

PREOPERATIVE PULMONARY EVALUATION

Clinically significant postoperative pulmonary complications are as common as postoperative cardiac complications. The most common complications include pneumonia, respiratory failure, bronchospasm, atelectasis, and exacerbation of underlying chronic lung disease.

Modifiable Patient-Related Risk Factors
Smoking
Operative risk has been shown to decline only after 8 wks of preoperative cessation [2]. 6 months of cessation may reduce the risk of pulmonary complications to nearly that of nonsmokers.

Chronic Obstructive Pulmonary Disease
The incidence of complications varies according to the severity of lung disease. Symptoms should be aggressively treated preoperatively. Combinations of bronchodilators, physical therapy, smoking cessation, and corticosteroids reduce the risk of postoperative pulmonary complications. Although not all patients with COPD respond to corticosteroid therapy, a 2-wk preoperative course is reasonable for symptomatic patients already on maximal bronchodilator therapy and who are not at their best personal baseline level as determined by exam, chest x-ray, and spirometry. Patients with recent sputum changes may benefit from an antibiotic course preoperatively.

Asthma
Before surgery, patients should be free of wheezing with a peak expiratory flow rate >80% of predicted or personal best level.

Procedure-Related Risk Factors

The surgical site is the most important predictor of pulmonary risk. Risk increases as the incision approaches the diaphragm. Upper abdominal and thoracic surgery carries the greatest risk of postoperative pulmonary complications.

Most studies have reported a lower risk of pulmonary complications for patients who undergo spinal or epidural anesthesia as compared to those who undergo general anesthesia. Regional anesthesia, such as an axillary block, carries even lower risk.

The use of **pancuronium** should be avoided in patients with chronic pulmonary disease, as there is a higher risk of postoperative hypoventilation due to neuromuscular blockade.

Preoperative Clinical Evaluation with Pulmonary Function Tests

Routine preoperative use of pulmonary function tests remains controversial. No data suggest that spirometry identifies a high-risk group with abnormal spirometric findings but no clinical evidence of pulmonary disease or other risk factors for pulmonary complications. There is also no identified level of airway obstruction that precludes surgery.

Clinicians may reserve preoperative spirometry for patients who are to undergo thoracic or upper abdominal surgery and who have symptoms of cough, dyspnea, or exercise intolerance that remain unexplained after careful history and physical exam.

Spirometry may be used for surveillance of lung volumes in patients with severe COPD or asthma in whom clinical assessment fails to elucidate the degree of airflow limitation.

Clinicians should not use ABG analysis to identify patients for whom the risk of surgery would be prohibitive. It may, however, guide postoperative ventilatory management so that minute ventilations are directed to maintain preoperative levels of carbon dioxide retention.

Reducing Pulmonary Risk Postoperatively

Lung Expansion Maneuvers
Postoperative use of incentive spirometry consistently reduces the relative risk of pulmonary complications by approximately 50% in repeated studies.

Continuous Positive Airway Pressure
Clinicians should restrict the use of continuous positive airway pressure to those patients who are unable to perform deep-breathing exercises or use an incentive spirometer.

Analgesia
The use of postoperative epidural analgesia is recommended in the setting of high-risk thoracic, abdominal, and major vascular surgery and has been shown to reduce the incidence of pulmonary complications.

HEMOSTASIS AND TRANSFUSION ISSUES IN SURGERY

Strategies to Reduce Homologous Blood Exposure

- Transfuse on a symptomatic basis only.
- Correct deficiencies in essential nutrients such as iron, folic acid, and vitamin B_{12}.
- Avoid pharmacologic coagulopathies.
- Pharmacologic stimulation of the bone marrow with recombinant erythropoietin.
- Arranging preoperative autologous blood donation.
- Hypothermia and positional blood pooling.
- Intraoperative blood salvage and autotransplantation.

General Transfusion Guidelines

The patient's own blood is still the safest, but this strategy can usually only be used when the patient is not anemic and is undergoing elective surgery in which adequate time (3 wks) is available for blood donation.

The arbitrary use of transfusion triggers (Hgb/Hct <10/30) should be abandoned, and estimates of operative blood loss should be based on appropriately timed Hct measurements.

Erythropoietin alone is not effective in reducing homologous blood transfusion in nonanemic or modestly anemic patients (Hgb <10) but has been approved for use perioperatively in mildly anemic patients (Hgb between 10–13) undergoing elective noncardiac surgery. Dose at 600 U/kg SC qwk starting 3 wks before surgery and last dose the day of surgery.

The combination of erythropoietin with iron is indicated in patients who are iron deficient. Oral iron supplementation suffices in patients whose serum ferritin is >100 ng/mL. For those patients whose ferritin level is <100 ng/mL, parenteral iron is indicated.

Patients with sickle cell anemia benefit from transfusion before surgery to reduce the percentage of Hgb S. Many physicians have set the target preoperative Hgb to 10 mg/dL in this situation, and it has been supported by at least one study [3].

SURGERY IN THE PATIENT WITH LIVER DISEASE

The risk of perioperative morbidity or mortality in patients with liver disease is related to the extent of hepatic dysfunction. The Child-Pugh score has been shown to correlate with perioperative mortality in patients undergoing nonportacaval shunt surgery and in cirrhotic patients undergoing abdominal procedures. In a retrospective analysis that assessed variables of survival after abdominal surgery in cirrhotic patients, the serum albumin level, leukocytosis, and an increased PT were the most sensitive indicators of perioperative mortality independent of the Child-Pugh score. In this study [4], patients with Child's class A, B, and C cirrhosis had mortality rates of 10%, 31%, and 76%, respectively.

Patients with acute symptomatic liver disease should have elective surgery postponed, if possible, until they have recovered. However, if surgery is emergent, the following steps should be taken to optimize preoperative status.

Coagulation Status

Correct vitamin K deficiency by a single IM dose of 10 mg. Further coagulation anomalies may require FFP, given as needed. If the PT remains prolonged, cryoprecipitate may be used. Plasma exchange has been used for refractory coagulopathy. Prophylactic platelet transfusions may be considered for thrombocytopenia (platelet count, <20 $K/\mu L$).

Renal and Electrolyte Abnormalities

Careful attention should be paid to volume status. Nephrotoxic substances, such as NSAIDs and aminoglycosides, should be avoided. Patients with cirrhosis often have hypokalemia and alkalosis, and these conditions should be corrected preoperatively to minimize the risks of cardiac arrhythmias and to diminish encephalopathy.

Ascites

The presence of ascites may influence respiratory mechanics and increase the risk of abdominal wound dehiscence. Thus, large-volume paracentesis may be indicated preoperatively. Careful attention is needed to prevent the excessive use of saline solutions and medications containing sodium. The use of albumin, blood products, or FFP is useful for intravascular volume expansion and slows ascites reaccumulation. If hyponatremia occurs, fluid restriction may be needed.

Encephalopathy

Lactulose may be administered at a dose of 30 mL PO q6h, titrated to 2–3 soft bowel movements per day. Protein restriction has been recommended for patients who respond poorly, but excessive restriction of protein can actually contribute to malnutrition and may be undesirable preoperatively. Encephalopathy is worsened or precipitated by the use of sedatives, and these should be avoided.

Nutrition

Malnutrition is common in patients with chronic liver disease and increases the risk of perioperative complications. Enteral nutrition is helpful in improving the patient's Child's class and reducing mortality in those with cirrhosis and malnutrition. A low-protein diet is only advised in those patients with active encephalopathy.

CLINICAL PEARLS

1. Remember to provide endocarditis prophylaxis when indicated.
2. Inquire about alcohol and drug use preoperative so as not to be surprised by a postoperative withdrawal delirium (see Chap. 47, Alcohol Withdrawal, and Chap. 48, Opioid Overdose and Withdrawal).
3. Do an accurate preoperative assessment of a patient's mental status to aid in evaluating delirium postoperatively (See Chap. 30, Approach to Mental Status Changes).
4. Remember to provide stress dose steroids in patients who have been on high-dose steroids.

5. Patients with mild to moderate hypothyroidism will have only a slight increase in minor perioperative complications and intraoperative hypotension. Patients with severe symptomatic hypothyroidism have an increased rate of cardiac complications and mortality.
6. For patients with renal failure, carefully follow postoperative potassium and serum HCO_3^- because tissue injury and intraoperative ischemia may result in hyperkalemia or acidosis that may not be easily handled when renal function is poor. Patients on hemodialysis should have an adequate dialysis session before surgery if feasible.

KEY POINTS TO REMEMBER

- The role of the medicine consultant is to stratify a patient's perioperative risk and provide recommendations on how to minimize the chance of complications.
- Perform additional tests only if it affects your preoperative intervention or medical management. Patients undergoing emergency procedures should therefore proceed to surgery without delay.

SUGGESTED READING

American College of Physicians. Guidelines for assessing and managing the perioperative risk from coronary artery disease associated with major noncardiac surgery. *Ann Intern Med* 1997;127:309–312.

Ashton CM, Petersen NJ, Wray NP, et al. The incidence of perioperative myocardial infarction in men undergoing noncardiac surgery. *Ann Intern Med* 1993;118:504–510.

Detsky AS, Abrams HB, McLaughlin JR, et al. Predicting cardiac complications in patients undergoing non-cardiac surgery. *J Gen Intern Med* 1986;1:211–219.

Eagle KA, Brundage BH, Chaitman BR, et al. Guidelines for perioperative cardiovascular evaluation for noncardiac surgery. Report of the American College of Cardiology/American Heart Association Task Force on Practice Guidelines (Committee on Perioperative Cardiovascular Evaluation for Noncardiac Surgery). *J Am Coll Cardiol* 1996;27:910–948.

Eagle KA, Coley CM, Newell JB, et al. Combining clinical and thallium data optimizes preoperative assessment of cardiac risk before major vascular surgery. *Ann Intern Med* 1989;110:859–866.

Garrison RN, Cryer HM, Howard DA, et al. Clarification of risk factors for abdominal operations in patients with hepatic cirrhosis. *Ann Surg* 1984;1999:648–655.

Gilbert K, Larocque BJ, Patrick LT. Prospective evaluation of cardiac risk indices for patients undergoing noncardiac surgery. *Ann Intern Med* 2000;133:356–359.

Mangano DT, Layug EL, Wallace A, et al. Effect of atenolol on mortality and cardiovascular morbidity after noncardiac surgery. Multicenter Study of Perioperative Ischemia Research Group. *N Engl J Med* 1996;335:1713–1720.

Osman DR. Antimicrobial prophylaxis in adults. *Mayo Clin Proc* 2000;75:98–109.

Patel T. Surgery in the patient with liver disease. *Mayo Clin Proc* 1999;74:593–599.

Pugh RN, Murray-Lyon IM, Dawson JL, et al. Transection of the esophagus for bleeding esophageal varices. *Br J Surg* 1973;60:646–649.

Smetana GW. Preoperative pulmonary evaluation. *N Engl J Med* 1999;340:937–944.

Vanzetto G, Machecourt J, Blendea D, et al. Additive value of thallium single-photon emission computed tomography myocardial imaging for prediction of perioperative events in clinically selected high cardiac risk patients having abdominal aortic surgery. *Am J Cardiol* 1996;77:143–148.

REFERENCES

1. Reilly DF, McNeely MJ, Doerner D, et al. Self-reported exercise tolerance and the risk of serious perioperative complications. *Arch Intern Med* 1999;159:2185–2192.
2. Warner MA. Role of preoperative cessation of smoking and other factors in postoperative pulmonary complications. *Mayo Clin Proc* 1989;64:609–616.
3. Vichinsky EP. A comparison of conservative and aggressive transfusion regimens in the perioperative management of sickle cell disease. *N Engl J Med* 1995;333:206–214.
4. Child CG III, Turcotte JG. Surgery and portal hypertension. *Major Probl Clin Surg* 1964;1:1–85.

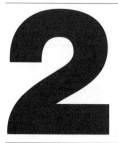

Approach to Edema

Christopher H. Kwoh

BILATERAL OR GENERALIZED EDEMA

In general, bilateral edema is the result of systemic conditions or obstruction at the inferior vena cava or above. Increased venous pressure and decreased oncotic pressure are the typical factors. Most common are right-sided heart failure, nephrosis, cirrhosis, or renal failure. See Table 2-1 for differential diagnosis.

Physical Exam for Bilateral Edema

- The exam should identify the type of edema (classic pitting vs. lipedema, etc.), as well as clues to the chronicity (the development of overlying skin changes).
- Look for signs of heart failure (hepatojugular reflex, cardiomegaly, elevated jugular venous pressure, S_3, S_4) or right-sided valvular disease. Look for stigmata of liver disease.
- Ascites can be present in severe heart failure, nephrosis, and various other disorders, as well as cirrhosis. An elevated jugular venous pressure aids in the differential diagnosis.
- Lymphedema is classically difficult to pit and involves the dorsal aspect of the feet and toes. In chronicity, one develops "lymphostatic verrucosis"—dark, wart-like projections over the skin.
- Periorbital edema suggests decreased oncotic pressure or superior vena cava obstruction.
- Chronic venous stasis typically has darkening of the skin (hemosiderosis) or medial malleolar ulceration (venous stasis ulcers).
- Myxedema will be rubbery and nonpitting, often with the texture and appearance of orange peel.
- Lipedema—fatty tissue in the lower extremities—is common in overweight women. It can have the appearance of classic edema but is nonpitting and spares the feet.
- Angioedema is typically rapid onset (within minutes to hours) and is frequently localized to the head or neck.
- Rapid onset of severe edema may result in pain, erythema, and warmth that mimics cellulitis.

Lab Evaluation

Lab evaluation should be guided by history and exam and should rule out systemic disease:

- One approach is to first evaluate for the presence of severe hypoalbuminemia (<2.5), which will lead one down the path of cardiac origin or decreased oncotic pressure.
- Initial evaluation of bilateral edema commonly includes electrolytes, liver function tests (focus on hypoalbuminemia), BUN/creatinine, and urinalysis. A TSH is not unreasonable.
- Consider ECG, echocardiography, and chest x-ray.

TABLE 2-1. DIFFERENTIAL DIAGNOSIS OF BILATERAL EDEMA (COMPILED FROM MULTIPLE SOURCES)

Increased venous pressure

Chronic venous insufficiency: the most common cause of trace edema.

Volume overload: renal failure, hepatic failure, or overaggressive IV hydration.

Increased right-sided heart pressure: heart failure, pulmonary HTN with cor pulmonale, right-sided valvular disease.

Venous (or lymphatic) obstruction: tumor (ovarian, uterine, bladder, prostate are most common), retroperitoneal fibrosis, or lymphadenopathy.

Decreased oncotic pressure

Nephrotic syndrome, cirrhosis, protein-calorie malnutrition, protein losing enteropathies.

Angioedema: hereditary, acquired, or medication induced (ACE inhibitors, NSAIDs, morphine, contrast).

Medications: calcium channel blockers, corticosteroids, sex hormones, NSAIDs, COX-2 inhibitors, other antihypertensives.

Myxedema: Graves disease, marked hypothyroidism.

Lipedema

Lymphedema: Lymphangioleiomyomatosis

Capillary leak syndromes

Any cause of localized edema may, rarely, occur bilaterally.

* 24-hr urine protein (if urinalysis shows significant proteinuria) and serum lipids can aid in the evaluation of the nephrotic syndrome.

    Imaging should be guided by results of history, physical, and lab evaluation:

* **Contrast venography** and **lymphangiography** are reliable in ruling out venous or lymphatic obstruction if necessary.
* **CT scan of the abdomen/pelvis** may identify retroperitoneal fibrosis or obstructing masses.

Management of Bilateral or Generalized Edema

* Treatment should be directed at the underlying disorder.
* **Compression stockings** or Ted hose may be used to limit swelling.
* Consider **leg elevation, calf exercises,** and the use of **diuretics** or a **low-salt diet.**

LOCALIZED EDEMA

Localized edema is usually due to obstructive processes of the veins or local inflammation. Most common are deep venous thrombosis (DVT) and surgical or radiation induced. See Table 2-2 for the differential diagnosis.

Presentation

History

Important in the history are risk factors for DVT, chronicity of the symptoms, presence of pain (localized obstruction and congenital forms are typically painless), prior surgeries or malignancies, previous injury, or emotional upset (suggests reflex sympathetic dystrophy).

TABLE 2-2. DIFFERENTIAL DIAGNOSIS OF LOCALIZED EDEMA

Deep venous thrombosis

Obstructive/inflammatory lymphedema: infections (filariasis, TB, recurrent lymphangitis), postsurgical, posttraumatic, radiation-induced, sarcoidosis.

Primary lymphedematous states: congenital lymphedema (Milroy's at birth, lymphedema praecox of women with onset puberty to ~30 yrs, lymphedema tarda after age 35 yrs).

Obstruction below the vena cava: tumors, lymph nodes.

Local trauma: Ruptured Baker's cyst, gastrocnemius muscle rupture.

Inflammation: cellulitis, underlying malignancy, superficial thrombophlebitis.

Reflex sympathetic dystrophy

Angioedema

Rare congenital: Klippel-Trenaunay (venovenous malformation with port wine nevus, extremity hypertrophy, unilateral varicose veins), Parke-Weber (arteriovenous with auscultated bruit).

Physical Exam

- As with bilateral edema, the exam should focus on the type of edema and evidence of chronicity.
- Patients with DVT may have warmth, tenderness, a palpable venous cord, pedal spasm, or tenderness when tapping the anterior shin (Lisker's sign).
- Reflex sympathetic dystrophy will usually have hyperesthesia with progression to hyperhydrosis, cool skin, induration, cyanosis, or livedo reticularis.
- A torn medial gastrocnemius head may have a palpable mass, purpura from tendinous/fascial bleeding, or a depression in the midcalf area. Tenderness is greatest at the medial midcalf.
- A ruptured Baker's cyst typically has a tender popliteal fossa and is often accompanied by signs of rheumatoid arthritis.
- Patients with angioedema can have marked localized circumferential swelling at sites of minor injury or often localized to the lips, head, or neck.

Imaging Evaluation

Imaging of unilateral edema commonly involves Doppler U/S, which may readily identify a DVT or a Baker's cyst. When results are equivocal, evaluation may involve contrast venography or magnetic resonance venography.

MANAGEMENT

Management is directed at the underlying disorder. Arteriovenous malformations and gastrocnemius ruptures may be best managed surgically.

KEY POINTS TO REMEMBER

- The history and physical exam should lead the physician to the diagnosis in most cases.
- In general, bilateral edema is the result of a systemic process or central lesion, whereas unilateral edema is usually the result of local pathology.
- Although benign orthostatic edema is a common condition, evaluation should rule out underlying disorders, most commonly right heart failure, renal failure/nephrotic syndrome, and liver failure.
- Patients with unilateral edema should be evaluated and treated for DVT in a timely manner to limit the risk of embolism.

REFERENCES AND SUGGESTED READINGS

Ciocon JO. Leg edema: clinical clues to the differential diagnosis. *Geriatrics* 1993;48:34–45.

Jensen NF. C1 esterase inhibitor deficiency, airway compromise, anesthesia. *Anesth Analg* 1998;87:480–488.

Schwartzman R. Reflex sympathetic dystrophy. *Arch Neurol* 1987;44:555–561.

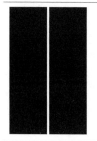

Cardiovascular

Approach to the Patient with Chest Pain

Eric F. Buch

INTRODUCTION

Chest pain is one of the most common reasons for ER visits and hospital admission: 4 million annually, including >1 million with acute MI.

Initial diagnostic approach includes a limited history and physical exam and emergent ECG, optimally completed within 10 mins of presentation. Results of the initial assessment guide further tests and treatments.

Despite the broad differential diagnosis of chest pain (Table 3-1), the immediate goal should be to exclude the four common life-threatening causes (bolded in Table 3-1).

High-risk patients (including those who appear ill or have abnormal vital signs or risk factors for coronary disease) need immediate IV access and cardiac monitoring.

PRESENTATION

History

Establish the location, quality, and severity of the chest discomfort, time course of symptoms, aggravating and alleviating factors, and any associated symptoms.

With this information, patients can be assigned to one of three categories based on the likelihood of cardiac ischemia (Table 3-2): (a) typical (definite) angina, (b) atypical (possible or probable) angina, or (c) nonanginal symptoms. Typical features may be lacking in acute coronary syndromes (e.g., precipitants, alleviating factors).

Estimate prior probability of coronary disease based on history of MI or cardiac arrest, history of percutaneous transluminal coronary angioplasty or coronary artery bypass graft, coronary artery disease documented by angiography, results of previous cardiac testing, and cardiac risk factors. Diabetic patients should be approached as if they had known coronary artery disease; their risk of cardiac events is similar to those with prior MI [1].

Other diagnoses that should not be missed are as follows:

- Pericarditis: pain typically worse with recumbency, relieved by sitting upright or leaning forward. Fever and persistence of pain may also be clues.
- Pulmonary embolism (PE): chest pain onset usually coincides with shortness of breath; may be pleuritic or accompanied by cough. Assess for predisposing factors: recent surgery, immobilization, malignancy, or hypercoagulability.
- Aortic dissection: typically presents with severe, tearing pain radiating to back.
- Pneumothorax: typically presents with sudden sharp pleuritic chest pain and dyspnea.

Physical Exam

An abbreviated exam, focusing on vital signs and arterial saturation, neck veins, lungs and heart, chest wall, abdomen, and pulses, may suggest a specific cause of chest pain (Table 3-3). However, physical exam is often unhelpful in reaching a diagnosis.

An **ECG** provides the most important initial data. 80% of patients with acute MI have ECG abnormalities; one-half of these are diagnostic. Table 3-4 lists the significance of common ECG abnormalities.

- Obtain ECG within 10 mins; repeat during pain or with any change in symptoms.
- Assume all abnormalities are new unless proven otherwise. Obtain old ECGs.

TABLE 3-1. DIFFERENTIAL DIAGNOSIS OF CHEST PAIN

Cardiac
  Coronary artery disease (angina pectoris, unstable angina, **MI**, coronary vasospasm)
  Pericarditis
  Aortic stenosis
  Hypertrophic cardiomyopathy
Vascular
  Aortic dissection
  Pulmonary embolism
  Pulmonary HTN
Pulmonary
  Pneumothorax or **tension pneumothorax**
  Pneumonitis, pleuritis (e.g., connective tissue disease or TB), or tracheobronchitis
  Pulmonary neoplasm
Gastrointestinal
  GERD, esophagitis
  Esophageal spasm, mucosal tear, rupture, or infection (e.g., esophageal candidiasis)
  Peptic ulcer disease
  Biliary colic or cholecystitis
  Pancreatitis
Musculoskeletal and neurologic
  Muscle strain (especially intercostal, interscalene, pectoralis)
  Costochondritis
  Subacromial bursitis
  Cervical spine disease with referred pain
  Herpes zoster
Psychiatric
  Emotional, anxiety-related, panic disorder

MANAGEMENT

Lab and Imaging Evaluation

Chest Radiography

- Although rarely diagnostic, chest radiography can help rule out less common causes of chest pain as well as complications of MI. It is more useful if comparison films are available.
- Pulmonary causes: may show focal infiltrate (pneumonia), unilateral radiolucency (pneumothorax), or wedge-shaped density (PE with infarction).
- Cardiovascular: cardiomegaly (pericardial effusion or MI complicated by left ventricular failure), mediastinal widening, or abnormal aorta (aortic dissection).
- Others: pneumomediastinum (esophageal rupture), rib fracture, or dislocation.

Tests of Myocardial Ischemia/Infarction

- Lab markers of myocardial injury, such as troponin and CK-MB assays, are sensitive and specific indications of cardiac muscle necrosis. See Chap. 4, Acute Coronary Syndromes, for further details.

TABLE 3-2. HISTORICAL FEATURES ASSOCIATED WITH ANGINA

Clinical feature	Typical angina	Atypical angina	Nonanginal symptoms
Location	Substernal ± radiation to neck, arm, shoulder	Epigastric, right-sided; to back, teeth, or ear	Radiation to lower abdomen or legs
Quality	Pressure, tightness, squeezing, heaviness	Burning, cramping, gas	Stabbing, sharp
Time course	Builds over 5–10 mins (sometimes sudden in MI)	Duration >30 mins without other signs of acute coronary syndrome	Lasts only seconds
Aggravating factors	Exercise, stress, cold weather	Occurs at rest (although MI, unstable angina, and Prinzmetal's may occur at rest)	Deep breathing, change in position
Alleviating factors	Rest, nitroglycerin	Belching, antacids	—
Associated symptoms	Dyspnea, diaphoresis, nausea and vomiting	—	—

- Echocardiography can show segmental myocardial dysfunction but cannot distinguish between acute MI, ischemia, and old infarction. The absence of regional wall motion defects does not rule out MI, but echocardiography can help when other data are equivocal.

Other Specific Confirmatory Tests

PERICARDIAL EFFUSION. Echocardiogram can show the presence of fluid in the pericardial sac as well as hemodynamic compromise from effusion. Pericarditis may be present without effusion.

TABLE 3-3. FEATURES FROM PHYSICAL EXAM SUGGESTING A SPECIFIC CAUSE

Physical finding	Diagnoses to consider
S_3, S_4, or MR murmur during pain	Myocardial ischemia
Friction rub or pericardial knock	Pericarditis
Tachycardia, tachypnea, hypotension, hypoxemia	Pulmonary embolism, MI with cardiogenic shock
Loud P_2 with fixed split of S_2	Pulmonary HTN, pulmonary embolism
Pleural friction rub	Pneumonia, pulmonary embolism
Aortic insufficiency murmur, asymmetric pulses or BPs	Aortic dissection
Unilateral decreased breath sounds and tympany	Pneumothorax
Chest wall tenderness and worse with movement	Musculoskeletal causes
Vesicular rash, dermatomal distribution	Herpes zoster

TABLE 3-4. SIGNIFICANT ECG FINDINGS IN CHEST PAIN

ECG finding	Likely diagnosis	Differential diagnosis
≥ 1 mm ST elevation in at least two contiguous leads	Acute MI	Coronary vasospasm Pericarditis Early repolarization Left ventricular aneurysm
≥ 1 mm ST depression	Myocardial ischemia or infarction	Normal variant LVH with strain Digitalis toxicity Electrolyte abnormalities
T-wave inversions in at least two contiguous leads	Myocardial ischemia or infarction	Normal variant CNS disease Hypertrophic obstructive cardiomyopathy
Q waves ≥ 1 mm and 0.04 sec in two contiguous leads	MI, age undetermined	Dilated cardiomyopathy LVH, hypertrophic obstructive cardiomyopathy, COPD Pulmonary embolism
Tall R waves $\pm$ T-wave inversions in V_1/V_2, right axis deviation, new right bundle branch block	Pulmonary embolism	Pulmonary HTN

LVH, left ventricular hypertrophy.

PULMONARY EMBOLISM. $\dot{V}/\dot{Q}$ scan or spiral CT with contrast with PE protocol are appropriate diagnostic tests. The gold standard, pulmonary angiography, should be reserved for cases in which less invasive studies are equivocal. For high suspicion, do not delay anticoagulation until testing is complete.

AORTIC DISSECTION. Transesophageal echocardiogram, CT, MRI, or aortography show details of aortic anatomy. If dissection is a possibility, one of these should be performed before initiating anticoagulation in suspected MI or PE.

ESOPHAGEAL DISEASE. Upper endoscopy is useful for diagnosing structural lesions of the esophagus and stomach, such as reflux esophagitis and peptic ulcer disease. 24-hr esophageal pH monitoring documents acid reflux. Esophageal manometry can demonstrate motility disorders or esophageal spasm.

SUSPECTED MYOCARDIAL ISCHEMIA. Once acute MI has been excluded by serial enzymes, patients with unstable angina should undergo further testing to identify anatomic abnormalities or inducible ischemia.

American College of Cardiology/American Heart Association guidelines recommend cardiac catheterization for patients with high-risk characteristics (prior revascularization, congestive heart failure, ventricular arrhythmias, recurrent angina, large defect on noninvasive test) [2]. Others should have a functional ischemia evaluation, such as an exercise or pharmacologic stress test.

KEY POINTS TO REMEMBER

• The initial evaluation should focus on conditions that are most dangerous and serious, including an acute coronary syndrome, pulmonary embolus, aortic dissection, and tension pneumothorax.

- An ECG should be rapidly obtained. The ECG is critical in risk stratifying a patient with the possibility of an acute coronary syndrome. History, physical exam, and cardiac risk factors should guide further evaluation for MI.

SUGGESTED READING

Jesse RL, Kontos MC. Evaluation of chest pain in the emergency department. *Curr Probl Cardiol* 1997;22:149–236.

Lee TH, Goldman L. Evaluation of the patient with acute chest pain. *N Engl J Med* 2000;342:1187–1195.

REFERENCES

1. Haffner SM, Lehto S, Ronnemaa T, et al. Mortality from coronary heart disease in subjects with type 2 diabetes and in nondiabetic subjects with and without prior myocardial infarction. *N Engl J Med* 1998;339:229–234.
2. Scanlon PJ, Faxon DP, Audet AM, et al. ACC/AHA guidelines for coronary angiography: executive summary and recommendations. A report of the American College of Cardiology/American Heart Association Task Force on Practice Guidelines (Committee on Coronary Angiography) developed in collaboration with the Society for Cardiac Angiography and Interventions. *Circulation* 1999;99:2345–2357.

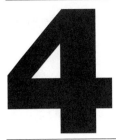

Acute Coronary Syndromes

Douglas R. Bree,
Chris Leach, and
Eric F. Buch

INTRODUCTION

Coronary artery disease (CAD) is the leading cause of death in the United States. 800,000 Americans suffer a coronary event annually, and >25% are fatal.

Acute MI (AMI) results from coronary artery occlusion by thrombus formed on an atheromatous plaque—usually immature plaque with a thin fibrous cap. Inflammation may contribute to its rupture, initiating a sequence of platelet aggregation, fibrin deposition, and vasoconstriction that eventually occludes the artery.

Unstable angina often results from an unstable ruptured plaque, resulting in intermittent ischemia.

CAUSES

Differential Diagnosis

For a detailed discussion on the differential diagnosis of chest pain, see Chap. 3, Approach to the Patient with Chest Pain.

PRESENTATION

History

Rapid recognition is the key to outcome: targeted history, physical, and 12-lead ECG should be completed within 5 mins of arrival. Assess the patient for thrombolysis or revascularization.

Typical chest pain is crushing discomfort; substernal or left-sided, and may radiate to left arm, neck, shoulder, back, or jaw. Onset may be during exertion or at rest. Pain lasting only seconds or pain localizable with one finger is unlikely to be of cardiac origin. Ischemic chest discomfort is often accompanied by dyspnea, diaphoresis, nausea, vomiting, palpitations, or an overwhelming sense of doom. AMI may also occur with atypical chest discomfort or none at all, particularly postoperatively in the elderly, in women, and in diabetic patients.

Unstable angina and MI are usually differentiated from stable angina by lack of relief with rest and/or nitroglycerin (NTG) and prolonged discomfort lasting >20 mins.

In patients with previous MI, inquire whether current pain is similar to prior episodes.

Physical Exam

The goals of the physical exam are as follows:

- Determine hemodynamic stability: assess for cardiogenic pulmonary edema and shock.
- Detect mechanical complications of MI (papillary muscle dysfunction, free wall rupture, ventricular septal defect).
- Evaluate for other possible etiologies of chest discomfort.

TABLE 4-1. CARDIAC ENZYMES WITH TIMING AND SPECIFICITY

Cardiac enzyme	Time to positive (hrs)	Time to peak (hrs)	Time to normal	Specificity
Troponin I/T	4–6	24–48	7–10 d	Very high
CK-MB	4–6	18–24	72 hrs	High (95%)
Myoglobin	1–4	—	—	Intermediate

Lab Evaluation

Diagnosis of AMI requires two of the following three criteria:

- Prolonged chest discomfort or anginal equivalent
- ECG changes consistent with ischemia or infarction
- Elevated cardiac enzymes

ECG

- Definitive ECG diagnosis of ST-elevation MI (STEMI) requires ≥ 1 mm of ST elevation in at least two contiguous leads.
- New left bundle branch block (LBBB) with acute chest symptoms is managed like STEMI (suggests proximal left anterior descending [coronary artery] occlusion). Ischemia can still be identified in patients with known old LBBB [1].
- The distribution of ST elevation or other ischemic changes is helpful in determining location of the occluded vessel, assessing prognosis, and predicting complications.

Lab markers document damaged myocardial tissue, but ECG is crucial to assigning patients to one of the following three groups for further management:

- STEMI
- Non-STEMI (NSTEMI)
- Undifferentiated chest pain syndrome, with normal cardiac enzymes, requiring further cardiac ischemia evaluation

Cardiac Enzymes

Troponin I has the highest sensitivity and specificity and is often positive when the others are negative. Frequently, the clinician will rule out an MI with troponins obtained at baseline and 12 hrs after the last episode of chest pain. CK-MB may be falsely positive with myopathies or other muscle injury. Myoglobin is not specific for cardiac muscle and a positive result requires more clinical interpretation. Myoglobin's use is based on the fact that it is the first enzyme to rise (Table 4-1).

MANAGEMENT

Treatment of Unstable Angina/Non-ST Elevation MI

Site of Treatment

Admit all patients with recurrent ischemic symptoms, ECG changes (ST depression or T-wave inversions), or elevated myocardial enzymes. Patients with continuing symptoms or hemodynamic instability should be admitted to a coronary care unit with continuous rhythm monitoring, high nurse-patient ratio, frequent assessment, and quick access to defibrillation. Patients who are symptom-free should be admitted to the hospital floor with continuous monitoring (e.g., step-down unit).

Goals of Treatment

- Control ischemia
- Provide antiplatelet and anticoagulation therapy
- Revascularize when appropriate

- Risk stratify
- Prevent future events (risk factor modification)

Antiischemic Therapy

Antiischemic therapy involves measures to improve the balance of myocardial oxygen supply and demand. Nonpharmacologic measures include bed rest and supplemental O_2.

NITROGLYCERIN. The mechanism of action of NTG includes venous, coronary, and systemic arterial vasodilation. It reduces preload and afterload, resulting in lower myocardial O_2 demand and dilates coronary arteries to improve myocardial O_2 supply.

Use of NTG is based more on pathophysiologic rationale and uncontrolled observations than high-level evidence [2].

Start with a 0.4-mg sublingual tablet or NTG spray, monitoring for hypotension. If ischemic symptoms are not completely relieved, repeat q5mins until 3 doses given. Provide IV NTG if symptoms persist after 3 doses of immediate-release NTG. Initiate IV NTG at 10 μg/min and increase by 10 μg/min q3–5mins until symptoms resolve or BP falls. Use with caution when SBP ≤ 110 mm Hg or has fallen by ≥ 25%. Remember that readministration of SL NTG will deliver much more NTG (400 μg) in a short time than increasing the IV drip rate. Therefore, if recurrent ischemia develops, then use SL NTG before increasing the drip.

Once a patient has been symptom-free for 12–24 hrs, change to topical or long-acting oral nitrates. If there are no recurrent ischemic symptoms, initiate a daily nitrate-free interval to prevent nitrate tolerance. Nitrates are contraindicated if sildenafil (Viagra) was used in the previous 24 hrs.

MORPHINE SULFATE. The mechanism of action is reduced preload via venodilation and also reduced heart rate and SBP, decreasing myocardial O_2 demand. Morphine sulfate is also a potent analgesic and anxiolytic.

Give 1–5 mg IV for symptoms refractory to 3 doses of immediate-release NTG. Repeat dose q5–30mins if necessary.

BETA BLOCKERS. By inhibiting beta-1 receptors, beta blockers reduce the cardiac rate and contractility and therefore myocardial O_2 demand. Also, diastole is prolonged, improving coronary perfusion and myocardial O_2 supply.

The evidence by metaanalysis suggests beta blockers in unstable angina (UA)/ NSTEMI reduce progression to AMI by 18% [3], but no mortality benefit has been demonstrated.

There is no clear evidence that any of the beta blockers is superior, but avoid those with intrinsic sympathomimetic activity (e.g., pindolol [Visken], acebutolol [Sectral]). Choice is usually based on clinician familiarity. Commonly used agents in acute ischemia include metoprolol (Lopressor), propranolol (Inderal), esmolol (Brevibloc), and atenolol (Tenormin). If concerned about tolerability of beta blockers, use a short-acting agent such as metoprolol or esmolol. The goal is a heart rate in the 50s as BP tolerates.

Typical dosing regimens are as follows:

- Metoprolol: 5 mg IV q5mins × 3, then 25–50 mg PO q6h × 48 hrs.
- Esmolol: start 0.1 mg/kg/min IV, titrating up by 0.05 mg/kg/min q10mins to max 0.3 mg/kg/min, as heart rate and BP tolerate.
- Propranolol: 0.5–1.0 mg IV loading dose, then in 1–2 hrs start 40–80 mg PO q6h.

Contraindications are as follows:

- Bradycardia or heart block: avoid beta blockers if heart rate ≤ 50, PR interval >240 msec, or any type of second- or third-degree heart block.
- Bronchospastic lung disease: most patients with a history of COPD will still tolerate a cardioselective beta blocker at low doses. Consider a trial of a very short-acting cardioselective agent, such as esmolol.

CALCIUM CHANNEL BLOCKERS. Metaanalyses have shown no significant mortality benefit for calcium channel blockers (CCBs) in UA/NSTEMI [3,4]; use is limited primarily to symptomatic relief. There is no role for immediate-release dihydropyridine CCBs (e.g., nifedipine) in acute coronary syndromes (ACS); studies have shown higher mortality in the absence of beta blockade [5,6].

In general, CCBs are second-line agents whose use is limited to the following situations:

- Refractory ischemia in patients already receiving nitrates and beta blockers
- Patients with contraindications to nitrates and/or beta blockers
- Patients with "variant" or Prinzmetal's angina from coronary vasospasm

CCBs are contraindicated in severe left ventricular (LV) dysfunction, Wolf-Parkinson-White syndrome (in IV form), or high-degree heart block.

Antiplatelet and Anticoagulation Therapy

ORAL ANTIPLATELET AGENTS. *Aspirin.* ASA should be administered immediately to all patients with suspected ACS unless contraindicated. It should be continued indefinitely.

- Mechanism: COX inhibitor that prevents thromboxane-mediated platelet aggregation.
- Evidence: multiple large studies [7–10] have consistently demonstrated reduction in death or MI, independent of dosage, formulation, or timing of administration. Pooled data suggest a relative risk reduction of 35% for the combined end point of cardiovascular death, MI, or stroke at 6 mos [11], with a number needed to treat of 20.
- Dosage: The initial dose (162–325 mg) should not be coated and may be chewed to speed absorption. Subsequent doses (81–325 mg PO daily) may be enteric coated.

Contraindications include serious active bleeding, active peptic ulcer disease or gastritis, and severe uncontrolled HTN (risk of intracranial hemorrhage).

Clopidogrel (Plavix)

- Mechanism: adenosine triphosphate antagonist that acts as an irreversible platelet inhibitor.

Clopidogrel is indicated for patients unable to tolerate ASA, those in whom an early noninvasive strategy is planned, and those undergoing percutaneous coronary intervention (PCI) [12].

The CURE trial [13] showed that clopidogrel added to ASA in selected patients with UA/NSTEMI reduced a composite end point of cardiovascular death, MI, or stroke. Give a loading dose of 300 mg PO followed by 75 mg PO daily. See Appendix A, Review of Selected Clinical Trials, for details of the CURE trial, including inclusion and exclusion criteria.

Avoid clopidogrel if the patient will have urgent coronary artery bypass graft (CABG) (clopidogrel must be withheld for 5–7 days preoperatively due to increased risk of major bleeding) or if the patient has had a recent intracranial hemorrhage.

HEPARINS. Heparin agents affect clotting factors, acting by a different pathway than oral antiplatelet agents. They should be added to ASA and/or clopidogrel in likely or definite ACS. No clear superiority of unfractionated or low-molecular-weight heparin (LMWH) has been proved.

Unfractionated Heparin. Several studies have compared the addition of unfractionated heparin (UFH) or placebo to ASA in UA, with most showing reductions in risk of MI and refractory angina that were not statistically significant. However, a metaanalysis combining data from 3 randomized clinical trials found a significant 56% reduction in risk of death or MI at 5 days [14].

Dosage should be weight-based, and most institutions have their own nomograms. Follow platelet count and Hct daily. The optimal duration of therapy is not established, but in most trials it was continued for 2–4 days.

Low-Molecular-Weight Heparins. Four large trials have compared LMWH to UFH in UA, with 2 showing no significant difference (using dalteparin and nadroparin) [15,16] and 2 showing significant reduction in death, MI, and recurrent ischemia in the group receiving LMWH (both used enoxaparin) [17,18] (see Appendix A for details of the ESSENCE trial). They are generally accepted to have similar efficacy, require less monitoring, and induce less thrombocytopenia than UFH. However, the level of anticoagulation is difficult to assess, and effects are harder to reverse. For this reason, some interventional cardiologists prefer UFH before PCI.

The dosage adjustments for renal failure (creatinine clearance, <30 mL/min) and obesity are unclear, limiting their use. Typical doses include enoxaparin (Lovenox),

1 mg/kg SC q12h up to 100 kg, and dalteparin (Fragmin), 120 U/kg SC q12h with a maximum dose of 10,000 U.

GLYCOPROTEIN IIB/IIIA INHIBITORS. *Mechanism.* Inhibit platelet aggregation by interfering with platelet binding to fibrinogen.

Evidence. The PRISM-PLUS trial [19] (tirofiban [Aggrastat]) and PURSUIT trial [20] (eptifibatide [Integrelin]) showed benefits of IIB/IIIA inhibitors in UA with ECG changes or enzyme elevation. See Appendix A, Review of Selected Clinical Trials, for details on PRISM-PLUS. CAPTURE [21] (abciximab [ReoPro]) showed benefit in association with PCI.

Summary. When using glycoprotein IIB/IIIA inhibitors, always add to the standard therapy of ASA and heparin (UFH better studied than LMWH). Eptifibatide and tirofiban are indicated in high-risk patients (continuing ischemia, dynamic ECG changes, abnormal cardiac enzymes) when PCI is not planned. Abciximab is the preferred agent in conjunction with PCI but should only be considered in patients for whom an early invasive strategy is planned.

Coronary Revascularization

There are 2 approaches to treatment of UA/NSTEMI: the early invasive and early conservative strategies.

EARLY INVASIVE APPROACH. The early invasive approach involves cardiac catheterization with possible revascularization in the absence of contraindications. This approach more quickly identifies patients at very low risk (e.g., no significant CAD) and very high risk (e.g., left main or 3-vessel CAD). It offers immediate revascularization of the culprit stenosis and prevention of angina.

The latest update to the ACC/AHA guidelines [22] recommends this strategy for patients with UA and any of the following **high-risk features**: recurrent angina at rest or low-level activity despite antiischemic therapy, elevated cardiac markers, new ST depression, angina with congestive heart failure symptoms or signs, high-risk stress test, LV ejection fraction ≤ 40%, hemodynamic instability, sustained ventricular tachycardia, PCI with stent in previous 6 mos, or prior CABG.

EARLY CONSERVATIVE APPROACH. The early conservative approach involves cardiac catheterization and percutaneous revascularization only for patients with refractory ischemia or a markedly abnormal stress test. This approach may avoid risks and costs associated with unnecessary coronary angiography, while achieving similar outcomes. It requires an echocardiogram to identify patients with LV dysfunction. If LV dysfunction is present, then angiography should be performed to rule out left-main or 3-vessel coronary disease (because CABG improves survival).

Risk Stratification

If the early conservative strategy is chosen, a noninvasive stress test can establish the presence of myocardial ischemia and identify high-risk patients who would benefit from angiography.

Two groups of patients may not require a noninvasive stress test:

- Those at highest risk (recurrent rest angina despite maximal therapy, severe LV dysfunction, hemodynamic instability) who will require angiography regardless of the results.
- Those at lowest risk (atypical symptoms without CAD risk factors) who would not be considered for angiography and revascularization regardless of the results, because the risk of adverse event is so low that angiography would not offer significant benefit.

For the selection of a noninvasive test, see Chap. 1, Approach to Perioperative Care, Perioperative Cardiac Evaluation.

Treatment of ST-Elevation MI

The initial goals in managing STEMI are as follows:

- Rapid confirmation of diagnosis with ECG and lab tests (as described earlier).
- Control of ischemic pain.
- Recognition and correction of hemodynamic abnormalities.

- Assessment and implementation of possible reperfusion strategies.
- Administration of antithrombotic and antiplatelet therapy and other adjunctive medications.

While awaiting ECG, give supplemental O_2 and initiate IV access and cardiac monitoring.

Once the diagnosis of STEMI has been established, consider the following adjunctive medications while evaluating for reperfusion (see earlier text for details): aspirin, beta blocker, NTG, and morphine sulfate.

Reperfusion

TIMING. Consider acute reperfusion within 12 hrs of symptom onset in patients with ST elevation or new LBBB. Patients with >12 hrs and <24 hrs of symptoms should still be considered for reperfusion (class IIb), particularly in the setting of continued ST elevation; persistent symptoms; LV dysfunction; widespread ECG changes; or prior MI, percutaneous transluminal coronary angioplasty (PTCA), or CABG.

The optimal reperfusion strategy remains controversial, and management varies by center and available resources. The intervention should not be delayed due to indecision on method.

THROMBOLYSIS. Advantages of thrombolysis are widespread availability and fast administration:

- The benefit of early thrombolytic therapy (within 12 hrs) is well studied [8,23,24]. Pooled data from the Fibrinolytic Therapy Trialists' Group showed an 18% reduction in mortality [25].
- Agents: non–fibrin-specific (streptokinase) and fibrin-specific (t-PA, reteplase, anistreplase, tenecteplase) have similar efficacy [26,27].
- The target door-to-needle (thrombolysis) time is <30 mins.
- Indications for thrombolysis include symptoms consistent with acute MI, time of onset <12 hrs prior, and ECG changes (either ST segment elevation of at least 1 mm in two contiguous leads or new LBBB).
- Thrombolytics increase the risk of hemorrhage (including intracranial bleed in 0.5–0.7%). Predictive factors for stroke and intracranial hemorrhage include age ≥ 65 yrs, weight <70 kg, HTN on admission, and the use of t-PA rather than other agents [28].
- Contraindications should always be carefully considered (Table 4-2).

TABLE 4-2. CONTRAINDICATIONS TO THROMBOLYSIS

Absolute contraindications

Active internal bleeding (not including menstruation)

Suspected aortic dissection

Major trauma or surgery within previous 2 wks

History of hemorrhagic stroke

Recent head trauma or known intracranial neoplasm

Hemorrhagic retinopathy

Relative contraindications

Uncontrolled HTN (BP >180/110) or history of chronic, severe HTN

History of any stroke

Bleeding diathesis or use of anticoagulant medications

Prolonged, traumatic CPR

Active peptic ulcer disease

Pregnancy

- Rescue PTCA: 15–50% of patients [29] do not achieve coronary artery patency with thrombolytics; patients with ongoing symptoms and persistent ST elevation 90 mins after thrombolysis should be considered for rescue PTCA.

Emergent Percutaneous Transluminal Coronary Angioplasty

Emergent PTCA has the advantage of increased early efficacy in opening occluded arteries, lower rates of hemorrhagic stroke, and improved survival.

A systematic review of 10 randomized clinical trials [30] found primary PTCA vs. thrombolysis reduced 30-day mortality (32% relative risk reduction; number needed to treat, 48). Given a lower stroke risk and higher efficacy, PTCA is the reperfusion method of choice in larger centers with the capacity for emergent PTCA and adequate experience. If patients have contraindications to thrombolysis and PTCA is not available, then consider transfer to a facility capable of emergent PTCA (class IIa).

The SHOCK trial showed a 6-mo mortality benefit of PTCA vs. thrombolysis in patients with cardiogenic shock [31] if PTCA is performed within 18 hrs of onset of shock (class I).

KEY POINTS TO REMEMBER

- The ECG is the single most important test in risk stratifying patients with suspected acute coronary syndrome.
- Some patients, such as diabetics, females, and the elderly, may present with atypical symptoms. A high index of suspicion must be maintained in these patients.
- Early recognition and initiation of appropriate therapy is critical in improving outcomes. Time is myocardium.
- ASA, beta blockers, nitrates, and heparin are given to most patients with acute coronary syndromes in the absence of contraindications.
- In UA/NSTEMI, selected patients benefit from addition of glycoprotein IIB/IIIA antagonists, clopidogrel, and early angiography.
- In STEMI, most patients should undergo emergent mechanical (PTCA) or pharmacologic (thrombolysis) reperfusion.

SUGGESTED READING

Braunwald E, Antman EM, Beasley JW, et al. ACC/AHA guidelines for the management of patients with unstable angina and non-ST-segment elevation myocardial infarction: executive summary and recommendations. A report of the American College of Cardiology/American Heart Association Task Force on Practice Guidelines (Committee on the Management of Patients with Unstable Angina). *Circulation* 2000;102:1193–1209.

Ryan TJ, Antman EM, Brooks NH, et al. 1999 update: ACC/AHA Guidelines for the management of patients with acute myocardial infarction: executive summary and recommendations: a report of the American College of Cardiology/American Heart Association Task Force on Practice Guidelines (Committee on Management of Acute Myocardial Infarction). *Circulation* 1999;100:1016–1030.

Scanlon PJ, Faxon DP, Audet AM, et al. ACC/AHA guidelines for coronary angiography: executive summary and recommendations. A report of the American College of Cardiology/American Heart Association Task Force on Practice Guidelines (Committee on Coronary Angiography) developed in collaboration with the Society for Cardiac Angiography and Interventions. *Circulation* 1999;99:2345–2357.

REFERENCES

1. Wackers FJ. The diagnosis of myocardial infarction in the presence of left bundle branch block. *Cardiol Clin* 1987;5(3):393–401.
2. Braunwald E, Antman EM, Beasley JW, et al. ACC/AHA guidelines for the management of patients with unstable angina and non-ST-segment elevation myocardial infarction. A report of the American College of Cardiology/American Heart

Association Task Force on Practice Guidelines (Committee on the Management of Patients With Unstable Angina). *J Am Coll Cardiol* 2000;36(3):970–1062.

3. Yusuf S, Wittes J, Friedman L. Overview of results of randomized clinical trials in heart disease. II. Unstable angina, heart failure, primary prevention with aspirin, and risk factor modification. *JAMA* 1988;260(15):2259–2263.

4. Held PH, Yusuf S, Furberg CD. Calcium channel blockers in acute myocardial infarction and unstable angina: an overview. *BMJ* 1989;299(6709):1187–1192.

5. Furberg CD, Psaty BM, Meyer JV. Nifedipine. Dose-related increase in mortality in patients with coronary heart disease. *Circulation* 1995;92(5):1326–1331.

6. Gibson RS, Boden WE, Theroux P, et al. Diltiazem and reinfarction in patients with non-Q-wave myocardial infarction. Results of a double-blind, randomized, multicenter trial. *N Engl J Med* 1986;315(7):423–429.

7. Lewis HD Jr, Davis JW, Archibald DG, et al. Protective effects of aspirin against acute myocardial infarction and death in men with unstable angina. Results of a Veterans Administration Cooperative Study. *N Engl J Med* 1983;309(7):396–403.

8. Randomised trial of intravenous streptokinase, oral aspirin, both, or neither among 17,187 cases of suspected acute myocardial infarction: ISIS-2. ISIS-2 (Second International Study of Infarct Survival) Collaborative Group. *Lancet* 1988;2(8607):349–360.

9. Theroux P, Ouimet H, McCans J, et al. Aspirin, heparin, or both to treat acute unstable angina. *N Engl J Med* 1988;319(17):1105–1111.

10. Risk of myocardial infarction and death during treatment with low dose aspirin and intravenous heparin in men with unstable coronary artery disease. The RISC Group. *Lancet* 1990;336(8719):827–830.

11. Antiplatelet Trialists' Collaboration. Collaborative overview of randomised trials of antiplatelet therapy—I: prevention of death, myocardial infarction, and stroke by prolonged antiplatelet therapy in various categories of patients. *BMJ* 1994;308(6921):81–106.

12. Mehta SR, Yusuf S, Peters RJ, et al. Effects of pretreatment with clopidogrel and aspirin followed by long-term therapy in patients undergoing percutaneous coronary intervention: the PCI-CURE study. *Lancet* 2001;358(9281):527–533.

13. Yusuf S, Zhao F, Mehta SR, et al. Effects of clopidogrel in addition to aspirin in patients with acute coronary syndromes without ST-segment elevation. *N Engl J Med* 2001;345(7):494–502.

14. Cohen M, Adams PC, Parry G, et al. Combination antithrombotic therapy in unstable rest angina and non-Q-wave infarction in nonprior aspirin users. Primary end points analysis from the ATACS trial. Antithrombotic Therapy in Acute Coronary Syndromes Research Group. *Circulation* 1994;89(1):81–88.

15. Klein W, Buchwald A, Hillis SE, et al. Comparison of low-molecular-weight heparin with unfractionated heparin acutely and with placebo for 6 weeks in the management of unstable coronary artery disease. Fragmin in unstable coronary artery disease study (FRIC). *Circulation* 1997;96(1):61–68.

16. Comparison of two treatment durations (6 days and 14 days) of a low molecular weight heparin with a 6-day treatment of unfractionated heparin in the initial management of unstable angina or non-Q wave myocardial infarction: FRAX.I.S. (FRAxiparine in Ischaemic Syndrome). *Eur Heart J* 1999;20(21):1553–1562.

17. Cohen M, Demers C, Gurfinkel EP, et al. A comparison of low-molecular-weight heparin with unfractionated heparin for unstable coronary artery disease. Efficacy and Safety of Subcutaneous Enoxaparin in Non-Q-Wave Coronary Events Study Group. *N Engl J Med* 1997;337(7):447–452.

18. Antman EM, McCabe CH, Gurfinkel EP, et al. Enoxaparin prevents death and cardiac ischemic events in unstable angina/non-Q-wave myocardial infarction. Results of the thrombolysis in myocardial infarction (TIMI) 11B trial. *Circulation* 1999;100(15):1593–1601.

19. Inhibition of the platelet glycoprotein IIb/IIIa receptor with tirofiban in unstable angina and non-Q-wave myocardial infarction. Platelet Receptor Inhibition in Ischemic Syndrome Management in Patients Limited by Unstable Signs and Symptoms (PRISM-PLUS) Study Investigators. *N Engl J Med* 1998;338(21):1488–1497.

20. Inhibition of platelet glycoprotein IIb/IIIa with eptifibatide in patients with acute coronary syndromes. The PURSUIT Trial Investigators. Platelet Glycoprotein IIb/IIIa in Unstable Angina: Receptor Suppression Using Integrilin Therapy. *N Engl J Med* 1998;339(7):436–443.

21. Randomised placebo-controlled trial of abciximab before and during coronary intervention in refractory unstable angina: the CAPTURE Study. *Lancet* 1997;349(9063):1429–1435.

22. American College of Cardiology Foundation Web site. Clinical statements/guidelines. Available at: http://www.acc.org/clinical/statements.htm. Accessed February 26, 2003.

23. Anderson HV, Willerson JT. Thrombolysis in acute myocardial infarction. *N Engl J Med* 1993;329(10):703–709.

24. An international randomized trial comparing four thrombolytic strategies for acute myocardial infarction. The GUSTO investigators. *N Engl J Med* 1993;329(10):673–682.

25. Indications for fibrinolytic therapy in suspected acute myocardial infarction: collaborative overview of early mortality and major morbidity results from all randomised trials of more than 1000 patients. Fibrinolytic Therapy Trialists' (FTT) Collaborative Group. *Lancet* 1994;343(8893):311–322.

26. ISIS-3: a randomised comparison of streptokinase vs tissue plasminogen activator vs anistreplase and of aspirin plus heparin vs aspirin alone among 41,299 cases of suspected acute myocardial infarction. ISIS-3 (Third International Study of Infarct Survival) Collaborative Group. *Lancet* 1992;339(8796):753–770.

27. GISSI-2: a factorial randomised trial of alteplase versus streptokinase and heparin versus no heparin among 12,490 patients with acute myocardial infarction. Gruppo Italiano per lo Studio della Sopravvivenza nell'Infarto Miocardico. *Lancet* 1990;336(8707):65–71.

28. Simoons ML, Maggioni AP, Knatterud G, et al. Individual risk assessment for intracranial haemorrhage during thrombolytic therapy. *Lancet* 1993;342(8886–8887):1523–1528.

29. Goldman LE, Eisenberg MJ. Identification and management of patients with failed thrombolysis after acute myocardial infarction. *Ann Intern Med* 2000;132(7):556–565.

30. Weaver WD, Simes RJ, Betriu A, et al. Comparison of primary coronary angioplasty and intravenous thrombolytic therapy for acute myocardial infarction: a quantitative review. *JAMA* 1997;278(23):2093–2098.

31. Hochman JS, Sleeper LA, Godfrey E, et al. SHould we emergently revascularize Occluded Coronaries for cardiogenic shocK: an international randomized trial of emergency PTCA/CABG-trial design. The SHOCK Trial Study Group. *Am Heart J* 1999;137(2):313–321.

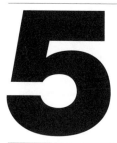

Approach to the Patient with Syncope

Eric F. Buch

INTRODUCTION

Syncope is defined as a sudden, brief loss of consciousness with loss of postural tone, followed by rapid and complete recovery, as a result of cerebral hypoperfusion.

A study of unselected patients with syncope and matched controls without syncope showed no increase in mortality from syncope itself but showed higher mortality in both groups for patients with underlying heart disease [1]. The risk of recurrence in unselected patients with syncope is 34% over 3 yrs.

The goals of the diagnostic workup are first to determine whether the event was truly syncope (vs. seizure or sudden death) and then to choose further diagnostic tests based on patient characteristics and results of initial assessment (Table 5-1). History, physical exam, and ECG will reveal a probable diagnosis in up to 45% of patients and should guide further evaluation.

Neurocardiogenic

Neurocardiogenic (also called **vasodepressor** or **reflex-mediated**) **syncope** is caused by alterations in vascular tone or heart rate, resulting in cerebral hypoperfusion. The source of autonomic instability may be central (emotional fainting) or peripheral (bladder, digestive tract, carotid sinus).

Orthostatic Hypotension

Orthostatic hypotension is commonly caused by hypovolemia (diuretics, poor intake, blood loss), vasodilatation (hyperthermia, alcohol), drug effects (antihypertensives, antidepressants, nitrates, opiates, sedatives), and autonomic insufficiency, either primary (Shy-Drager syndrome, Parkinson's disease) or secondary (diabetes, connective tissue diseases, amyloidosis, infections, nutritional deficiencies).

Cardiovascular

Cardiovascular causes have a worse prognosis than noncardiovascular causes (18–36% 1-yr mortality vs. <6%). They include the following:

- **Arrhythmias** such as bradyarrhythmias, ventricular tachyarrhythmias, and supraventricular tachyarrhythmias.
- **Anatomic/mechanical:** aortic stenosis is important to diagnose because the prognosis is poor if untreated. Hypertrophic obstructive cardiomyopathy causes syncope in 30% of patients with dynamic outflow obstruction.

CNS

Cerebrovascular disease is an uncommon cause of syncope, usually instead causing dizziness (vertebrobasilar circulation) or focal neurologic deficits (anterior circulation).

TABLE 5-1. DIFFERENTIAL DIAGNOSIS OF SYNCOPE

Neurocardiogenic (vasomotor instability)

Vasovagal (18%)

Situational (5%): micturition, cough, deglutition, defecation

Carotid sinus hypersensitivity (1%)

Psychiatric disorders (10%)

Others: neuralgia, postexercise

Orthostatic hypotension (10%)

Cardiovascular (20%)

Arrhythmias

Bradyarrhythmias

Sinus bradycardia

Atrioventricular block (second or third degree)

Drug-induced

Pacemaker malfunction

Tachyarrhythmias

Ventricular tachycardia, torsades de pointes

Supraventricular tachycardia

Anatomic/mechanical

Left ventricular outflow/inflow obstruction: aortic stenosis, hypertrophic obstructive cardiomyopathy, mitral stenosis, atrial myxoma

Right ventricular outflow/inflow obstruction: pulmonary stenosis, pulmonary embolism, pulmonary HTN

Pump failure: MI, cardiac ischemia, decompensated congestive heart failure

Other: tamponade, aortic dissection, subclavian steal

CNS (10%)

Transient ischemic attack/stroke

Seizure (technically not syncope)

Migraine

PRESENTATION

History

Establish whether the event was actually syncope. The following are distinct clinical entities, and individuals with these should **not** be labeled as having syncope:

- **Sudden cardiac death:** includes any arrest requiring CPR or electrical or chemical cardioversion. Prognoses differ, and these should not be confused.
- **Seizure:** may cause loss of consciousness, but usually with prolonged recovery, postictal confusion, and/or focal neurologic symptoms. Suspect seizure if loss of consciousness is ≥ 5 mins. Rhythmic jerking can occur in syncope or seizure.

Details surrounding events sometimes yield a diagnosis (see Table 5-2 for historical clues). Establish number and timing of episodes, associated symptoms and activities, manner of recovery, presence of coexisting medical illnesses (especially cardiovascular disease), and complete drug history.

TABLE 5-2. FEATURES FROM HISTORY SUGGESTING A SPECIFIC CAUSE

Clinical feature or symptom	Diagnoses to consider
Following pain, fear, emotional distress	Vasovagal syncope
Preceded by yawning, nausea, diaphoresis	Vasovagal syncope
During coughing, micturition, defecation	Situational syncope
Post-defecation	Pulmonary embolism
Associated with multiple vague somatic complaints	Psychiatric syncope
Immediately after standing	Orthostatic hypotension
Patient dehydrated or taking antihypertensives	Orthostatic hypotension
Triggered by exertion	Aortic stenosis, hypertrophic obstructive cardiomyopathy, pulmonary HTN, pulmonary embolism, mitral stenosis, cardiac ischemia
While shaving, during head rotation, or during pressure on neck	Carotid sinus hypersensitivity
Post-episode confusion, duration >5 mins	Seizure
Associated vertigo, diplopia, dysarthria	Migraine, transient ischemic attack
During or after arm exercise	Subclavian steal
Sudden loss of consciousness without prodrome	Arrhythmias

Physical Exam

Assess for orthostatic hypotension (drop of SBP by ≥ 20 mm Hg 2–5 mins after standing), BP difference between arms (≥ 20 mm Hg suggests aortic dissection or subclavian steal), physical signs of congenital or valvular heart disease, focal neurologic deficits, and occult blood loss, including stool guaiac.

Lab and Imaging Evaluation

Only history, physical exam, and ECG are routinely indicated. Routine lab testing is not recommended because it rarely yields a cause. Initial assessment will reveal a probable etiology without further testing in 45%.

ECG is abnormal in 50% of cases but yields a diagnosis in only 5%. ECG should be performed on all patients for risk stratification. Significant findings include atrioventricular block, bundle branch block, prolonged QT, left ventricular hypertrophy, and signs of prior infarction.

After the initial assessment, **divide patients into three groups:** diagnosis made, diagnosis suggested, or unexplained syncope.

- **Diagnosis made: treat the underlying disorder** without further testing.
- **Diagnosis suggested: choose** from among the following **specific confirmatory tests.** None is part of the routine syncope workup.
  - **Electroencephalogram (EEG)** is indicated only for those with **possible seizure** or witnessed seizure-like activity. An EEG produces useful information in <2% of unselected patients with syncope.
  - **Neurologic imaging** (head CT, MRI/magnetic resonance angiography, Doppler flow studies, and cerebral angiography): indicated only to confirm suspected **CNS etiology**, with focal neurologic deficits or significant head trauma.
  - **V̇/Q̇ scan or spiral CT** of lungs is used for suspected **pulmonary embolism.**

- **Carotid sinus massage** can be performed at bedside in those with suspected **carotid sinus hypersensitivity** and no evidence of carotid artery disease on physical exam. Vigorous pressure is applied unilaterally with a circular movement to the carotid artery just below the angle of the jaw for 6–10 secs, preferably with ECG and noninvasive BP monitoring. Considered positive if symptoms reproduced or pause of ≥ 3 secs provoked. Complications: serious but rare, with neurologic complications in <0.3% in a recent study.
- **Markers of myocardial injury** can be considered if there are multiple risk factors for MI or a suggestive history.
- **Cardiac stress testing** is used for suspected ischemic event.
- **Echocardiography** is indicated when **structural heart disease** resulting in flow obstruction is suspected (e.g., aortic stenosis, hypertrophic obstructive cardiomyopathy). The diagnostic yield is only 3%, but it reveals an undiagnosed abnormality in 5–10%.
- **Unexplained syncope:** in the 55% of patients still undiagnosed, further testing reveals a diagnosis in approximately one-half. The presence of underlying heart disease on history, physical exam, or ECG should guide the selection of further tests. Echocardiography and stress testing are recommended for all patients with suspected but unconfirmed heart disease. A cause is never diagnosed in up to 30%.

Patients with structural heart disease or suggestive history should be considered for evaluation for arrhythmia. Patients without structural heart disease and recurrent syncope should be evaluated for neurocardiogenic syncope.

Evaluation for Arrhythmia
Extended ECG monitoring can identify arrhythmia as the cause of syncope [2]:

- **Ambulatory ECG (Holter) monitoring:** usually continuous monitoring of heart rhythm and rate for 24–72 hrs, with mechanism for patient to signal occurrence of symptoms. Often nondiagnostic due to lack of correlation: 4% show arrhythmic syncope, 17% symptoms but no arrhythmia, and 13% arrhythmias but no symptoms. 79% have no symptoms during a 24-hr observation period [3].
- **Event (loop) monitoring:** allows longer period of observation (usually 30 days), with two electrodes worn for ≥ 1 mo, and a patient-triggered recorder that stores ≤ 5 mins of rhythm strip before the event and 30–60 secs after. Requires patient to activate device immediately on awakening. Recommended if infrequent, multiple episodes; yields diagnosis in 8–20% [4].
- **An implantable recorder** is an SC monitor that remains in place for >1 yr, storing a rhythm strip when activated by an abnormal heart rate or manually by application of a magnet. They are expensive and invasive but may be the only effective test when other methods fail. One study followed 85 patients with unexplained syncope—implantable recorders revealed arrhythmia in 42%.

Electrophysiologic studies involve invasive testing that uses electrical stimulation to uncover conduction system disease and inducible arrhythmias. The most **useful findings** suggesting **bradyarrhythmia** as the cause of syncope are prolonged sinus node recovery and His-ventricle interval. For **tachyarrhythmia,** induced supraventricular tachycardia (with hypotension) and sustained monomorphic ventricular tachycardia are more specific than nonsustained or polymorphic ventricular tachycardia or ventricular fibrillation.

In general, electrophysiologic study should be **reserved for those with structural heart disease** when less invasive tests fail. In this setting, electrophysiologic study yields diagnostically useful information in >50% (21% with inducible tachycardia and 34% with bradycardia). By contrast, diagnostic yield in the absence of structural heart disease is only 10%.

Evaluation for Neurocardiogenic Syncope: Upright Tilt Table Testing
Upright tilt table testing is a **provocative test for vasovagal syncope,** involving a table that quickly brings the patient from supine to head-up and holds this position for 10–60 mins [5]. ECG and noninvasive BP monitoring are performed throughout the test, and pharmacologic agents (isoproterenol, nitrates, adenosine) can be administered if there is no response initially. The test is positive if there is loss of consciousness or posture with a significant fall in BP or heart rate.

TABLE 5-3. COST-EFFECTIVENESS OF TESTS USED TO EVALUATE SYNCOPE

Diagnostic test	Cost per diagnosis (1993 dollars)
External loop recorder	529
Upright tilt table test	1024
Holter monitor	1562
Implantable loop recorder	5586
Electrophysiology study (patient with structural heart disease)	7044
Echocardiography	34,433
Electrophysiology study (patient without structural heart disease)	73,260

Data from Krahn AD, Klein GJ, Yee R, et al. The high cost of syncope: cost implications of a new insertable loop recorder in the investigation of recurrent syncope. *Am Heart J* 1999;137:870.

Upright tilt table testing should be considered for **evaluation of recurrent unexplained syncope** in which cardiac causes are unlikely, especially in younger and healthier patients. It is more dangerous and less useful in patients with structural heart disease and elderly patients.

Results among patients with unexplained syncope are that 50% have a positive tilt table test (66% with isoproterenol). In a review of many studies using a clinical diagnosis of vasovagal syncope as the gold standard, sensitivity was 67–83%, and specificity averaged 90% (75% with isoproterenol).

Psychiatric Evaluation
Many psychiatric illnesses can cause syncope, including panic disorder, anxiety disorders, major depressive disorder, somatization disorder, and substance abuse/dependence. Psychiatric evaluation should be considered in young patients in otherwise good health with recurrent syncope. Psychiatric syncope is not associated with increased mortality, but does have a high rate of recurrence.

Cost Issues
The cost-effectiveness of diagnostic tests was calculated in a cohort simulation using estimated costs and published diagnostic yields, showing a wide range of cost-effectiveness (Table 5-3).

Indications for Hospital Admission
There are no controlled trials to elucidate which patients benefit most from admission and/or telemetry monitoring; commonly used criteria are based on risk of arrhythmic syncope or cardiac death—known structural heart disease, symptoms suggesting cardiac syncope, abnormal ECG, and age >65 yrs. Other indications include focal neurologic findings and severe orthostatic hypotension. Using these criteria, most patients with syncope can be evaluated and treated as outpatients.

MANAGEMENT
Treat the underlying disorder if identified. Further specific therapies are as follows:

Vasovagal Syncope

Nonpharmacologic Measures
Avoid inciting factors such as long periods standing, dehydration, heat, fasting, alcohol, and other drugs. Have patients with prodromal symptoms sit or lie down immediately.

Pharmacologic Therapy

Pharmacologic therapy is usually reserved for recurrent or refractory syncope.

- **Beta blockers:** may work by suppressing afferent arm of Bezold-Jarisch reflex.
  - **Studies:** randomized, double-blind trial of atenolol vs. placebo showed 5% tilt table positive vs. 62% in the control group at 1 mo [6]. An uncontrolled study using propranolol found no recurrent syncope in 90% of patients over a mean follow-up of 28 mos.
  - Atenolol (Tenormin) and metoprolol (Lopressor, Toprol-XL) are used most often, although pindolol (Visken) may be especially useful for patients with low baseline pulse or BP, due to intrinsic sympathomimetic effect.
- **Other agents:** if beta blockers fail or are not tolerated, second-line agents may be tried: fludrocortisone (Florinef) with increased salt intake, disopyramide (Norpace), scopolamine (Transderm Scop, Scopace), theophylline (Uniphyl, Theodur), ephedrine, midodrine (ProAmatine), SSRIs.

Pacemaker Therapy

Pacemaker therapy is usually reserved for pharmacologic failure. Although the mechanism for vasovagal syncope is a combination of bradycardia and loss of vasomotor tone, encouraging results have been seen with pacing alone. These trials were limited to patients with **documented bradycardia:**

- **North American Vasovagal Pacemaker Study (VPM):** randomized 54 patients with recurrent syncope to pacemaker or no pacemaker. Intervention group had a much lower rate of syncope (22% vs. 70%) [7].
- **Vasovagal Syncope International Study (VASIS):** randomized 42 patients with recurrent syncope and positive tilt table test and found less recurrent syncope (5% vs. 61%) over a mean 3.7-yr follow-up [8].

Orthostatic Hypotension

Avoid volume depletion and medications that can exacerbate orthostasis (alpha and beta blockers, vasodilators, opiates, sedatives). Have patients arise slowly and in stages, wear fitted stockings to reduce venous stasis, and advise them to sit or lie down with any presyncopal symptoms. Consider **pharmacologic therapy** if these conservative measures fail:

- Volume expansion: high salt and fluid intake ± mineralocorticoid (e.g., fludrocortisone starting at 0.1 mg PO qd and titrating upwards).
- Other agents: alpha-1 agonists (e.g., ephedrine, midodrine [ProAmatine]), caffeine, NSAIDs, fluoxetine (Prozac).

KEY POINTS TO REMEMBER

- History, physical exam, and ECG will reveal a probable diagnosis in up to 45% of patients and should guide further evaluation.
- It is important in the initial evaluation to distinguish an episode of syncope, characterized by loss of consciousness and postural tone with rapid recovery, from sudden cardiac death or seizure.
- Those with structural heart disease or left ventricular dysfunction presenting with syncope are far more likely to have an arrhythmia as a cause, have a poorer prognosis, and should be evaluated more aggressively.
- Vasovagal syncope can usually be treated effectively with beta blockers. Failure of pharmacologic therapy of arrhythmic syncope warrants subspecialty referral.

SUGGESTED READING

Heaven DJ, Sutton R. Syncope. *Crit Care Med* 2000;28:N116–N120.
Kapoor WN. Syncope. *N Engl J Med* 2000;343:1856–1862.

Linzer M, Yang EH, Estes NA 3rd, et al. Diagnosing syncope. Part 1: value of history, physical examination, and electrocardiography. Clinical Efficacy Assessment Project of the American College of Physicians. *Ann Intern Med* 1997;126:989–996.

Nyman JA, Krahn AD, Bland PC, et al. The costs of recurrent syncope of unknown origin in elderly patients. *Pacing Clin Electrophysiol* 1999;22:1386–1394.

Simpson CS, Krahn AD, Klein GJ, et al. A cost effective approach to the investigation of syncope: relative merit of different diagnostic strategies. *Can J Cardiol* 1999;15:579–584.

REFERENCES

1. Kapoor WN, Hanusa BH. Is syncope a risk factor for poor outcomes? Comparison of patients with and without syncope. *Am J Med* 1996;100:646–655.
2. Crawford MH, Bernstein SJ, Deedwania PC, et al. ACC/AHA guidelines for ambulatory electrocardiography: executive summary and recommendations. A report of the American College of Cardiology/American Heart Association task force on practice guidelines (Committee to Revise the Guidelines for Ambulatory Electrocardiography). *Circulation* 1999;100:886–893.
3. Linzer M, Yang EH, Estes NA, 3rd, et al. Diagnosing syncope. Part 2: unexplained syncope. Clinical Efficacy Assessment Project of the American College of Physicians. *Ann Intern Med* 1997;127:76–86.
4. Linzer M, Pritchett EL, Pontinen M, et al. Incremental diagnostic yield of loop electrocardiographic recorders in unexplained syncope. *Am J Cardiol* 1990;66:214–219.
5. Kapoor WN, Smith MA, Miller NL. Upright tilt testing in evaluating syncope: a comprehensive literature review. *Am J Med* 1994;97:78–88.
6. Mahanonda N, Bhuripanyo K, Kangkagate C, et al. Randomized double-blind, placebo-controlled trial of oral atenolol in patients with unexplained syncope and positive upright tilt table test results. *Am Heart J* 1995;130:1250–1253.
7. Connolly SJ, Sheldon R, Roberts RS, et al. The North American Vasovagal Pacemaker Study (VPS). A randomized trial of permanent cardiac pacing for the prevention of vasovagal syncope. *J Am Coll Cardiol* 1999;33:16–20.
8. Sutton R, Brignole M, Menozzi C, et al. Dual-chamber pacing in the treatment of neurally mediated tilt-positive cardioinhibitory syncope: pacemaker versus no therapy: a multicenter randomized study. The Vasovagal Syncope International Study (VASIS) Investigators. *Circulation* 2000;102:294–299.

Management of Congestive Heart Failure

Michael J. Riley
and Eric F. Buch

INTRODUCTION

Acute heart failure (HF) is the sudden development of symptoms and signs of reduced cardiac output. It may occur in a previously normal heart or superimposed on chronic compensated HF. Precipitating factors should be identified and addressed rapidly—patients with acute HF have high mortality and may deteriorate quickly.

Potential inciting factors include acute myocardial ischemia, arrhythmias (e.g., atrial fibrillation), infective endocarditis or any acute valvular dysfunction, hypertensive crisis, overly aggressive IV fluid administration, renal failure, myocardial toxins, peripartum state or postcardiac surgery, and various inflammatory processes. Acute right-sided HF may develop in the setting of pulmonary embolism. In the context of chronic, compensated pump dysfunction, acute HF may also occur because of noncompliance with the prescribed dietary (low salt) or medical regimen.

MANAGEMENT OF CARDIOGENIC PULMONARY EDEMA

Pulmonary edema is often the most intense and frightening symptom of acute left ventricular dysfunction. Elevated pulmonary pressures cause fluid to accumulate in interstitial and alveolar spaces, impairing oxygenation.

Lab and Imaging Evaluation

Obtain an ECG to evaluate for ischemia or arrhythmia; measure cardiac enzymes to rule out infarction. Brain natriuretic peptide is almost always elevated and may be useful if the diagnosis is unclear. A chest x-ray should be obtained to evaluate the extent of edema and to rule out other conditions resulting in dyspnea.

Treatment

Immediately administer supplemental O_2 and initiate continuous pulse oximetry; sit the patient upright to shift fluid location as well as maximize use of accessory muscles. If a precipitating arrhythmia is found, consider electrical cardioversion.

In the setting of renal failure, consider hemodialysis or ultrafiltration in addition to pharmacologic management.

Pharmacologic Management

Nitroglycerin

Nitroglycerin (NTG) is the agent of choice for treating acute pulmonary edema. NTG dilates arteries and veins, reducing afterload and preload and unloading the pulmonary vasculature.

Sublingual NTG in pill or spray form can be administered quickly, before obtaining IV access. The usual dose is 0.3–0.6 mg q5mins, not to exceed 1.2 mg in 15 mins. The spray is preferred over tablets in patients with dry mucous membranes. Topical NTG is slow acting and not a good first step in treating acute edema.

IV NTG can be started at 5–10 μg/min and increased every few minutes to desired effect or a maximum of 300 μg/min.

Nitrate tolerance (declining effectiveness with continuous administration) develops by 24 hrs but can be avoided with nitrate-free intervals.

Morphine Sulfate
Morphine has a rapid venodilatory effect and curbs anxiety associated with dyspnea. Administer in doses of 2–5 mg, slow IV push, with close observation for adverse effects (hypotension, respiratory depression).

Loop Diuretics
Besides reducing total body salt and water, furosemide (Lasix) acts as a direct venodilator, reducing preload within minutes. Give a single IV dose of 40–80 mg for acute pulmonary edema (or higher if the patient receives chronic high-dose diuretics or has renal failure). A second dose can be given after 15–20 mins, with close attention to urine output and volume status. Double subsequent doses if no effect to the previous dose, up to a maximum single dose of 200 mg.

Nitroprusside
Nitroprusside (Nipride) is a powerful vasodilator. It can further reduce afterload and preload when agents previously discussed are inadequate.

Start at 0.1 μg/kg/min IV and titrate to a maximum dose of 5 μg/kg/min. Given the potency and risk of hypotension, titration should be guided by peripheral arterial catheterization.

In hepatic or renal impairment, patients may develop cyanide or thiocyanate toxicity, respectively. Nitroprusside may also worsen myocardial ischemia via coronary steal.

Bronchodilators
Consider nebulized albuterol (Proventil, Ventolin) in doses of 2.5 mg if bronchospasm is present.

Inotropic Agents
Inotropic agents may be used in refractory pulmonary edema:

- Dose titration is often guided by pulmonary artery catheterization.
- Inotropes are proarrhythmic and may increase myocardial O_2 demand; use with extreme caution in the setting of arrhythmia or ischemia.
- **Dobutamine (Dobutrex)** may be initiated at 2–3 μg/kg/min IV and titrated to maximum of 20 μg/kg/min.
- **Milrinone (Primacor)** bolused with 0.25–0.75 μg/kg over 10–15 mins, then infused at 0.375–0.75 μg/kg/min may also be used. It is a potent vasodilator; avoid in cases of systemic hypotension. A dose reduction is required in renal failure.

MANAGEMENT OF CHRONIC HEART FAILURE

Chronic HF affects approximately 2% of the adult population in the United States (4.5 million), and undiagnosed asymptomatic left ventricular dysfunction likely affects millions more.

Chronic HF management has several goals: improve long-term survival, reduce symptoms, increase functional capacity, reduce hospitalizations, and prevent or potentially reverse cardiac remodeling.

Although a large number of pharmacologic agents and nonpharmacologic approaches are used to manage chronic HF, the most appropriate combination depends to a great extent on the patient's functional class (Table 6-1).

Physical Exam

Exam may reveal pulmonary edema on chest auscultation, a displaced point of maximal impulse, or a gallop. Auscultation in the left lateral decubitus may accentuate

TABLE 6-1. NEW YORK HEART ASSOCIATION FUNCTIONAL CLASSIFICATION OF CHRONIC HEART FAILURE

Class I	Symptoms of heart failure only at levels that would limit healthy individuals
Class II	Symptoms of heart failure with ordinary exertion
Class III	Symptoms of heart failure on less than ordinary exertion
Class IV	Symptoms of heart failure at rest

left-sided gallops and mitral regurgitation. Wide open mitral regurgitation from valve annular dilatation is frequently inaudible. Daily evaluation of jugular venous pressure (JVP) and peripheral edema should be used to judge volume status. Edema collects first in the most dependent areas, which in hospitalized, bed bound patients is over the sacrum. Physical exam may not reliably distinguish systolic from diastolic dysfunction.

The hepatojugular reflex (HJR) should be performed by watching the jugular venous pulsation while applying pressure for 20–30 secs to the right upper quadrant. A positive test is a sustained increase in JVP or a rapid fall **after** pressure is released. An early rise and subsequent fall is **not** a positive test. A positive HJR is a sensitive exam technique for poor cardiac output and identifies patients who may be sensitive to volume infusions. The changing location of the JVP during the HJR is also useful in helping to identify venous pulsations in difficult exams.

Treatment

The role of the consultant is to maintain appropriate volume status, as well as ensure that the patient is receiving appropriate medical therapy.

- Daily weights, ins and outs, and physical exam, focusing on JVP, peripheral edema, and evidence of pulmonary edema, should be used to monitor volume status. Frequent evaluation of electrolytes and renal function should be performed if diuretic doses or other medications are adjusted.
- Adjust diuretic doses based on volume status.
- Ensure that an adequate Hct is maintained. For the patient with HF, a goal of Hct >30 is frequently used to ensure adequate O_2 delivery and to minimize ischemia.

Nonpharmacologic Treatments

- Low-salt diet: All patients should restrict salt intake to reduce fluid retention and vascular congestion. Required doses of diuretics are reduced with a low-salt diet.
- Identify and treat comorbid conditions like HTN, diabetes mellitus, hyperlipidemia, obesity, and alcohol use.
- Regular exercise, consisting of mild-to-moderate amounts of regular aerobic activity, improves functional capacity and reduces symptoms.
- Close follow-up is vital to encourage compliance with the treatment regimen.
- Patients with low LVEF and continued class III or IV symptoms despite appropriate medical management who have a wide native QRS complex (>130–140) may benefit from biventricular pacing ± an automated implantable cardio-defibrillator.
- Patients with LVEF <35% from ischemic cardiomyopathy with nonsustained ventricular tachycardia should be evaluated for an electrophysiology study and possible automated implantable cardio-defibrillator [1].

Pharmacologic Treatments

ACE INHIBITORS. ACE inhibitors are **first-line agents** and a mandatory part of any HF regimen, if tolerated. Numerous studies have demonstrated the ability of ACE inhibitors to reduce morbidity and mortality in HF.

ACE inhibitors reduce afterload and preload, decreasing vascular congestion and symptoms. They may also attenuate the deleterious effect of angiotensin on cardiac myocytes, including hypertrophy, apoptosis, remodeling, and progressive dysfunction.

Patients are usually started at low dose and titrated up slowly, with careful attention to serum creatinine, electrolytes, and BP. A frequent initiation regimen is captopril (Capoten), 12.5 mg PO q6–8h, increased by 12.5 mg/dose as tolerated until the maximal dose is reached. A longer-acting agent may then be substituted.

HYDRALAZINE AND NITRATE COMBINATION THERAPY. VheFT-I trial showed relief of symptoms with this regimen and modest mortality reduction (but less than ACE-inhibitors) [2]. Hydralazine (Apresoline), 75–100 mg PO tid-qid, may be combined with isosorbide dinitrate (Iso-Bid, Isordil) at a dose of 10–30 mg PO tid. Most commonly, they are used in patients intolerant of ACE inhibitors.

ANGIOTENSIN II RECEPTOR BLOCKERS. Angiotensin II receptor blockers are often substituted for ACE inhibitors in those intolerant because of cough. Like ACE inhibitors, they can cause hyperkalemia and acute worsening of renal function.

Trials are ongoing to evaluate angiotensin II receptor blockers as substitutes for or adjuncts to ACE inhibitors. The ELITE II study (losartan vs. captopril) showed no difference in mortality or hospitalization [3]. Currently, these agents are considered second-line in treatment of HF.

SPIRONOLACTONE. Spironolactone (Aldactone) is recommended for the treatment of severe HF. The Randomized Aldactone Evaluation Study (RALES) showed a 30% mortality reduction in patients with New York Heart Association class III-IV HF, as well as substantial reductions in HF symptoms and hospitalizations [4]. The recommended dose is 25 mg PO daily, increased to 50 mg or decreased to 12.5 mg as renal function and serum potassium levels allow.

BETA BLOCKERS. Beta blockers, once thought deleterious in HF management, are now considered **first-line treatment.** Numerous studies (including MERIT-HF, MOCHA, and CIBIS II [5–7]) have demonstrated the ability of beta-blocking agents to reduce mortality in class II-III HF. The COPERNICUS trial showed mortality reduction in class IV patients [8].

Initiate beta blockade only in patients with well-compensated HF already on optimal doses of standard HF medication (including ACE inhibitors and diuretics). Start at a low dose and advance as tolerated to doses proven beneficial in clinical trials (e.g., start with carvedilol [Coreg], 3.125 mg PO bid; metoprolol, 12.5 mg PO bid; or bisoprolol (Zebeta), 1.25 mg PO qd).

DIURETICS. Diuretics reduce intravascular volume and help to control symptoms of volume overload. Besides spironolactone, no diuretic has been shown to reduce mortality. Use the lowest dose of diuretic that maintains euvolemia, to reduce side effects. PO furosemide has approximately one-half the bioavailability of the IV form.

Diuretic resistance is a common problem with prolonged use. It is often due to interfering medications (e.g., NSAIDs, probenecid) or failure to adhere to a low-salt diet. Sometimes dose and/or frequency must be increased or a thiazide diuretic added for synergy (e.g., metolazone to furosemide).

DIGOXIN. Digitalis glycosides were among the first medications used in HF. By inhibiting Na^+K^+ adenosine triphosphatase in myocytes, digoxin (Lanoxin) increases force of ventricular contraction. Digoxin has not been shown to reduce mortality in HF but does reduce symptoms, improve functional status, prevent hospitalizations, and improve quality of life. Digoxin is useful in controlling ventricular rate in atrial fibrillation among patients with HF.

PROVED [9] and RADIANCE [10] studies showed worsening of symptoms and increased hospitalizations after withdrawing digoxin from regimen of HF patients previously tolerating the drug.

To load digoxin, give 0.5 mg PO, then 0.25 mg q6h to a total dose of 1.25 mg, followed by maintenance dose of 0.125–0.25 mg/day. Adjust the dose to keep serum levels 0.5–2 mg/dL, with a trough of 0.5–1 mg/dL to reduce side effects.

Digoxin has a narrow therapeutic range; toxicity may occur even at therapeutic levels. Toxicity is enhanced in the setting of renal failure, hypokalemia, hypomagnesemia, and in the presence of drugs that increase serum digoxin levels.

DVT PROPHYLAXIS. Patients hospitalized with CHF are at high risk for DVT, especially if bed bound. Consider heparin (5,000 SC q8–12h) or enoxaparin (Lovenox), 40 mg SC qd, to decrease the risk of deep venous thrombosis and pulmonary embolism while hospitalized.

KEY POINTS TO REMEMBER

- One important role of the consultant is to maintain euvolemia to prevent complications of pulmonary or peripheral edema from volume overload or renal failure from hypovolemia. Accurate inputs and outputs and daily evaluations of volume status on physical exam are critical in maintaining euvolemia.
- The consultant should be familiar with medications that decrease mortality, including ACE inhibitors, spironolactone, and beta blockers. Patients who cannot tolerate ACE inhibitors or ARBs should be treated with nitrates and hydralazine.

SUGGESTED READING

ACC/AHA guidelines for evaluation and management of chronic heart failure in the adult: executive summary 2001 revision. Available at: http://www.acc.org/clinical/guidelines/failure/exec_summ/pdfs/hf_execsumm.pdf. Accessed February 27, 2003.

REFERENCES

1. Moss AJ. Improved survival with an implantable defibrillator in patients with coronary disease at high risk for ventricular arrhythmia. *N Engl J Med* 1996;335:1933–1940.
2. Cohn JN, Archibald DG, Ziesche S, et al. Effect of vasodilator therapy on mortality in chronic congestive heart failure. Results of a Veterans Administration Cooperative Study. *N Engl J Med* 1986;314:1547–1552.
3. Pitt B, Poole-Wilson PA, Segal R, et al. Effect of losartan compared with captopril on mortality in patients with symptomatic heart failure: randomised trial—the Losartan Heart Failure Survival Study ELITE II. *Lancet* 2000;355:1582–1587.
4. Pitt B, Zannad F, Remme WJ, et al. The effect of spironolactone on morbidity and mortality in patients with severe heart failure. Randomized Aldactone Evaluation Study Investigators. *N Engl J Med* 1999;341:709–717.
5. Hjalmarson A, Goldstein S, Fagerberg B, et al. Effects of controlled-release metoprolol on total mortality, hospitalizations, and well-being in patients with heart failure: the Metoprolol CR/XL Randomized Intervention Trial in congestive heart failure (MERIT-HF). MERIT-HF Study Group. *JAMA* 2000;283:1295–1302.
6. The Cardiac Insufficiency Bisoprolol Study II (CIBIS-II): a randomised trial. *Lancet* 1999;353:9–13.
7. Bristow MR, Gilbert EM, Abraham WT, et al. Carvedilol produces dose-related improvements in left ventricular function and survival in subjects with chronic heart failure. MOCHA Investigators. *Circulation* 1996;94:2807–2816.
8. Packer M, Coats AJ, Fowler MB, et al. Effect of carvedilol on survival in severe chronic heart failure. *N Engl J Med* 2001;344:1651–1658.
9. Uretsky BF, Young JB, Shahidi FE, et al. Randomized study assessing the effect of digoxin withdrawal in patients with mild to moderate chronic congestive heart failure: results of the PROVED trial. PROVED Investigative Group. *J Am Coll Cardiol* 1993;22:955–962.
10. Packer M, Gheorghiade M, Young JB, et al. Withdrawal of digoxin from patients with chronic heart failure treated with angiotensin-converting-enzyme inhibitors. RADIANCE Study. *N Engl J Med* 1993;329:1–7.

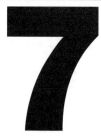

Atrial Fibrillation

Michael J. Riley,
Peter A. Crawford,
and Eric F. Buch

INTRODUCTION

Atrial fibrillation (A-fib) is the most common sustained arrhythmia, affecting up to 1% of the general population, 0.5% of the population aged 50–59 yrs, and almost 10% of the population older than 80. A-fib confers a fivefold increase in the **risk of stroke** and doubles the mortality rate.

CAUSES

Differential Diagnosis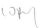

- **Structural heart disease:** valvular heart disease (i.e., mitral valve stenosis or prolapse, mitral annular calcification), hypertrophic or dilated cardiomyopathy, coronary artery disease (CAD).
- **Other arrhythmias:** sick sinus (tachy-brady) syndrome, Wolff-Parkinson-White syndrome.
- **Acute conditions:** acute MI, pulmonary embolism, pericarditis, alcohol intoxication ("holiday heart"), cardiac surgery, infections.
- **Systemic illnesses:** HTN, diabetes mellitus, hyperthyroidism, or hypothyroidism.
- **Drugs:** anticholinergic and sympathomimetic drugs, theophylline.
- **Echocardiographic correlates:** left ventricular hypertrophy, left atrial enlargement, reduced left ventricular ejection fraction, mitral valve abnormalities.
- **"Lone atrial fibrillation":** 10–15% of patients have no identifiable risk factors for thromboembolism or cardiac structural abnormality. The risk factors include **age >65, previous stroke or transient ischemic attack, HTN, diabetes mellitus, congestive heart failure, coronary artery disease, and thyrotoxicosis.** In addition, echocardiographic risk factors include **left atrial enlargement** and a **reduced left ventricular ejection fraction.**

PRESENTATION

History

Patients present with a **wide variety of symptoms,** determined to a large extent by underlying cardiac function, comorbidities, and patient perception; they may also be asymptomatic. **Common complaints** include palpitations, dizziness, fatigue, chest pain, dyspnea, or presyncope. Most symptoms result from tachycardia. It is unusual for patients to have dizziness or dyspnea from rate-controlled A-fib alone, and these patients should be evaluated for other causes of their symptoms.

Patients may present with **unstable angina** in the setting of significant CAD, heart failure with **pulmonary edema** (with underlying LV dysfunction, mitral stenosis, or a tachycardia-induced cardiomyopathy), focal **neurologic deficits** (in the setting of an embolic stroke), severe **abdominal or extremity pain** (in the setting of peripheral embolization with mesenteric or limb ischemia), or frank **syncope.**

Physical Exam

BP and heart rate are of prime concern in management. Usually, there is a rapid, **irregularly irregular** pulse, S1 of varying intensity, and absence of S4 or A waves. Also look for signs of heart failure. **Other possible findings** include goiter, hyperthyroid signs, focal neurologic deficits, or evidence of peripheral embolization (a cold extremity or absent pulse).

Lab and Imaging Evaluation

ECG reveals the absence of P waves and coarse, undulating baseline. An irregularly irregular ventricular rhythm is usually at a **rate** of **110–170 bpm.** The QRS complexes are narrow, except in the setting of underlying bundle branch block, with Ashman's phenomenon (aberrant conduction of the atrial impulses due to a difference in refractory period between the right and left bundle branches), or with concomitant ventricular ectopy.

Besides a 12-lead ECG, initial workup should include **echocardiography** to evaluate for valvular or other cardiac structural abnormality, **thyroid function tests,** and **pulse oximetry.**

Other testing should be performed as history and physical exam dictates (e.g., serial cardiac enzymes if acute MI suspected, known CAD, or multiple CAD risk factors; cardiac stress testing; ABG sampling, lower-extremity Doppler studies, and a ventilation/perfusion scan if acute pulmonary embolism is suspected; brain imaging with neurologic deficits; theophylline level).

MANAGEMENT

The **therapeutic approach** to A-fib is best **divided** into 3 broad areas: (a) control of the ventricular rate, (b) reduction of the risk of thromboembolic complications (anticoagulation), and (c) restoration and maintenance of sinus rhythm.

Ultimately, the specific **approach** to management of A-fib **will vary** for individual patients and will depend, to a large extent, on concomitant illnesses/conditions, patient preferences, and severity of symptoms/complications.

If symptoms are severe or if the patient is **hemodynamically unstable,** the treatment of choice is immediate **direct current cardioversion (DCC).**

Rate Control

Usually the **ventricular rate is 110–170 bpm** in the absence of drug therapy or conduction system disease.

Rapid ventricular response accounts for most symptoms due to decreased ventricular filling and increased myocardial demand. If the rapid rate persists, patients may develop **tachycardia-induced cardiomyopathy** with left ventricular (LV) systolic dysfunction.

Remember to **reassess the adequacy of the rate control** with **activity and ambulation,** not just at rest.

Pharmacologic Rate Control

In the **absence of significant symptoms,** IV medications are unnecessary and best avoided in favor of **oral preparations,** which carry less risk of hypotension and symptomatic bradycardia.

Beta blockers blunt atrioventricular (AV) nodal conduction and slow ventricular response. **They are the agents of choice** when A-fib is associated with thyrotoxicosis, acute MI, or postoperatively (where beta blockers have been shown to improve mortality). If acutely needed, metoprolol (Lopressor, Toprol-XL) may be given starting at 5 mg IV over 2–3 mins and repeated twice more until desired heart rate is achieved. This should be followed by an oral dose of metoprolol, 25–50 mg PO bid.

Calcium channel blockers are available in both IV and PO preparations. The **dihydropyridine** subtype (e.g., amlodipine, felodipine, nifedipine) has **minimal effect** on AV nodal conduction and is not useful for rate control in A-fib. The **nondihydropyridines** (e.g., diltiazem, verapamil) are **effective rate control** agents. Consider verapamil (Isoptin), 2.5–5 mg IV over 2–3 mins. A repeat double dose may be given in 15–30 mins if needed to achieve the desired ventricular rate. Alternatively, diltiazem (Cardizem), 20–25 mg IV over 2 mins, may be given and repeated in 15 mins if desired rate is not achieved. Avoid calcium channel blockers with Wolff-Parkinson-White syndrome or with severe heart failure. Oral preparations may be used for long-term rate control.

Digoxin (Lanoxin) slows the ventricular response by increasing vagal tone and blunting AV nodal conduction:

- The onset of **action is significantly delayed** compared to other agents, and rate control is often lost with increased **sympathetic tone** (e.g., exercise). It is therefore most effective in controlling **resting** heart rate. Unlike its ionotropic effects, rate control is not seen until serum levels are >1.4 ng/mL.
- It is **best suited** for patients with coexisting **LV dysfunction** (given its positive inotropic effect), as an **adjunct** to beta blocker or calcium channel blocker therapy or an **alternative** for intolerant patients.
- The optimal dose depends on renal function. See Chap. 6, Management of Congestive Heart Failure, for details on dosing.

Nonpharmacologic Rate Control

In patients who are persistently tachycardic or who remain **symptomatic despite treatment** with pharmacologic agents, or for whom serious **contraindications to drug therapy** exist, rate control can be accomplished by **ablation** of the AV node and implantation of a **permanent pacemaker.** Patients who undergo AV nodal ablation carry the same risk of thromboembolic complications and still require anticoagulation.

Thromboembolic Risk Reduction

When anticoagulating for A-fib, target INR of 2.0–3.0 with warfarin (Coumadin). It is acceptable to anticoagulate patients with "lone A-fib" (see Differential Diagnosis for definition) with daily ASA, 325 mg PO qd, instead of warfarin. Patients with rheumatic heart disease have an extremely high rate of thromboembolic events and should be fully anticoagulated with warfarin.

In early studies, patients who underwent cardioversion for A-fib without anticoagulation had a 7% overall incidence of thromboembolism. With anticoagulation with warfarin, the incidence dropped to <1%.

The American Heart Association recommends that patients undergoing cardioversion, whether electrical or pharmacologic, receive systemic anticoagulation for 3–4 wks before and at least 4 wks after restoration of sinus rhythm, unless an absolute contraindication exists.

If A-fib has clearly been present for <48 hrs, it is generally considered safe to cardiovert during this period without anticoagulation.

The Assessment of Cardioversion Using Transesophageal Echocardiography (ACUTE) study has demonstrated the safety and efficacy of TEE to dictate anticoagulation. In this strategy, patients are systemically anticoagulated with heparin and then undergo TEE to evaluate for intraatrial thrombus. If the TEE is clear, then patients are electrically cardioverted, followed by at least 4 wks of warfarin therapy, eliminating the need for, and risk of, preprocedural anticoagulation. See Appendix A for details of the ACUTE trial.

Postoperative A-Fib (e.g., after coronary artery bypass graft) requires anticoagulation but often resolves spontaneously or with cardioversion. 1 mo after the last episode of A-fib, anticoagulation with warfarin can usually be ceased.

Patients with atrial flutter should be anticoagulated as if they had A-fib.

Restoration and Maintenance of Sinus Rhythm

No studies have demonstrated a survival benefit or a reduction in thromboembolic events with chronic rhythm control over the alternate strategy of ventricular rate control and long-term anticoagulation, particularly in patients prone to persistent or chronic A-fib, rate control and anticoagulation are sufficient, assuming the patient tolerates the rhythm.

TABLE 7-1. PHARMACOLOGIC AGENTS USED TO TREAT ATRIAL FIBRILLATION

Medication	Indication	Dosing
Amiodarone (Cordarone, Pacerone)	Conversion and maintenance in patients with normal ventricles or systolic dysfunction	Oral load: 300 mg PO bid to tid for 1–3 wks, then maintain at 200–300 mg PO qd. Check baseline thyroid, liver, and pulmonary function tests. IV load: 150 mg IV over 10 min, then 1 mg/min for 6 hrs, then 0.5 mg/min for 18 hrs, followed by oral maintenance.
Flecainide (Tambocor)	For paroxysmal atrial fibrillation with normal left ventricular function and no coronary artery disease	Maintenance: start 50 mg PO bid.
Propafenone (Rythmol)	For structurally normal hearts and no coronary artery disease	Conversion: 600 mg PO once. Maintenance: start 150–300 mg PO bid.
Sotalol (Betapace, Betapace AF)	For maintenance only	Starting dose: 80 mg PO bid. Follow QT interval for excessive prolongation (daily for ≥ 3 days) and should be initiated as an inpatient with monitoring. Must have renal dosing.

DCC may be attempted at 200 J (synchronized) followed by increasing joules until sinus rhythm is established. Unless the procedure is emergent, it should be administered under some sedation in a controlled setting with hemodynamic monitoring and the assistance of anesthesia personnel, if necessary, for airway protection.

Several **pharmacologic agents** for restoration and maintenance of sinus rhythm are shown in Table 7-1. Although the conversion rate with drugs is significantly lower than with electrical cardioversion, these agents are commonly used as either alternatives to DCC, adjuncts to DCC, or as salvage therapy in case of failed DCC. **Do not pharmacologically cardiovert a patient whom you would not be comfortable electrically cardioverting based on embolic risk.**

Amiodarone has significant cumulative toxicities that may be of concern when used in young patients with a long life expectancy. Dofetilide (Tikosyn) is an option in refractory cases, but should be administered by a cardiologist or electrophysiologist.

Nonpharmacologic methods of restoring/maintaining sinus rhythm exist. The **Maze** procedure is a cardiac operation in which a sternotomy is performed and a series of carefully placed incisions are made in the atria to channel the erratic electrical activity to the AV node. Percutaneous approaches, including **pulmonary vein isolation** and **ablation**, are used in specialized settings.

The focus of **atrial flutter** may be destroyed by **radiofrequency ablation,** often resulting in restoration of normal sinus rhythm. Many of these patients will be left with A-fib, however.

KEY POINTS TO REMEMBER

- The three components of the management of A-fib are **rate control, anticoagulation, and rhythm control.** Whether paroxysmal, persistent, or permanent, most patients should be given some form of long-term anticoagulation (unless contraindicated). Assess the adequacy of rate control with activity.

- Patients who are **known** to have recent (<48 hrs) onset of A-fib can be cardioverted safely without anticoagulation. Anticoagulation is still necessary for at least 4 wks **after** cardioversion (unless contraindicated).
- It is **not advisable** to cardiovert patients who present to the office or ER in A-fib (because the duration of the arrhythmia cannot be determined) without TEE clearance or at least 3 wks of anticoagulation. The **exception** is hemodynamically unstable patients.

REFERENCES AND SUGGESTED READINGS

Assessment of Cardioversion Using Transesophageal Echocardiography (ACUTE) Investigators. Use of transesophageal echocardiography to guide cardioversion in patients with atrial fibrillation. *N Engl J Med* 2001;344:1411–1420.

Cardiac Arrhythmia Suppression Trial (CAST) Investigators. Preliminary report on effect of encainide and flecainide on mortality in a randomized trial of arrhythmia suppression after myocardial infarction. *N Engl J Med* 1989;321:406–412.

Fuster V, Ryden LE, Asinger RW, et al. ACC/AHA/ESC guidelines for the management of patients with atrial fibrillation: executive summary. *Circulation* 2001;104: 2118–2150.

Mason JW. A comparison of seven antiarrhythmic drugs in patients with ventricular tachyarrhythmias. Electrophysiologic Study vs. Electrocardiographic Monitoring Investigators. *N Engl J Med* 1993;329:452–458.

Prytowsky EN, Benson DW, Fuster V, et al. Management of patients with atrial fibrillation. A statement for health care professionals. From the Subcommittee on Electrocardiography and Electrophysiology, American Heart Association. *Circulation* 1996;93:1262–1277.

Stroke Prevention in Atrial Fibrillation Investigators. Stroke Prevention in Atrial Fibrillation Study. Final results. *Circulation* 1991;84:527–539.

Stroke Prevention in Atrial Fibrillation Investigators. Warfarin vs. aspirin for prevention of thromboembolism in atrial fibrillation: Stroke Prevention in Atrial Fibrillation II Study. *Lancet* 1994;343:687–691.

Wyse DG. A comparison of rate control and rhythm control in patients with atrial fibrillation (AFFIRM trial). *N Engl J Med* 2002;347:1825–1833.

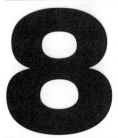

Anticoagulation and Surgery

Alan Zajarias
and Eric F. Buch

INTRODUCTION

Leading indications for anticoagulation are venous thromboembolic disease [deep venous thrombosis (DVT) or pulmonary embolism (PE)], atrial fibrillation (A-fib), and mechanical heart valves. The role of the consultant is to weigh the risk of thrombotic complications associated with discontinuing oral anticoagulation (OAC) against the risk of bleeding complications.

Discontinuation of warfarin causes a theoretical procoagulant milieu; however, this has not been proven clinically.

Regional or epidural anesthesia carries risk of hematoma formation and resultant cord compression. Low-molecular-weight heparins (LMWHs) are not currently FDA–approved for patients receiving epidural anesthesia.

PERIOPERATIVE MANAGEMENT OF ANTICOAGULATION WITH PROSTHETIC HEART VALVES

Factors that increase the risk of thromboembolic events include A-fib, severe left ventricular dysfunction, prior embolic event, mitral vs. aortic valve, and hypercoagulable states. OAC reduces thromboembolic risk by 75% (Table 8-1).

Fluctuations in anticoagulant levels may increase thrombus formation (when subtherapeutic) and decrease clot adherence when therapeutic levels are reached. Discontinuation of anticoagulation is associated with 3.7-fold increased risk of thromboembolic events [1].

American College of Chest Physicians (ACCP) guidelines for anticoagulation [2] for prosthetic heart valves are as follows:

- **St. Jude** valve, **Carbomedics** valve, **Medtronic-Hall** tilting disk in **aortic position** in patient with normal sinus rhythm and no left atrial enlargement: target **INR** range, 2.0–3.0. If patient has A-fib, then target INR 2.5–3.5 or add ASA, 80–100 mg/day.
- **St. Jude** valve, **Carbomedics** valve, **Medtronic-Hall** tilting disk in **mitral position:** target **INR 3.0** (range, 2.5–3.5).
- **Caged-ball** or **caged-disk** valve or **prior embolic event** despite adequate anticoagulation: target **INR 3.0** (range, 2.5–3.5) **and ASA,** 80–100 mg/day.
- **Bioprosthetic valves:** target **INR 2.5** (range, 2.0–3.0) for first 3 mos, then daily **ASA** 80 mg/day for life if no other risk factors for thromboembolism.

No consensus on **perioperative management** with prosthetic heart valves exists due to a lack of randomized trials. **Recommendations** of Kearon and Hirsh [4] and Tiede et al. [5] conclude that the embolic risk in most patients with A-fib or a prosthetic valve is not sufficient to warrant perioperative IV heparin:

- **No prior history** of embolism: stop OAC, operate when INR 1.3–1.5, **no IV heparin** unless INR <2.0 for 5 days.
- **High risk or history** of embolism: discontinue warfarin preoperatively. **Bridge with IV heparin** while INR <2.0, keeping PTT 2–2.5 times upper limit of normal. Discontinue heparin 4 hrs before surgery. Resume heparin and warfarin as soon as possible. Discontinue heparin once INR >2.0.

TABLE 8-1. SYSTEMIC EMBOLIZATION RISKS FOR REPRESENTATIVE PROSTHETIC HEART VALVES WITHOUT ANTICOAGULATION

Björk-Shiley	St. Jude
Aortic: 23% per yr	Aortic: 12.3% per yr
Bioprosthetic	Mitral: 22.2% per yr
Mitral: 17.6% for first 3 mos	

- **Subcutaneous or LMWH** is recommended for DVT prophylaxis in high-risk patients.
- After an **arterial embolic event,** postpone elective surgery for the first month. For urgent surgery, use IV heparin pre- and postoperatively if bleeding risk is acceptable.
- For **dental surgery,** continue anticoagulation. Patients with bleeding can use mouthwash containing tranexamic or epsilon-aminocaproic acid.

PERIOPERATIVE MANAGEMENT OF ANTICOAGULATION AND DEEP VENOUS THROMBOSIS

DVT risk factors include advanced age, immobility, stroke, prior DVT/PE, trauma, obesity, cardiac dysfunction, intravascular catheters, inflammatory bowel disease, nephrotic syndrome, pregnancy, estrogen administration, and smoking. **Risk of recurrence** depends on risk factors, circumstances precipitating initial DVT, and time treated with OAC:

- Recurrence at 3 mos without anticoagulation is 50%. Hypercoagulable state (e.g., neoplasm) with recurrent DVT: 15% per year even with anticoagulation.
- In the first month after a DVT: each day not anticoagulated increases absolute recurrence risk by 1%.

The ACCP delineates **risk stratification for postoperative DVT:**

- **Low risk:** age <40 yrs, undergoing minor surgery.
- **Moderate risk:** age <40 yrs with risk factors (as above) undergoing minor surgery or without risk factors undergoing major surgery; age 40–60 yrs without risk factors not going to major surgery.
- **High risk:** age >60 yrs, patients with risk factors or >40 yrs undergoing major surgery.
- **Very high risk:** age >40 yrs with prior DVT, hypercoagulable state, or cancer; patients undergoing hip or knee surgery; major trauma or spinal cord injury.
- For **patients with known DVTs: delay surgery** if possible—at least 3 mos or until OAC has been completed.

Kearon et al. [3,4] recommend the following anticoagulation management:

- **DVT <1 mo prior** and surgery necessary: full anticoagulation with IV heparin until 4–8 hrs preoperatively; restart at previous maintenance rate without bolus 12 hrs postoperatively.
- **DVT 1–3 mos prior:** no preoperative heparin unless other risk factors (debilitating illness, neoplasia, immobilization) present; postoperative IV heparin until INR >2.0.
- If **DVT >3 mos prior:** no preoperative heparin; postoperative DVT prophylaxis until INR >2.0.

ACCP Guidelines [5] recommend the following anticoagulation management:

- **DVT <3 mos prior:** preoperative heparin for 2 days before surgery while INR drifts down, then stop 4–8 hrs preoperatively; postoperative heparin until INR therapeutic.
- **DVT >3 mos prior:** let INR drift down preoperatively. Begin DVT prophylaxis postoperatively if intervention increases the risk of DVT.

- **Gynecologic and urologic surgery**: decrease warfarin dose to obtain INR 1.3–1.5 before surgery; restart full-dose warfarin and 5,000 U SC heparin twice daily after surgery.

PERIOPERATIVE MANAGEMENT OF ANTICOAGULATION AND ATRIAL FIBRILLATION

Embolization Risk

Nonvalvular A-fib has a 4.5% risk per year of systemic embolization. Risk increases with ventricular dysfunction, age >75 yrs, HTN, previous stroke or transient ischemic attack (12% risk per year), and diabetes mellitus. In the 30 days after an **arterial embolic event**, there is a 0.5% risk per day. **OAC provides a 66% relative risk reduction** of systemic embolization with nonvalvular A-fib.

Bleeding Risk with Oral Anticoagulation

- **Risk of major bleeding (Stroke Prevention in Atrial Fibrillation II) [6]:** 2.3% per year in patients older than 75 yrs with INR 2.0–4.5.
- **Risk of intracranial hemorrhage (Stroke Prevention in Atrial Fibrillation III) [7]:** 0.5% per year in high-risk patients (mean age 71 yrs) with INR 2.0–3.0. See Appendix A for details of this trial.

Recommendations per Albers et al.

Discontinue OAC before surgery, letting INR drift to <1.5 [8]. **The risk** of bleeding **outweighs the benefit** of OAC perioperatively because the incidence of embolic events is small on a daily basis. **Resume OAC** when the patient tolerates PO intake and the risk of bleeding has diminished.

DVT prophylaxis with LMWH or SC heparin should still be provided for high-risk patients.

KEY POINTS TO REMEMBER

- The decision to anticoagulate perioperatively for patients with A-fib and prosthetic valves should be based on embolization risk. Those at high risk should be bridged perioperatively with heparin. Most patients will not need perioperative heparin for A-fib alone.
- Similarly, patients receiving warfarin (Coumadin) for DVT or PE should be evaluated for risk of recurrence. Time since DVT/PE and duration of anticoagulation are the most important risk factors for recurrence, and those with recent DVTs should receive IV heparin preoperatively.

SUGGESTED READING

Ansell J, Hirsh J, Dalen J, et al. Managing oral anticoagulant therapy. *Chest* 2001;119 (Suppl 1):22S–38S.

Hirsh J, Dalen J, Anderson D, et al. Oral anticoagulants: mechanism of action, clinical effectiveness and optimal therapeutic range. *Chest* 2001;119(Suppl 1):8S–21S.

Jacobs L, Nusbaum N. Perioperative management and reversal of antithrombotic therapy. *Clin Geri Med* 2001;17:189–203.

REFERENCES

1. Cannegieter SC, Rosendaal FR, Briet E. Thromboembolic and bleeding complications in patients with mechanical heart valve prostheses. *Circulation* 1994;89:635–641.
2. Stein PD, Alpert JS, Bussey HI, et al. Antithrombotic therapy in patients with mechanical and biological prosthetic heart valves. *Chest* 2001;119:220S–227S.

3. Kearon C, Hirsh J. Management of anticoagulation before and after elective surgery. *N Engl J Med* 1997;336:1506–1511.
4. Tiede DJ, Nishimura RA, Gastineau DA, et al. Modern management of prosthetic valve anticoagulation. *Mayo Clin Proc* 1998;73:665–680.
5. Geerts WH, Heit JA, Clagett GP, et al. Prevention of venous thromboembolism. *Chest* 2001;119:132S–175S.
6. Warfarin versus aspirin for prevention of thromboembolism in atrial fibrillation: Stroke Prevention in Atrial Fibrillation II Study. *Lancet* 1994;343:687–691.
7. Adjusted-dose warfarin versus low-intensity, fixed-dose warfarin plus aspirin for high-risk patients with atrial fibrillation: Stroke Prevention in Atrial Fibrillation III randomised clinical trial. *Lancet* 1996;348:633–638.
8. Albers GW, Dalen JE, Laupacis A, et al. Antithrombotic therapy in atrial fibrillation. *Chest* 2001;119:194S–206S.

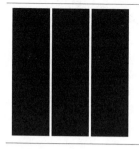

Pulmonary

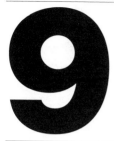

Approach
to Dyspnea

Christopher H. Kwoh

INTRODUCTION

Dyspnea is the sensation of difficulty breathing and is distinct from hypoxia. The main cause is either decreased delivery of O_2 to the tissues, impaired removal of carbon dioxide from the blood, increased work of breathing, or is psychogenic. Of chief consideration is distinguishing cardiac from pulmonary causes. The list of specific disease entities is tremendous.

DIFFERENTIAL DIAGNOSIS

Table 9-1 reviews the differential diagnosis in general terms. Further details on many of the elements in the differential are discussed in other chapters.

The medical consultant is frequently called to evaluate an inpatient who experiences the sudden onset of dyspnea. In this situation, consider pulmonary embolism, pneumothorax, aspiration pneumonitis/pneumonia, acute coronary syndrome, pulmonary edema, and arrhythmias.

Psychogenic dyspnea should also be in the differential in acute dyspnea. Often, patients have associated it with anxiety, depression, or pain. Patients may describe progressive anxiety culminating in dyspnea (rather than progressive dyspnea resulting in anxiety). They may also describe perioral or extremity numbness.

Metabolic acidosis is compensated by a tachypnea with large tidal volumes and a respiratory alkalosis. This rarely leads to dyspnea, unless the acidosis is severe or there is underlying pulmonary pathology.

PRESENTATION

Physical Exam

Exam should focus on the cardiovascular and respiratory systems. Respiratory rate, effort, and pattern of breathing should also be carefully evaluated.

Lab and Imaging Evaluation

Further testing should be directed based on results of history, physical exam, and vital signs (including pulse oximetry). Anemia is rapidly ruled out with a Hgb and Hct. A chest x-ray and ECG should also be obtained. Most causes of acute onset dyspnea are apparent after these evaluations.

The ABG can provide a great deal of information. A patient can have a normal SaO_2, but an ABG may reveal a wide A-a gradient—an indication of lung pathology. A simple but useful approach to the blood gas is to consider a low PO_2 to be the result of pulmonary parenchymal or airspace disease, right to left shunts, $\dot{V}/\dot{Q}$ mismatching, or a dramatic increase in oxygen consumption with respect to delivery. An elevated PCO_2 is almost invariably the result of decreased alveolar ventilation or decreased exchange of gas between atmosphere and the alveolus. Most commonly, this is due to disease of the airways (COPD or asthma) but may also be caused by chest wall disease or weakness of the respiratory muscles. Central causes of elevated PCO_2 include CNS lesions, obesity,

TABLE 9-1. DIFFERENTIAL DIAGNOSIS OF DYSPNEA

Pulmonary: diseases leading to hypoxia, increased effort of breathing (obstructive), pulmonary HTN, chest wall or respiratory muscle diseases.

Cardiac: causes of decreased cardiac output, right to left shunts, pulmonary edema.

Hematologic: significant anemia, toxins resulting in impaired O_2-Hgb association or dissociation (e.g., CO).

CNS (rare): increased intracranial pressure (Cushing's response) or other CNS lesions.

Respiratory alkalosis as a response to severe metabolic acidosis.

Deconditioning.

Psychogenic (a diagnosis of exclusion).

hypoventilation, and hypothyroidism. In psychogenic causes, the ABG often reveals respiratory alkalosis in the face of normal O_2 transfer.

Consider pulmonary function testing with diffusing capacity for CO of the lung, echocardiography, and CT scan of the chest. Often, exercise cardiopulmonary testing and ABG may reveal abnormalities that are not apparent at rest.

Maintain a high degree of suspicion for pulmonary embolism or you will miss the diagnosis. It is unusual for a pulmonary embolism to result in an elevated PCO_2 without severe hemodynamic compromise.

MANAGEMENT

Management should focus on identifying and treating the underlying cause. Further details regarding management are discussed in other chapters.

Psychogenic dyspnea can be controlled with lorazepam (Ativan) or with haloperidol (Haldol) (which will not cause respiratory depression). Many patients achieve symptomatic improvement by having air blowing on their face from a fan.

KEY POINTS TO REMEMBER

- A normal O_2 saturation, even 100%, on room air does not exclude a significant alveolar-arterial oxygen gradient and significant pulmonary disease.
- Maintain a high index of suspicion for pulmonary embolism given its high mortality rate and significant benefit from therapy.
- A careful history and physical exam will usually suggest the diagnosis. Common things being common, the initial evaluation should focus on the lungs, heart, and blood.

REFERENCES AND SUGGESTED READINGS

ATS board. Dyspnea. Mechanisms, assessment, and management: a consensus statement. American Thoracic Society. *Am J Respir Crit Care Med* 1999;159:321–340.

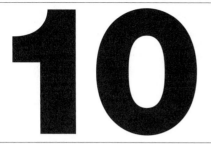

Chronic Obstructive Pulmonary Disease

Jeanie Park and
Steven L. Leh

INTRODUCTION

COPD is a progressive disease state characterized by airflow obstruction due to chronic bronchitis or emphysema.

Chronic bronchitis is defined as the presence of chronic productive cough on most days for 3 mos in each of 2 consecutive years.

Emphysema is a pathologic diagnosis characterized by destruction of the lung parenchyma and enlargement of air spaces, with loss of lung elasticity and obstruction of small airways.

Genetic factors, which remain to be determined, must play an intricate role, as only 15% of tobacco smokers develop clinically significant COPD.

Chronic, irreversible, airflow obstruction results from the combination of a mononuclear inflammatory process, ciliary dysfunction, mucus hypersecretion, and the loss of alveolar septal tethering due to emphysema.

In the United States, COPD is the fourth leading cause of death behind heart disease, cancer, and cerebrovascular accidents.

PRESENTATION

History

Classic symptoms include chronic daily productive cough, shortness of breath, and dyspnea on exertion. Cough is usually the initial symptom, occurring in the fifth decade of life. Dyspnea on exertion generally presents in the sixth to seventh decades of life. Obstructive lung disease in the absence of a significant smoking history should bring to consideration other pathologies (i.e., alpha-1 antitrypsin deficiency, cystic fibrosis, asthma). Weight loss may occur with severe COPD, but malignancy should be excluded.

Acute exacerbations of COPD consist of increasing dyspnea, an increase in cough or sputum production, and an increase in sputum purulence.

Physical Exam

Vital signs are critical. Tachypnea is common. Fever may be a clue to an infection as the underlying source of an exacerbation. An alteration in mental status may represent hypoxia or hypercarbia. Observation of respiratory status includes pursed-lip breathing, accessory muscle use, nasal flaring, and paradoxic abdominal movements.

Pulmonary exam may reveal a prolonged expiration, expiratory wheezes, rales, or bronchial breath sounds on auscultation. With severe exacerbations, breath sounds may be nearly inaudible.

Look for evidence of cor pulmonale, including right ventricular heave, jugular venous distension, and lower extremity edema.

Lab Evaluation

Draw an ABG to assess PaO_2 and $PaCO_2$. Obtain an ECG to look for signs of cor pulmonale.

In stable patients, diagnosis and severity of COPD are confirmed by pulmonary function tests. Patients will have an increase in total lung capacity, residual volume, and functional residual capacity. The diffusing capacity of CO is reduced in proportion to the severity of COPD. FEV_1 is decreased, with a decrease in the FEV_1/forced vital capacity ratio. Staging systems generally use FEV_1 as an indicator of the severity of COPD.

Imaging Evaluation

Findings of posteroanterior/lateral chest x-ray include flattened diaphragms, bullae, increased retrosternal clear space (unless right ventricular enlargement is present), and a long, narrow heart shadow. In acute exacerbations, it is important to evaluate for other causes of dyspnea, including pulmonary edema, pneumonia, and pneumothorax.

MANAGEMENT OF ACUTE EXACERBATIONS OF COPD

First and foremost, identify the underlying cause of the exacerbation. Most often it is a respiratory tract infection or change in the flora of the airway. It may also be due to another respiratory insult.

Cautious use of **supplemental O_2** is required to increase the pulse oximetry to 88–93% or PaO_2 to 60–70 mm Hg. Hypercarbia is a potential hazard of oxygen therapy, and therefore arterial blood gases should be followed to assess PaO_2 and $PaCO_2$. If hypercarbia occurs secondary to overzealous O_2 administration, do not abruptly remove supplemental O_2, as this may lead to significant hypoxemia.

Bronchodilators administered via nebulizer [albuterol (Proventil; Ventolin), 2.5 mg q30–60mins, and ipratropium (Atrovent), 500 μg every 2–4 hrs] or metered-dose inhalers are the mainstays of therapy.

Systemic steroids are recommended during acute exacerbations of COPD. A recent randomized, placebo-controlled trial involving methylprednisolone (Medrol), 125 mg IV q6h for 3 days, followed by oral prednisone (Deltasone) taper for 2 wks, was shown to decrease morbidity primarily through a reduction in intensification of drug therapy.

Antibiotics are indicated in patients with history/physical exam findings consistent with acute exacerbation of chronic bronchitis or pneumonia. The most common bacterial pathogens implicated include *Streptococcus pneumoniae, Haemophilus influenzae,* and *Moraxella catarrhalis.* Treatment of these pathogens is based on local resistance patterns. Some options are trimethoprim/sulfamethoxazole (Bactrim; Septra), azithromycin (Zithromax), or a quinolone. Duration of therapy is typically 10–14 days.

Methylxanthines (aminophylline and theophylline) are not indicated in the acute exacerbation.

Noninvasive positive pressure ventilation, such as bilevel positive airway pressure, has been shown to decrease endotracheal intubations and may decrease mortality and length of hospital stay. Indications include respiratory rate >25, worsening dyspnea despite the appropriate management previously described, and pH <7.35 with $PaCO_2$ >45. Try to find results of old ABGs obtained during clinical stability. This provides valuable information on the presence and degree of CO_2 retention at their baseline and may be used to determine whether CO_2 retention is worse than usual. Contraindications include maxillofacial trauma, inability to protect the airway, cardiorespiratory instability, uncooperative patient, and extreme obesity.

Mechanical ventilation is indicated when the above therapies have failed to relieve the patient's symptoms, there is a failure to correct hypoxemia/hypercarbia/acidosis, or there are signs of impending respiratory failure. As mechanical ventilation is beyond the scope of this discussion, important factors to remember include the following:

- Avoid hyperventilation and respiratory alkalosis, especially in patients with chronic respiratory acidosis.
- Avoid excessive positive end-expiratory pressure. Be cautious of auto–positive end-expiratory pressure and its adverse consequences, including hypotension, barotrauma, and impaired inspiratory effort.

- Allow for adequate expiratory time. This can be accomplished by increasing inspiratory flow rates or decreasing respiratory rate.

Long-term O_2 therapy on discharge has been shown to improve survival and quality of life. Indications for long-term O_2 therapy include $PaO_2 \leq 55$ or O_2 saturation $\leq 88\%$, or PaO_2 of 56–59 or O_2 saturation of 89% with signs of cor pulmonale or polycythemia.

Encourage smoking cessation. Hospitalization affords an excellent opportunity to alter smoking habits.

Refer to a smoking cessation group or counselor, if available. The Nicoderm patch may be used to limit nicotine cravings. Start with the 21-mg/day patch for 4–8 wks if the patient smokes 0.5–1.0 packs per day or more. If the patient smokes less, then start at 14 mg/day for 4–6 wks. Taper by 7 mg/day q2–4wks. Alternatively, nicotine gum may be used (chew one piece prn up to 30/day). Bupropion (Zyban; 150 mg PO qd × 3 days, then 150 mg PO bid × 7–12 wks) is a useful adjunct to smoking cessation.

Pulmonary rehabilitation has been shown to improve quality of life and exercise tolerance. Make sure that vaccines are kept up to date (pneumovax q5yrs, flu vaccine qyr).

KEY POINTS TO REMEMBER

- Chronic bronchitis is a clinical diagnosis based on daily cough and sputum production. Emphysema may also be a clinical diagnosis based on physical exam findings but is often found on imaging.
- Only 15–20% of smokers ever develop COPD. Therefore, do not assume that every smoker has COPD or that dyspnea in a smoker is due to COPD.

Patients with COPD with $PaO_2 \leq 55$, or with cor pulmonale or polycythemia and $PaO_2 \leq 60$ should have O_2 supplementation to decrease mortality. Patients should also be counseled on smoking cessation.

REFERENCES AND SUGGESTED READINGS

American Library Association Web site. Available at http://www.ALA.org. Accessed September 2003.

Bach JR, Brougher P, Hess DR, et al. Consensus conference: noninvasive positive pressure ventilation. *Resp Care* 1997;42(4):364–369.

Bach PB, Brown C, Gelfand SE, et al. Management of acute exacerbations of chronic obstructive pulmonary disease: a summary and appraisal of published evidence. *Ann Intern Med* 2001;134:600–620.

Barnes J. Chronic obstructive pulmonary disease. *N Engl J Med* 2000;343(4):269–280.

Ferguson G. Recommendations for the management of COPD. *Chest* 2000;117(2):23S–28S.

Global strategy for the diagnosis, management, and prevention of chronic obstructive pulmonary disease: National Heart, Lung, and Blood Institute and World Health Organization Global Initiative for chronic obstructive lung disease (GOLD): executive summary. *Resp Care* 2001;46(8):798–825.

Medical Research Council Working Party. Long-term domiciliary oxygen therapy in chronic hypoxic cor pulmonale complicating chronic bronchitis and emphysema. *Lancet* 1981;1:681–686.

Niewoehner DE, Erbland ML, Deupree RH, et al. Effect of systemic glucocorticoids on exacerbations of chronic obstructive pulmonary disease. *N Engl J Med* 1999;340(25):1941–1947.

Nocturnal Oxygen Therapy Trial Group. Continuous or nocturnal oxygen therapy in hypoxemic chronic obstructive lung disease: a clinical trial. *Ann Intern Med* 1980;93:391–398.

Snow V, Lascher S, Mottur-Pilson C. Joint Expert Panel on Chronic Obstructive Pulmonary Disease of the American College of Chest Physicians and ACP-ASIM. Evidence base for management of acute exacerbations of chronic obstructive pulmonary disease. *Ann Intern Med* 2001;134:595–599.

Standards for the diagnosis and care of patients with chronic obstructive pulmonary disease: American Thoracic Society. *Am J Respir Crit Care Med* 1995;152(suppl):S77–S121.

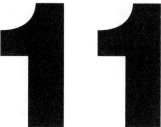

Asthma

Elizabeth Friedman
and Steven L. Leh

INTRODUCTION

The National Asthma Education and Prevention Program Expert Panel II consensus statement defines *asthma* as "a chronic inflammatory disorder of the airways resulting in recurrent episodes of wheezing, breathlessness, chest tightness, and cough, particularly at night and/or in the early morning. These episodes are usually associated with widespread but variable airflow obstruction that is often reversible either spontaneously or with treatment. These changes are associated with an increase in the existing bronchial hyperresponsiveness to a variety of stimuli."

Airflow obstruction is the result of a combination of inflammation mediated predominantly through eosinophils, airway smooth muscle spasm, bronchial hyperresponsiveness, mucosal edema, and mucus plugging.

In the United States, approximately 14 million people are affected by asthma.

PRESENTATION

History

Classic symptoms include wheezing, chest tightness, and a sensation of "not getting air in." Cough may be the sole presenting symptom in cough-variant asthma. Symptoms only after vigorous activity are indicative of exercise-induced asthma.

In determining the severity of asthma, pertinent history includes the frequency of symptoms and "rescue" metered-dose inhaler (MDI) use, presence of nocturnal symptoms, and peak expiratory flow rates (PEFRs). Other factors include a history of frequent ER visits, prior ICU admissions/mechanical ventilation, recent oral corticosteroid therapy, and history of psychosocial problems, including medical noncompliance.

It is important to identify aggravating factors or "triggers" for asthma. A careful allergy history should be obtained, including the presence of atopy, pets, active or passive smoke inhalation, and home/work/school environments. Know the common triggers for your geographic area during each session.

Physical Exam

Between exacerbations, the exam may be completely normal. Vital signs may reveal tachypnea and tachycardia (often from high doses of beta agonists). A decreasing respiratory rate may indicate respiratory muscle fatigue rather than improvement in airway obstruction. A decreasing mental status may represent hypercarbia or hypoxia.

HEENT exam can assess for signs of chronic allergic disease, including conjunctivitis, nasal polyps, rhinorrhea, and sinus tenderness.

Observe for signs of respiratory fatigue or failure. These include inability to speak (words, phrases, sentences), inability to lie down, accessory muscle use, paradoxic abdominal movements, and pulsus paradoxus.

Auscultation may reveal inspiratory/expiratory wheezing, prolonged expiratory phase, and diminished general air movement. In patients with audible inspiratory/expiratory wheezes over the upper airways or neck, rule out other causes of airway obstruction, including vocal cord dysfunction, foreign bodies, and upper-airway tumors.

Beware of the patient with no wheezing and poor air movement, as these findings may signify severe asthma and respiratory failure.

Assess for signs of chronic steroid use such as thin skin, easy bruising, cushingoid facies, central obesity, and proximal muscle weakness.

Lab Evaluation

In stable patients, diagnosis and severity of asthma are confirmed by pulmonary function tests. In general, there is evidence of obstructive lung disease with a reduced FEV_1 to forced vital capacity ratio. In addition, a postbronchodilator improvement in FEV_1 should be seen, indicative of reversible airway disease. No definitive criteria have been established; however, a positive bronchodilator response is generally indicated by an improvement in FEV_1 by 12% and 200 mL. Lung volumes will often show increased residual volume and a normal diffusion capacity of CO. The latter differentiates asthma from COPD.

Bronchial challenge testing can be used to identify patients with abnormal airway hyperresponsiveness. Pharmacologic testing using methacholine has varying sensitivity and specificity based on the state of symptoms at the time of testing. In general, a positive test is indicated by a reduction in the FEV_1 of 20% at methacholine concentrations of <8 mg/mL. Many asthmatics have exercise-induced airway changes, even in the absence of exercise-induced symptoms. Pulmonary function tests obtained before and after treadmill testing may therefore reveal the variability in FEV_1.

During acute exacerbations, PEFR should be routinely checked before and 15–20 mins after administration of bronchodilators to assess efficacy of therapy. Hypokalemia may occur as a result of high doses of beta-agonist.

Imaging Evaluation

Posteroanterior and lateral chest x-ray should be obtained to rule out other etiologies of dyspnea such as pneumonia, pneumothorax, and pneumomediastinum.

ABG is not routinely indicated in acute exacerbations of asthma. However, in patients who fail to respond to initial therapy with persistently diminished PEFR <25% of predicted, or in patients unable to perform PEFR, an ABG should be performed. Early in the course, the tachypnea usually results in a below normal $PaCO_2$. The presence of normal or increased $PaCO_2$ may indicate impending respiratory failure.

MANAGEMENT

Acute Exacerbations of Asthma

An algorithm for the management of acute exacerbations has been published by the National Heart, Lung, and Blood Institute. Treatment guidelines are based on the PEFR. In general, severe exacerbations are defined as PEFR <50% of predicted. An inadequate response to therapy is defined as a <10% improvement in PEFR after bronchodilator therapy.

- Avoidance of triggers or allergens is mandatory.
- Provide supplemental O_2 to achieve O_2 saturation ≥ 90%.
- Provide inhaled beta$_2$-bronchodilators via nebulizer or MDI, as MDI use with spacer is as efficacious. Recommended doses include albuterol nebulizer, 2.5 mg q20mins × 3 doses, then every hour. An MDI dose of 4–6 puffs is equivalent to one nebulizer treatment. An alternative regimen includes a 10- to 15-mg continuous albuterol nebulizer over 1 hr.
- In patients not responding to albuterol therapy, the addition of ipratropium (Atrovent), 0.5-mg nebulizer every 2–4 hrs, is indicated. Trials have shown enhanced bronchodilation with the combination.
- Corticosteroids are indicated to reduce the inflammatory component of asthma exacerbations and have been shown to reduce morbidity and mortality. The onset of activity in parenteral steroids is approximately 60 mins, with maximal effect at

approximately 5 hrs. Oral steroids show onset of effect within 3 hrs, with maximal effect at 8–12 hrs. Typical regimens include IV methylprednisolone (Solu-Medrol), 1 mg/kg every 6 hrs, with a maximum dose of 60 mg every 6 hrs. Patients are then tapered on oral prednisone (Deltasone) over 10–14 days in divided doses.

- Inhaled corticosteroids are indicated for all hospitalized patients after discharge. Because their onset of action is not for several days, initiate therapy as soon as patients are able to use MDI.
- In refractory cases, the use of SC epinephrine (0.3 mg of 1:1,000 dilution), q20mins × 3 doses, may be used.
- IV magnesium and the methylxanthines are not indicated in the acute exacerbation.
- In patients refractory to the above treatments, or in whom worsening fatigue, hypoxemia, hypercapnia, or mental status changes are evident, mechanical ventilation is indicated.

Long-Term Management and Follow-Up

The mainstay of therapy is inhaled corticosteroids at the appropriate dosage, dependent on severity of symptoms. The National Heart, Lung, and Blood Institute uses a stepwise algorithm for the management of chronic asthma. Four categories of asthma are defined with their recommended treatment regimen:

- **Mild intermittent:** defined by occasional symptoms <1 time/wk, rare nocturnal symptoms <2 times/mo, normal lung function between exacerbations, and PEFR >80% predicted. Use of prn albuterol MDI (Proventil; Ventolin) ("rescue therapy") is indicated.
- **Mild persistent:** defined by symptoms >1 time/wk but <1 time/day, nocturnal symptoms >2 times/mo, exacerbations may affect activity, and PEFR >80% predicted. Use of a low-dose inhaled corticosteroid such as fluticasone (Flovent), 44 μg 2 puffs bid; beclomethasone (Qvar; Vanceril), 84 μg 2 puffs bid; or triamcinolone (Azmacort), 100 μg 4 puffs bid, is indicated. Albuterol MDI can be used prn for breakthrough symptoms, not to exceed 3–4×/day.
- **Moderate persistent:** defined by daily symptoms, nocturnal symptoms >1 time/wk, exacerbations affect daily activities, daily use of "rescue" MDI is necessary, and PEFR between 60–80% predicted. Moderate doses of inhaled steroids such as fluticasone, 110 μg 2–4 puffs bid; beclomethasone, 84 μg 4 puffs bid; or budesonide, 200 μg one inhalation bid, is indicated. If there is a predominance of nocturnal symptoms, salmeterol (Serevent) (a long-acting beta$_2$-agonist), 2 puffs bid, can be added.
- **Severe persistent:** defined by continuous symptoms, frequent nocturnal symptoms, daily, limiting exacerbations, and PEFR <60% predicted. High doses of inhaled steroids such as fluticasone, 220 μg two puffs bid, or budesonide, 200 μg, 2 inhalations bid, are indicated. Use of salmeterol is also indicated. A combination salmeterol/fluticasone diskus is available for ease of dosing. The lowest possible dose of oral steroid or alternate day dosing of PO steroids may be necessary.

Long-acting beta$_2$-agonists such as salmeterol have been shown to improve nocturnal symptoms and reduce inhaled steroid requirements. Standard dosing of salmeterol is 2 puffs bid.

Nedocromil (Tilade) MDI, 2 puffs qid, or cromolyn sodium, 20 mg nebulizer qid, may be used in mild persistent asthma.

Leukotriene antagonists such as zafirlukast (Accolate) (20 mg PO bid) and montelukast (Singulair) (10 mg PO qhs) are more effective than placebo but less effective than inhaled corticosteroids. Instances in which they are particularly useful include ASA-induced asthma, exercise-induced asthma, and inability to use an MDI.

KEY POINTS TO REMEMBER

- A normal diffusing capacity for carbon monoxide helps to distinguish asthma from emphysema.

- Management of the acute asthma exacerbation involves reducing inflammation with PO and inhaled corticosteroids, bronchodilation, and identification and reversal of any underlying triggering infection.
- The highest yield long-term intervention for asthmatics is identification and avoidance or removal of triggers and allergens.

REFERENCES AND SUGGESTED READINGS

Beasley R, Keil V, vonMutius E, et al. Worldwide variation in prevalence of symptoms of asthma, allergic rhinoconjunctivitis, and atopic eczema: ISAAC. *Lancet* 1998;351:1225–1232.

Busse WW, Lemanske RF. Advances in immunology: asthma. *N Engl J Med* 2001; 344(5):350–362.

Castro M. Estimated comparative daily dosages for inhaled corticosteroids. Handout. Washington University School of Medicine Lecture, 2001.

Corbridge TC, Hall JB. The assessment and management of adults with status asthmaticus. *Am J Resp Crit Care Med* 1995;151(5):1296–1316.

Greenberger PA, Patterson R. Diagnosis and management of allergic bronchopulmonary aspergillosis. *Ann Allergy* 1986;56:444–452.

Hartert TV, Peebles RS. Epidemiology of asthma: the year in review. *Curr Opin Pulm Med* 2000;6(1):4–9.

Lemanske RF, Busse WW. Asthma. *JAMA* 1997;278(22):1855–1873.

Madison JM, Irwin RS. Status asthmaticus. In: Irwin RS, Rippe JM, eds. *Intensive care medicine*, 3rd ed. Boston: Little, Brown, 1996:605–618.

Middleton E, Reed CE, Ellis EF, eds. *Allergy: principles & practice*, 5th ed. St. Louis: Mosby, 1998.

National Asthma Education and Prevention Program Expert Panel Report 2: guidelines for the diagnosis and management of asthma. National Institutes of Health, National Heart, Lung, and Blood Institute, Publication No. 97-4051, 1997.

National Heart, Lung, and Blood Institute. *Data fact sheet: asthma statistics 1999*. Bethesda, MD: National Heart, Lung, and Blood Institute, 1999.

National Heart, Lung, and Blood Institute. *Executive summary: guidelines for the diagnosis and management of asthma*. Bethesda, MD: U.S. Department of Health and Human Services; 1991. NIH publication 91-3042.

Sly RM. Decreases in asthma mortality in the United States. *Ann Allergy Asthma Immunol* 2000;85:121–127.

Smith LJ. Comparative efficacy of inhaled corticosteroids and antileukotriene drugs in asthma. *BioDrugs* 2001;15(4):239–249.

Suissa S, Ernst P. Inhaled corticosteroids: impact on asthma morbidity and mortality. *J Allergy Clin Immunol* 2001;107(6):937–944.

Turner MO, Noertjojo K, Vedal S, et al. Risk factors for near-fatal asthma: a case control study in hospitalized patients with asthma. *Am J Resp Crit Care Med* 1998;157:1804–1809.

12

Solitary Pulmonary Nodule

Christopher H. Kwoh

INTRODUCTION

The solitary pulmonary nodule (SPN), or coin lesion, is defined as a <3 cm isolated spherical lesion on chest radiologic imaging without associated parenchymal changes or adenopathy. Lesions >3 cm are so frequently malignant that they are not considered SPNs and are usually referred to as **masses.**

The prevalence of SPNs is reported to be up to 0.2% of adult radiographs. Roughly 20% of these will be malignant nodules, depending on the population studied. The role of the physician is to assess the probability of malignancy and weigh the benefits of diagnosis with the risks of invasive evaluation.

Most of the likelihood ratios (LRs) reported here are based on Bayesian analysis of numerous solitary nodules [1].

PRESENTATION

History

Age is critical. SPNs in patients <30 yrs are rarely malignant (LR, 0.05), but in patients >50 yrs are commonly malignant (LR, >2.0).

A history of hemoptysis suggests malignancy (LR, >5), as does current or past cigarette smoking or prior malignancy.

Imaging Evaluation

Radiologic factors suggesting malignancy are as follows:

- Likelihood of malignancy increases rapidly with size. Less than 1 cm is not usually malignant, but >2 cm usually is.
- Most important is growth rate. Nodules with a doubling time of ≥ 465 days or that double in <1–2 wks are nearly always benign (LR <0.01).
- Smooth, well-defined borders suggest benign nodules. Spiculated nodules are usually malignant. Popcorn, laminated, or heavy calcifications suggest benign nodules (malignant calcifications are eccentric and few).
- Less helpful is the observation that cavitations in benign lesions are regular and thin, unlike the irregular thick walls commonly seen in malignant SPNs. Walls <4 mm in thickness are rarely malignant (LR, 0.07), whereas walls >1.5 cm are usually malignant (LR, 38).

In patients with intermediate risk, one may further image the nodule with a high-resolution CT to clarify the radiographic factors suggesting malignancy. When considering resection, obtain a staging CT of the chest to ensure that there is no lymphadenopathy, metastases, or other lesions.

One may also consider PET scanning (reported accuracy ~90%), if available, in patients with intermediate malignant risk. The combination of CT and PET scanning is reported to be highly accurate (up to 96%) [2].

MANAGEMENT

Obtain old radiologic studies. Nodules unchanged over 1.5–2 yrs, having benign calcifications, or SPNs in patients <35 yrs with no other risk factors, may be managed with watchful waiting.

When pursuing watchful waiting, it is common to obtain chest x-rays q3mos for 1 yr and then q6mos for 1 yr, unless existing studies confirm stability of the nodule size.

Any solitary lesion >3 cm, SPNs in patients with known prior malignancy, or SPNs in smokers of old age should be resected unless the surgical risk is prohibitively high or there is evidence of spread.

Patients with high risk of malignancy should be biopsied or resected, with the decision based on operative morbidity and likelihood of malignancy.

Tissue may be obtained in multiple ways:

- Thoracotomy is most decisive but with operative mortality in the range of 3%. It results in resectable cures of 80–90% if the lesion proves malignant.
- Video-assisted thoracotomy (VATS) has lower mortality than traditional thoracotomy and maintains its high success rate. Approximately 20% of video-assisted thoracotomies, however, are converted to open thoracotomies.
- Transthoracic needle aspiration biopsy is useful in peripheral lesions (yield >90%) and smaller lesions (<2 cm with 60% yield). One-third develop pneumothorax. Transthoracic needle aspiration biopsy is for diagnosis only.
- Bronchoscopy may be useful in large lesions (>2 cm with 50% yield) and central lesions or lesions adjacent to a bronchus per CT (~70% yield). Mortality is <0.5%, and morbidity is far less than with thoracotomy, but bronchoscopy lacks the curative potential.

KEY POINTS TO REMEMBER

- The role of the consultant is to determine the malignant potential of any pulmonary nodule and weigh the benefits of diagnosis of malignancy versus the risks of biopsy.
- The most important risk factors are age, smoking history, size of nodule, hemoptysis, history of malignancy, and progression in the size of the nodule over time.

SUGGESTED READING

Ost D. Evaluation and management of the solitary pulmonary nodule. *Am J Respir Crit Care Med* 2000;162:782–787.

REFERENCES

1. Gurney JW. Determining the likelihood of malignancy in solitary pulmonary nodules with Bayesian analysis (2 parts). *Radiology* 1993;186:405–422.
2. Vansteenkiste JF. Mediastinal lymph node staging with FDG-PET scan in patients with potentially operable non-small cell lung cancer: a prospective analysis of 50 cases. *Chest* 1997;112:1480–1486.

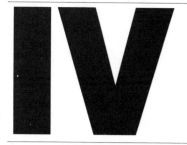

Gastroenterology

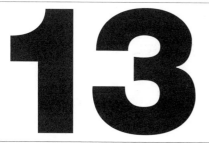

Approach to Nausea and Vomiting

Rajesh Shah and
Christopher H. Kwoh

INTRODUCTION

Nausea and vomiting leading to dehydration is a common reason for admission to the hospital. In addition, many inpatients under severe metabolic stress and with many new medications experience severe nausea while in the hospital.

The vomiting center is in the dorsal lateral reticular formation, in which emesis is initiated and integrated. Signals come to the vomiting center from various sources, including the vestibular system (labyrinthine apparatus, cerebellum, and vestibular nucleus), the GI tract (via vagal nerve), and the chemoreceptor zone of the area postrema. See Table 13-1 for a differential diagnosis.

PRESENTATION

History

A medication history is critical in identifying nausea as a side effect of a new drug. Ask about bowel movements and flatus, the absence of which suggests a more serious bowel pathology.

Acute vomiting (onset 1–2 days) suggests infection, medication, or toxin. Viral gastroenteritis is the most common cause of acute nausea and vomiting in the outpatient setting.

Vomiting within minutes of a meal suggests gastric outlet obstruction or other gastric/duodenal pathology.

Inflammatory conditions result in vomiting approximately 1 hr after meals. Gastroparesis results in vomiting several hours after a meal.

Pregnancy and uremia commonly cause **early-morning** nausea and vomiting.

Vomiting of undigested foods suggests achalasia or other esophageal pathology.

Bilious vomiting proves that obstruction is distal to the duodenal papilla. Malodorous or feculent emesis suggests distal obstruction, bacterial overgrowth, or fistula.

Physical Exam

Assessment of volume status and orthostatic hypotension/tachycardia is important for gauging volume resuscitation. Absent bowel sounds are consistent with ileus. High-pitched, hyperactive bowel sounds suggest bowel obstruction. A succussion splash may be found in severe gastroparesis. Also examine for signs of peritoneal inflammation (involuntary guarding and rebound tenderness).

Lab Evaluation

Serum chemistries may reveal hypokalemia and contraction metabolic alkalosis from loss of gastric fluids. Hyponatremia and elevated BUN and creatinine may result from volume depletion.

Rule out pregnancy with a urine beta-hCG and pancreatitis with amylase/lipase in the appropriate settings.

TABLE 13-1. DIFFERENTIAL DIAGNOSIS OF NAUSEA AND VOMITING (PARTIAL LIST)

Medications

Viral gastroenteritis

  Rotavirus, Norwalk, reovirus, adenovirus

Bacterial food poisoning

  Staphylococcus aureus, Bacillus cereus, Salmonella, Clostridium perfringens

Other infections

  Meningitis, acute hepatitis, otitis media

GI disorders

  Gastroparesis, intestinal obstruction, gastric outlet obstruction, pancreatitis, appendicitis, gallbladder, GERD, peptic ulcer disease, functional motility disorder, cyclical vomiting

Metabolic disorders

  Ketoacidosis, uremia, hypercalcemia, hypothyroidism/hyperthyroidism, adrenal insufficiency, parathyroid disease

CNS

  Increased intracranial pressure, vestibular and labyrinthine disorders (vertigo), migraine, psychiatric

Pregnancy

A CBC and liver chemistries should be obtained on all patients. An obstructive series may show evidence of a bowel obstruction (air fluid levels and proximal bowel dilatation) or may reveal an ileus.

A small bowel follow-through may be more revealing if a partial small bowel obstruction is suspected. CT of the abdomen and pelvis may help evaluate the entire GI tract and accessory organs. Gastric emptying studies may be useful with suspected gastroparesis. Endoscopy may also be considered to evaluate the mucosa and to rule out other mechanical causes.

MANAGEMENT

Correct Any Treatable Underlying Disorders

Provide IV fluids for the hypovolemic patient. With significant symptoms, limit oral intake to clear liquids or keep NPO. If symptoms are severe, consider nasogastric intubation and low intermittent suction.

See Chap. 31, Approach to the Patient with Vertigo, for therapy for vertiginous disorders.

Nausea Pharmacotherapy (Antiemetics)

- Antihistamines
  - Meclizine (Antivert), 25 mg PO qid (useful for labyrinthitis)
  - Promethazine (Phenergan), 12.5–25 mg PO/IV q6h (useful for uremia)
- Anticholinergics: scopolamine (Transderm-Scop) (comes in a convenient patch format with hyoscine)
- Dopamine receptor antagonists: prochlorperazine (Compazine) (5–10 mg PO tid to qid), chlorpromazine (Thorazine)
- 5-HT$_3$ receptor antagonists: ondansetron (Zofran) (useful for chemotherapy induced) at 4 mg IV q4–8h. May give as much as 32 mg IV in a day.

- Corticosteroids may benefit patients with CNS lesions or with chemotherapy. Some physicians give a 10–20 mg dose of dexamethasone (Decadron) as a trial with continued therapy at 2–4 mg q6h.

Prokinetic Agents

Metoclopramide (Reglan), 10 mg PO qid (or qAC and qhs) is useful for gastroparesis or chemotherapy-induced nausea.

KEY POINTS TO REMEMBER

- Rule out serious pathology such as a metabolic derangement, diabetic ketoacidosis, or mechanical obstruction first. Provide ample fluid resuscitation in the dehydrated patient.
- Medical management should be directed toward correcting the underlying disorder and then toward symptomatic relief.

REFERENCES AND SUGGESTED READINGS

Sleisenger MH, ed. *Gastrointestinal disease: pathophysiology, diagnosis, management*, 5th ed. Philadelphia: Saunders, 1993:509–523.

Yamada T. *Handbook of gastroenterology*. Philadelphia: Lippincott–Raven, 1998:41–48.

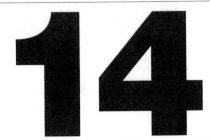

Approach to Gastrointestinal Bleeding

Aaron Shiels

INTRODUCTION

Upper GI (UGI) bleeding is generally defined as bleeding that occurs in the digestive tract proximal to the ligament of Treitz. Lower GI bleeding is distal to the ligament of Treitz.

Mortality rates range from 3.5–7% for UGI bleeds and <5% for lower GI bleeds. Approximately 80% of all acute episodes of upper and lower GI hemorrhage will resolve without intervention. Thus, the consultant must place emphasis on determining which patients will require intervention to stop bleeding or prevent rebleeding.

DIFFERENTIAL DIAGNOSIS

See Table 14-1 for a listing of etiologies of UGI bleeding, as well as relative frequencies of each.

See Table 14-2 for the differential diagnosis and the relative frequencies of lesions found during evaluation for lower GI bleeding.

Occult GI bleeding is defined as a positive fecal occult blood test without other evidence of blood in the stool. Although these patients require further evaluation, most may be managed as outpatients, and that discussion is beyond the scope of this chapter.

PRESENTATION

History

The history should focus on determining the severity of bleeding, identifying whether it is an upper or lower source, and then narrowing down a specific etiology.

Abrupt hematochezia or hematemesis (<24 hrs) associated with hemodynamic instability and symptoms of orthostasis, dizziness, or dyspnea suggests major blood loss and the need for rapid resuscitation and intervention.

A careful history should include any hematemesis, melena, or hematochezia. Also ask about frequency and volume. Use of color-coded cards is helpful in determining the actual color of patients' stools.

- **Hematemesis,** the vomiting of blood, invariably indicates bleeding above the ligament of Treitz. When vomitus is red, recent bleeding should be suspected. With degradation in the stomach, it may take on the appearance of coffee grounds.
- **Melena** is black, tarry, sticky stool that has a characteristic odor, produced when blood comes into contact with hydrochloric acid. As little as 60 cc of blood can result in melena. Only one-half of patients with melena will have concurrent hematemesis, but most have a UGI source.
- **Hematochezia,** or bright red blood per rectum, usually denotes a lower GI bleed. However, brisk UGI bleeding can produce hematochezia. In a recent series, 11% of patients with hematochezia were later found to have a lesion in the UGI tract.

Associated symptoms, including abdominal pain (see Chap. 15, Approach to Abdominal Pain), recent change in bowel habits, fever, or weight loss, may point to specific diagnoses.

Relevant medical history includes previous bleeding (diverticulosis, hemorrhoids, ulcers, varices, and angiodysplasia); results of previous endoscopies; recent polypec-

TABLE 14-1. CAUSES OF ACUTE UPPER GI BLEEDING

Cause	Frequency (%)
Peptic ulcer disease (gastric and duodenal)	45
Gastric erosions	23
Varices (esophageal/gastric)	10
Mallory-Weiss tear	7
Esophagitis	6
Upper GI tract tumors	3
Others: atrioventricular malformations, Dieulafoy's ulcer, erosive duodenitis, aortoenteric fistula, hemobilia, portal HTN gastropathy, gastric antral vascular ectasia, Osler-Weber-Rendu, hemosuccus pancreaticus, postoperatively	13

tomy; past abdominal surgeries; inflammatory bowel disease; cirrhosis (and portal hypertension); coagulation abnormalities; malignancy; and history of radiation therapy to the chest, abdomen, or pelvis.

Review medications including NSAIDs and ASA (which are associated with erosions and ulcerations throughout the GI tract) and anticoagulants. Corticosteroids also promote gastric erosions and peptic ulcers. Alcohol use is also associated with bleeding through multiple mechanisms.

Peptic ulcer disease may present as bleeding without prior dyspepsia, especially in the elderly.

Mallory-Weiss tears typically present as repeated retching or vomiting followed by hematemesis. The hemorrhage is self-limiting, and the tear itself usually heals within 2 days. Comorbid portal hypertension confers a risk of more massive bleeding from Mallory-Weiss tears.

Approximately one-third of patients with cirrhosis will have at least one variceal hemorrhage. However, up to 25% of cirrhotics who present with a UGI bleed have a source of bleeding other than varices.

Painless faucet-like hematochezia is the classic presentation of diverticular bleeds. Although most diverticuli are left sided, 70% of episodes of diverticular bleeding occur in the right colon. Recurrence among patients who spontaneously cease bleeding is 25–35%.

Recent anorexia, weight loss, or change in the caliber of stools may indicate an underlying malignancy.

The typical presentation of ischemic colitis is crampy left lower quadrant abdominal pain, followed within 24 hrs by hematochezia or bloody diarrhea.

TABLE 14-2. LESIONS IN LOWER GI BLEEDING

Lesion	Frequency (%)
Diverticulosis	17–40
Angiodysplasia	2–30
Colitis (radiation, ischemic, infectious, inflammatory)	9–21
Colonic neoplasm/postpolypectomy	4–10
Anorectal source	4–10
Upper GI source	0–11
Small bowel source	2–9

Physical Exam

Vital signs are the most immediately important item of the physical exam:

- Orthostatic hypotension, defined as a 10-mm decrease in SBP when going from supine to upright position, denotes a 20% loss of intravascular volume.
- Severe, rapid, or unrelenting bleeding may produce **shock** (approximately 40% loss of volume) with the resultant signs of tachycardia, supine hypotension, and pallor.
- Increased vagal tone to the heart caused by shock or concomitant use of beta blockers may produce bradycardia and confuse the clinician.

Verify stool characteristics with a rectal exam. Look for hemorrhoids. The abdominal exam is critical for looking for masses and areas of tenderness. Stigmata of chronic liver disease and portal HTN (i.e., telangiectasias, ascites, splenomegaly) should be sought.

Lab Evaluation

The Hgb and Hct must be followed throughout the hospital stay. Do not expect the initial Hgb and Hct to reflect the degree of blood loss until the intravascular volume is restored with crystalloid or from the extravascular space.

Type and cross, platelet count, PT/PTT, and a complete metabolic panel should be performed. BUN is often elevated out of proportion to creatinine, a finding that is classically more extreme in a UGI source.

The **nasogastric tube** should be placed in all cases of UGI bleed. Also place an NG tube in probable lower GI bleeds if UGI bleeding is a possibility:

- A positive **gastric aspirate** (fresh blood or Gastroccult-positive coffee grounds) indicates that bleeding has occurred proximal to the jejunum. **A negative aspirate does not preclude UGI bleeding.** Do not use Hemoccult testing on gastric aspirates.
- **Gastric lavage** should be performed by instilling water into the stomach and then aspirating it back. It serves two functions:
  - Assesses rapidity, severity, and current activity of bleeding by determining how much water is required to clear the aspirate. In brisk bleeds the aspirate may not clear.
  - Clears the endoscopic field of blood, clots, and particulate matter.

An ECG should be obtained in those who have hemodynamic changes or ischemic cardiac symptoms. **Ischemic organ damage** can be precipitated by blood loss, and cardiac ischemia may be precipitated by the low Hct.

MANAGEMENT

The first and foremost issue is to stabilize the patient hemodynamically:

- Place two large bore (18-gauge or larger) peripheral IV lines.
- Restore volume with crystalloid. Follow vital signs to determine rate and volume of infusion. Try to avoid vasopressors because these patients are hypovolemic.
- If bleeding is brisk, then restoration of volume with packed RBCs may be necessary. Administer O-negative blood products without delay.
- Depending on the rapidity of the blood loss, make sure that several units of packed red blood cells are ready in the lab in case their administration becomes emergently necessary.

Correct coagulopathies with vitamin K, platelet, or FFP transfusions as necessary. Consider endotracheal intubation for brisk UGI bleeds. The risk of aspiration is high, especially when the patient is not alert.

In most cases, endoscopy is the diagnostic and therapeutic modality of choice. Therapeutic interventions may be performed during endoscopy, including injection of vasoconstricting agents, photocoagulation, sclerotherapy, and banding of varices. Lower GI bleeds will have intervenable lesions 25% of the time.

Patients with UGI bleeds and positive nasogastric aspirates should undergo urgent esophagogastroduodenoscopy, especially if the lavage fails to clear.

TABLE 14-3. RISK OF RECURRENT UGI BLEEDING BASED ON ESOPHAGOGASTRODUODENOSCOPY FINDINGS

Endoscopic finding	Rebleeding risk (%)
Arterial spurting	90
Visible nonbleeding vessel	50
Adherent clot	25–30
Oozing without visible vessel	10–20
Flat spot	7–10
Clean ulcer base	3–5

Patients with UGI bleeds and negative aspirates may undergo elective upper endoscopy. A negative esophagogastroduodenoscopy should be followed by lower endoscopy looking for a lower GI source or push enteroscopy to evaluate the small bowel. 24% of patients with melena will have no diagnosis by upper endoscopy.

See Table 14-3 for the risk of rebleeding on medical management based on endoscopic findings.

Colonoscopy is usually performed for suspected lower GI sources. The overall diagnostic yield for colonoscopy in this setting is 70–80%. Approximately 25% of patients with lower GI bleeds have lesions that are amenable to endoscopic therapy. A negative colonoscopy should be followed by upper endoscopy and possibly enteroscopy.

Further imaging to localize bleeding should be considered in patients with ongoing blood loss and no source identified by endoscopy. If surgical intervention becomes necessary, then localization decreases surgical morbidity and mortality. Various imaging modalities are available:

- **Arteriography** is rarely indicated but can be helpful in localizing the source of bleeding if blood loss into the GI tract is too brisk to allow for endoscopy. They may also identify arteriovenous malformations. The rate of the bleeding must be >0.5 mL/min. Selective abdominal arteriography by an interventional radiologist also allows for therapeutic capabilities in the form of arterial embolization or intraarterial vasopressin.
- **Tagged RBC scan** may be used in the evaluation of an active lower GI bleed. Bleeding must exceed a rate of 0.1 mL/min to be detected. Unfortunately, they are positive less than one-half of the time. Ideally, they may be used to further localize bleeding for further diagnostic studies, such as angiography.
- **Pill endoscopy** probably has more of a role in occult GI bleeding. Its role in acute bleeds has not been well defined.

Additional therapeutics vary according to etiology:

- In peptic ulcer disease with certain stigmata, high-dose proton pump inhibitors [e.g., omeprazole (Prilosec), 40 mg PO bid] are frequently used to reduce rebleeding and, according to a recent trial, reduce mortality. Proton pump inhibitors may also be used for gastric erosions.
- In variceal bleeding, octreotide acetate (Sandostatin) may be administered to reduce portal HTN and improve hemostasis in conjunction with endoscopic therapy. It should be given as a 50–100 μg IV bolus followed by an infusion at 25–50 μg/hr.
- In intractable esophageal variceal bleeds, a **Sengstaken-Blakemore or Minnesota tube** may be used to tamponade the bleeding varices. This is only a temporizing measure, and rebleeding usually occurs when the tube is removed.
- **Transjugular intrahepatic portosystemic shunts or surgical shunts** may be placed in refractory cases of variceal bleeding.
- After a Mallory-Weiss tear, **ranitidine** (Zantac) (150 mg PO bid), **omeprazole** (20 mg PO qd), and **sucralfate** (Carafate) (1 g PO tid) can help promote healing.

The best management for GI tract erosions and ulcers is prevention: Use proton pump inhibitors or H_2 blockers in ICU patients or others who are critically ill or at high risk.

In bleeding from diverticulosis and hemorrhoids, consider high-fiber diets and supplements to slow formation and progression of diverticuli long term.

Intractable cases may require surgical removal of the segment of the intestine or stomach that is the source of the bleeding. Notify the surgeons early.

KEY POINTS TO REMEMBER

- Initiate resuscitative measures and appropriate level of monitoring before starting diagnostic testing and therapeutic intervention. Ensure adequate IV access. Intensive care monitoring is appropriate for patients with unstable vital signs (not responding to resuscitative therapy) and those with comorbid conditions.
- Approximately one-third of patients with cirrhosis will have at least one variceal hemorrhage. However, up to 25% of cirrhotics who present with a UGI bleed have a source of bleeding other than varices.
- A negative nasogastric aspirate does not preclude UGI bleeding.
- Patients with persistent or recurrent lower GI bleeding may require surgical intervention. The accurate localization of bleeding before surgery will decrease morbidity and mortality.
- Melena is highly associated with an upper GI source. Although hematochezia usually indicates a lower GI source, 11% of patients presenting with hematochezia are found to have an upper GI source.

REFERENCES AND SUGGESTED READINGS

Epstein A, Isselbacher K. Gastrointestinal bleeding. In: Fauci A, et al., eds. *Harrison's principles of internal medicine,* 14th ed. New York: McGraw-Hill, 1998:246–249.

Peter DJ, Dougherty JM. Evaluation of the patient with gastrointestinal bleeding: an evidence based approach. *Emerg Med Clin North Am* 1999;17:239–261.

Yamada T. *Textbook of gastroenterology*. Philadelphia: Lippincott Williams & Wilkins, 1999.

Zuccaro G Jr. Management of the adult patient with acute lower gastrointestinal bleeding. *Am J Gastroenterol* 1998;93:1202–1208.

Zuckerman GR, Prakash C. Acute lower intestinal bleeding part I: clinical presentation and diagnosis. *Gastrointest Endosc* 1998;48:606–616.

Zuckerman GR, Prakash C. Acute lower intestinal bleeding part II: etiology, therapy, and outcomes. *Gastrointest Endosc* 1999;49:228–238.

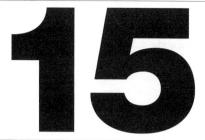

Approach to Abdominal Pain

Aaron Shiels

INTRODUCTION

Abdominal pain represents one of the most common complaints for which patients seek medical attention. Because there are hundreds of disorders that can result in the perception of pain in the abdomen, an orderly approach is critical to avoid unnecessary testing and potentially harmful delays in diagnosis. Table 15-1 lists some important items on the differential diagnosis of abdominal pain.

PRESENTATION

History

The two most important mechanisms of pain are parietal pain and visceral (somatic) pain.

Parietal pain is caused by irritation of the parietal peritoneum, which may be caused by inflammation from an adjacent organ. The presence of blood, stool, or gastric contents against the peritoneum also causes parietal pain.

Visceral pain is due to noxious stimuli to the visceral organs and has such causes as traction on the peritoneum, distension of a hollow viscus, or muscular contraction, often against an obstructed lumen.

The distinguishing features between the two are demonstrated in Table 15-2.

Other important mechanisms of pain include ischemia, musculoskeletal pain, referred pain, metabolic derangements, neurogenic pain, and functional pain.

Location of the pain helps to identify likely etiologies. Table 15-3 lists commonly affected organs and their perceived areas of pain.

Pain that begins abruptly suggests possible intraabdominal catastrophe, including ruptured abdominal vasculature or perforated viscus. Pain that develops rapidly over minutes suggests inflammation or obstruction of a viscus. Gradual onset over a few hours also suggests inflammation.

Pain from peptic ulcer disease often improves with eating or antacids, but worsens 1–2 hrs after eating.

Hematemesis, hematochezia, melena, obstipation, hematuria, and fever may further focus the diagnostic evaluation. Always take a menstrual history in women of child-bearing age. Do not miss an ectopic pregnancy or other obstetric catastrophes.

Physical Exam

Vital Signs

The presence of tachycardia or orthostatic hypotension suggests significant volume depletion and should prompt an immediate search for the underlying cause (hemorrhage, vomiting, diarrhea, third-spacing). Tachycardia may be the only sign of impending hemodynamic collapse in a patient with a vascular catastrophe. Fever suggests an inflammatory process, often infectious.

Patients with peritonitis will often lie very still, whereas those with renal colic will often writhe in bed.

TABLE 15-1. DIFFERENTIAL DIAGNOSIS OF ABDOMINAL PAIN

Inflammatory conditions
  Cholecystitis
  Pancreatitis
  Appendicitis
  Diverticulitis
  Hepatitis
  Pelvic inflammatory disease
  Peptic ulcer
  Gastroenteritis
  Spontaneous bacterial peritonitis
  Acute colitis
  Pyelonephritis
  Acute cholangitis
Mechanical causes
  Small or large bowel obstruction
  Volvulus
  Biliary obstruction
  Ureteral stones
  Ruptured aortic aneurysm
  Ruptured ectopic pregnancy

Ischemic causes
  Mesenteric ischemia
  Splenic infarction
  Testicular torsion
  Ovarian cyst torsion
Metabolic causes
  Diabetic ketoacidosis
  Uremia
  Porphyria
  Lead poisoning
Other causes
  Thoracic disorders
  Herpes zoster
  Systemic lupus erythematosus
  Musculoskeletal disorders
  Functional abdominal pain
  Acute angle closure glaucoma
  Ectopic pregnancy

Abdominal Exam

The abdomen should be visually inspected for surgical scars, distention, bulging flanks, or other obvious abnormalities. Auscultate for the presence or absence of bowel sounds. Gentle pressure with the stethoscope allows assessment of tenderness without alarming the patient. Palpation should begin furthest from the area of pain.

Peritoneal inflammation is best determined by light percussion on the abdomen, gently shaking the bed, or asking the patient to cough. "Rebound tenderness" is less specific for peritoneal inflammation, whereas involuntary guarding and rigidity are more specific.

All patients with acute abdominal pain should have a rectal and pelvic (women) exam performed.

Severe pain with a benign exam suggests mesenteric ischemia.

TABLE 15-2. PARIETAL PAIN VS VISCERAL PAIN

	Parietal pain	Visceral pain
Localization	Well localized and lateralizing	Often midline or diffuse
Character	Constant, worse with movement or coughing	Often dull, colicky or intermittent, but may be constant
Associated symptoms	Pain with bed shaking	Autonomic symptoms such as nausea, vomiting, diaphoresis, pallor
Exam findings	Involuntary and voluntary guarding; abdominal rigidity	Voluntary guarding, soft abdomen

TABLE 15-3. ORGAN INVOLVEMENT AND PERCEIVED LOCATION OF PAIN

Organ	Perceived location of pain
Esophagus	Chest, epigastrium
Stomach	Epigastrium
Small intestine	Periumbilical region
Colon	Lower abdomen
Gallbladder	Right upper quadrant or epigastric, radiation to right scapula or shoulder
Liver	Right upper quadrant
Kidney or ureter	Costovertebral angle, flank, radiation to groin
Bladder	Suprapubic region
Aorta	Mid-back region
Spleen	Left upper quadrant or epigastric, radiation to left shoulder
Pancreas	Epigastric, radiation to the back
Colonic diverticula	Typically left lower quadrant
Ovaries	Lower quadrants

Lab Evaluation

As most patients with acute abdominal pain can be diagnosed with a careful history and physical exam, further diagnostic evaluation should be targeted to the clinical scenario. Always obtain a urine beta-hCG in women of child-bearing age. Excessive undirected testing increases the costs and may cause unnecessary delays in diagnosis and treatment.

Some basic tests to consider include CBC, BMP, liver function tests, amylase/lipase, and UA.

Imaging Evaluation

Standard Radiography
Not all patients with acute abdominal pain require plain or upright films of the abdomen. However, abdominal x-rays are useful for diagnosing perforated viscus (identified as free air), ileus, or bowel obstruction.

U/S
Transabdominal U/S is useful for patients with suspected biliary tract disease, including acute cholecystitis, biliary pain, and choledocholithiasis. It is the initial test of choice for right upper quadrant pain. U/S also allows rapid diagnosis of abdominal aortic aneurysms.

CT
Abdominal CT, especially with rapid spiral scanning techniques, provides a powerful imaging tool. It is the most sensitive test for identifying a perforated viscus and is useful for suspected cases of bowel obstruction, intraabdominal abscess, appendicitis, ruptured aortic aneurysm, necrotizing pancreatitis, and diverticulitis. However, care must be used in selecting patients for abdominal CT. The test is time-consuming and costly and may unnecessarily delay diagnosis and treatment, especially in patients who require urgent surgery.

KEY POINTS TO REMEMBER

- A careful, detailed history and physical exam are the keys to efficient evaluation of the patient with abdominal pain. An accurate diagnosis can be made in the majority of patients with only a meticulous history and physical exam.

- The pain caused by irritation of the parietal peritoneum is usually well localized and lateralizes to the site of irritation.
- Visceral pain is dull and poorly localized. There are often associated autonomic symptoms, including nausea, vomiting, diaphoresis, or pallor.
- Peritoneal inflammation is best determined by light percussion on the abdomen, gently shaking the bed, or asking the patient to cough. "Rebound tenderness" is less specific for peritoneal inflammation.

REFERENCES AND SUGGESTED READINGS

Fauci AS, Hauser SL, Longo DL, et al., eds. *Harrison's principles of internal medicine*, 14th ed. New York: McGraw-Hill, 1998:65–68.

Sleisenger MH, Fordtran JS. *Gastrointestinal disease: pathophysiology, diagnosis, management*, 5th ed. Philadelphia: Saunders, 1993:150–162.

Wolfe MM. Therapy of digestive disorders. Philadelphia: Saunders, 2000:711–716.

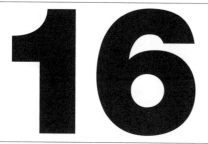

Approach to Abnormal Liver Enzymes

Christopher H. Kwoh
and Aaron Shiels

INTRODUCTION

The transaminases (AST/ALT) and alkaline phosphatase are commonly referred to as liver function tests (LFTs), although these are actually measures more of liver inflammation than function. Albumin, bilirubin, and PT are better tests for the synthetic function of the liver; however, abnormalities are not specific to liver disease.

DIFFERENTIAL DIAGNOSIS

Nonhepatic causes may result in elevations of many of the hepatic enzymes:

- Alkaline phosphatase may be elevated in diseases of the bone (fractures, metastatic lesions, Paget's disease, hyperparathyroidism), from intestinal disorders, or from the placenta (pregnancy, uterine disease).
- AST may be elevated in MI or other disorders with muscle damage (where creatine kinase may be elevated), dysthyroidemia, Addison's disease, and celiac sprue.
- Isolated hyperbilirubinemia may occur in hemolysis, resorption of a large hematoma, sepsis, or in enzyme deficiencies (Dubin-Johnson and Rotor causing direct hyperbilirubinemia, Gilbert's and Crigler-Najjar with indirect hyperbilirubinemia).
- PT is often prolonged with certain antibiotics, vitamin K malabsorption, or medications (warfarin). (See Chap. 35, Approach to a Prolonged Prothrombin Time/Partial Thromboplastin Time.)

Other **distinctive patterns** in liver enzymes have been noted:

- AST:ALT >2 is typical of alcoholic injury, whereas ALT>AST is typical of viral injury and nonalcoholic steatohepatitis.
- Transaminases in the thousands are seen with toxic, ischemic, or viral damage. Alcoholic hepatitis rarely causes transaminase elevations >450.
- ALT:LDH ratio of <1.5 is suggestive of ischemic hepatitis rather than viral hepatitis.

PRESENTATION

History

Symptoms of malaise, jaundice, nausea, vomiting, and weight loss are nonspecific but may aid in estimating the onset of disease. A change in the taste of cigarettes may be associated with viral hepatitis.

Hemochromatosis may be associated with diabetes, skin bronzing, congestive heart failure, arthritis, and hypogonadism. Wilson's disease may also present with movement disorders, psychiatric symptoms, and renal tubular disorders. Alpha-1 antitrypsin is associated with early emphysema (emphysema in nonsmokers should raise suspicion).

Venoocclusive disease of the liver is associated with several hematologic disorders and oral contraceptive use, often with hyperbilirubinemia as the only manifestation.

Exposure to blood products, IV drug abuse, tattoos, or close family members with hepatitis should raise suspicion of viral hepatitis. Raw oysters and other contaminated foods may spread hepatitis A. Travel history may be revealing.

Autoimmune hepatitis is most common in women <40 yrs old and may be associated with thyroid disease, rheumatoid arthritis, and other autoimmunities.

Primary biliary cirrhosis affects mostly women in their 50s and may be associated with several autoimmune disorders. Primary sclerosing cholangitis is seen in men in their 30s and is strongly associated with ulcerative colitis. Both disorders present with a cholestatic picture.

Ischemic hepatitis is usually in the setting of a hypotensive episode or cardiac arrest. Acute tubular necrosis and anoxic brain injury are often concomitant findings.

Nonalcoholic steatohepatitis is commonly seen in obese patients, diabetics, and patients with hypertriglyceridemia.

Medication use and toxins are an important cause of liver enzyme abnormalities. Do a thorough alcohol, medication, work, and environmental exposure history. Always consider acetaminophen toxicity, especially in alcoholics who may suffer toxicity at otherwise tolerable levels. Do not assume that liver disease in an alcoholic is due to alcohol alone!

Family history should include inquiries into Wilson's disease, alpha-1 antitrypsin deficiency, and hemochromatosis.

Physical Exam

The presence of stigmata of liver disease points to a significant hepatic process. Look for jaundice, spider telangiectasias, palmar erythema, testicular atrophy, gynecomastia, Dupuytren's contracture, and ascites. Asterixis and fetor hepaticus point to serious hepatic dysfunction and impending hepatic encephalopathy.

Extrahepatic manifestations of viral hepatitis include polyarteritis nodosa or glomerulonephritis with hepatitis B or membranoproliferative glomerulonephritis, polyarthritis, porphyria cutanea tardae, or cryoglobulinemia with hepatitis C.

Look for the copper discoloration of Descemet's membrane from Wilson's disease (Kayser-Fleischer rings) and the bronze discoloration of the skin from hemochromatosis.

Volume overload and severe congestive heart failure, especially with severe tricuspid regurgitation, may result in a congestive hepatopathy. Marked enlargement of the liver (>15 cm) and a pulsatile liver are suggestive physical findings (Tables 16-1, 16-2, and 16-3).

Lab Evaluation

Hepatocellular Pattern

Repeat transaminases to confirm elevation. If only AST is elevated, then consider aldolase or creatine kinase to confirm hepatic source vs. muscle source.

If history and physical exam do not point to an obvious cause, then initial lab evaluation should include an acute hepatitis panel [hepatitis A virus antibody (Ab), hepati-

TABLE 16-1. PATTERNS OF ENZYME CHANGES

Test	Hepatocellular	Cholestatic	Infiltrative
AST/ALT	Markedly elevated	Normal or mild elevation	Normal or mild elevation
Alkaline phosphatase	Normal to mild elevation	Markedly elevated	Markedly elevated
Bilirubin	Normal to marked elevation	Normal to prolonged	Normal
PT	Normal or prolonged	Normal or prolonged, but responds to vitamin K	Normal

TABLE 16-2. DIFFERENTIAL DIAGNOSIS OF HEPATOCELLULAR PATTERNS OF INJURY

Viral hepatitis	Medication induced	Alcohol use
Wilson's disease	Hemochromatosis	Alpha-1 antitrypsin deficiency
Various toxins	Nonalcoholic steatohepatitis	Ischemic hepatitis
Celiac sprue	Congestive hepatopathy	Autoimmune hepatitis
Various bacterial infections	Hyperthyroidism	Venoocclusive disease

tis C virus Ab, hepatitis B virus (HBV) surface antigen, HBeAb, HBV surface Ab], serum ceruloplasmin (if patient <40), serum iron and total iron-binding capacity, and serum protein electrophoresis (to evaluate for autoimmune hepatitis pattern or alpha-1 antitrypsin deficiency, which may have a decrease in alpha globulin bands).

In acute cases, an acetaminophen level should be obtained if appropriate.

Additional tests may include antiendomysial or antigliadin antibodies, alpha-1 antitrypsin phenotyping, other specific hepatitis virus tests (consider hepatitis E, herpes simplex virus, cytomegalovirus, Epstein-Barr virus, etc.), or other tests for autoimmune hepatitis (ANA, antismooth muscle antibodies, anti–kidney-liver microsome antibodies).

Right upper quadrant U/S may help to identify steatosis in patients who may have nonalcoholic steatohepatitis.

If the above tests are unrevealing, then one may proceed to percutaneous liver biopsy. The approach of watchful waiting in patients with transaminase elevations <2 × normal has been supported in two studies and is advocated by many physicians.

Cholestatic Pattern

Obtain a beta-hCG in the appropriate clinical setting to exclude pregnancy as a cause.

Confirm a hepatic source using gamma-glutaryl transferase levels (concomitant elevation suggests a hepatic source) or 5' nucleotidase alkaline phosphatase isoenzymes (specific for liver source).

Consider antimitochondrial antibodies to evaluate for primary biliary cirrhosis. If elevation of the alkaline phosphatase is >3 × normal or persistently elevated, then a right upper quadrant U/S or CT of the abdomen should be obtained to evaluate for obstruction of the biliary system as indicated by dilated ducts. This may be followed by endoscopic retrograde cholangiopancreatography or percutaneous transhepatic cholangiography (PTC) to identify and treat obstruction.

TABLE 16-3. DIFFERENTIAL DIAGNOSIS OF CHOLESTATIC PATTERNS

Primary biliary cirrhosis

Autoimmune cholangiopathy

TPN

Sepsis and postoperative states

Extrahepatic obstruction: choledocholithiasis, cholangiocarcinoma, strictures, etc.

Sclerosing cholangitis

Medication induced

Acute liver injury (viral or alcoholic)

Granulomatous hepatitis

If no obstruction is identified, then further evaluation could depend on the appearance of the liver:

- Evidence of focal lesions suggests infectious causes (pyogenic or amebic abscess) or malignant causes (primary or metastatic), which should be evaluated by drainage or biopsy.
- Normal or diffusely affected liver may be evaluated by liver biopsy. Endoscopic retrograde cholangiopancreatography or PTC may be useful to rule out extrahepatic obstruction in the setting of brief duration of enzyme elevation in which the biliary system has not had time to dilate.

KEY POINTS TO REMEMBER

- Identifying the pattern of enzyme abnormality helps to focus the evaluation.
- Know which enzymes are elevated out of proportion in the hepatocellular (transaminases), cholestatic (alkaline phosphatase and bilirubin), and infiltrative (alkaline phosphatase) patterns.

REFERENCES AND SUGGESTED READINGS

Bernal W, Wendon J. Acute liver failure; clinical features and management. *Eur J Gastroenterol Hepatol* 1999;11(9):977–984.

Cassidy WM. Serum lactate dehydrogenase in the differential diagnosis of acute hepatocellular injury. *J Clin Gastroenterol* 1994;19:118.

Gill R, Sterling R. Acute liver failure. *J Clin Gastroenterol* 2001;33(3):191–198.

O'Grady J. Comprehensive clinical hepatology. St. Louis: Mosby-Year Book, 2000.

Pratt DS. Evaluation of abnormal liver enzyme results in asymptomatic patients. *N Engl J Med* 2000;342(17):1266–1271.

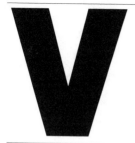

Nephrology

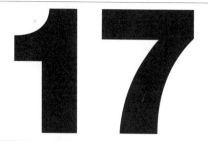

Approach to Acute Renal Failure

Georges Saab and
Christopher H. Kwoh

INTRODUCTION

Acute renal failure (ARF) is defined as an acute decline in glomerular filtration rate (GFR) from baseline. It can be divided into three broad categories:

1. **Prerenal azotemia** is defined as a decrease in the effective perfusion of the renal vasculature. Causes may be from hypovolemia, heart failure, or hypotension, among others. This is the most common cause of acute renal failure in the hospital. ACE inhibitors, angiotensin receptor blockers, and NSAIDs produce essentially a prerenal picture through their effects on the renal vasculature.
2. **Intrinsic azotemia** is characterized by disease affective in the renal parenchyma itself, the causes of which can be divided into the portion of the kidney affected.
   - **Vasculature:** Causes include atheroembolic disease, vasculitides, and arterial dissection.
   - **Tubules:** Acute tubular necrosis (ATN) is often seen as a continuum of prerenal azotemia and prolonged or severe renal hypoperfusion (renal infarct or ischemic ATN). ATN may also result from medications or endogenous or exogenous toxins. Urine sediment will contain coarse granular casts or large muddy brown casts.
   - **Interstitium:** Acute interstitial nephritis is seen most commonly in respect to medications. Common causes include the semisynthetic penicillins (methicillin and nafcillin) and sulfa drugs, but any medication can be a culprit. Onset may be days after drug initiation or may occur after months of use. This condition is often associated with rash, peripheral eosinophilia, and eosinophiluria.
   - **Glomeruli:** Acute glomerulonephritis is relatively uncommon but is characterized by hematuria, oliguria, and HTN. Examination of the urine sediment will usually reveal RBC casts and dysmorphic RBCs.
3. **Postrenal azotemia:** ARF due to postrenal causes must involve both kidneys (unless the patient has only a solitary kidney or the patient has baseline poor renal function). The most common sources are the prostate (benign prostatic hyperplasia and prostatic carcinoma), cervix (cervical carcinoma), bilateral stones, and retroperitoneal fibrosis.

PRESENTATION

History

One focus of the history is to determine whether renal failure is truly acute or chronic. Some clues to differentiating this include the following:

- **Previous creatinine** measurements.
- **Renal size:** Patients with chronic renal failure tend to have bilateral, shrunken kidneys, whereas renal size is usually normal in acute failure. Some exceptions are diabetic nephropathy, polycystic kidney disease, amyloidoses, and HIV nephropathy, in which renal size is normal or increased.
- **Anemia:** Patients with GFR <30 mL/min and chronic renal disease tend to be anemic secondary to decreased erythropoietin production. One exception is chronic renal failure from autosomal dominant polycystic kidney disease, in which patients are typically **not** anemic.

- **Renal osteodystrophy:** Patients with prolonged chronic renal failure may have evidence of renal osteodystrophy. The clavicles and wrists are common sites to see changes.

  Other key history includes the following:

- Recent IV contrast administration.
- Recent infections: pharyngitis (post-strep glomerulonephritis), upper respiratory infection (IgA nephropathy), sinusitis (Wegener's), bloody diarrhea (hemolytic uremic syndrome).
- Hemoptysis: lupus, Wegener's, Goodpasture's, endocarditis.
- Urine appearance: hematuria (glomerulonephritis or nephrolithiasis).
- Fluid balance: dehydration from vomiting, diarrhea, or poor oral intake.
- Rashes: allergic, interstitial nephritis, vasculitis, or autoimmune.
- Medication history: allergic interstitial nephritis, NSAID nephropathy, nephrotoxins. Anticholinergics (e.g., TCAs) may cause urinary retention and postrenal failure.
- Social history: IV drug abuse (HIV, hepatitis, endocarditis).
- Total ins and outs for the last few days: Is the patient markedly negative (suggesting prerenal) or positive?

Physical Exam

Determine whether the patient is oliguric (<500 cc of urine/day) or anuric (<100 cc/day). Anuria should raise the possibility of obstructive uropathy or severe ATN/cortical necrosis.

Volume status is critical for both diagnosis (to identify a prerenal state) and fluid management. Assess volume status with orthostatic vital signs, exam of jugular venous pressure, skin turgor, moistness of mucous membranes, and axillary sweat. Examine the fundus in diabetics with chronic renal insufficiency. It is unusual to develop diabetic nephropathy without retinopathy. Retinal exam may also reveal the bright orange arteriolar changes of atheroembolic disease. Listen for abdominal bruits, which may be audible with renal artery stenosis. Palpate for an enlarged bladder (from prostatic obstructive uropathy) or kidneys. Skin exam may reveal evidence of vasculitis, lupus, livedo reticularis (from cholesterol emboli), drug rash, or peripheral stigmata of endocarditis. A pelvic and prostate exam are needed to look for a source of obstruction. Look for signs of congestive heart failure as a cause of decreased renal perfusion.

Also, look for evidence of uremic encephalopathy with confusion and sometimes asterixis. Listen for a pericardial friction rub, which may indicate uremic pericarditis.

Lab and Imaging Evaluation

The UA is the single most important test in evaluating renal failure. Lab data also include electrolytes, CBC, UA with micro/macro, urine electrolytes, and creatine kinase. Peripheral eosinophilia should raise the possibility of allergic interstitial nephritis or atheroembolic disease.

Place a Foley catheter, especially in men, to rule out distal obstruction. A normal urine output does **not** exclude obstruction.

Obtain a renal U/S to assess kidney size and exclude obstruction.

Figure 17-1 is a simple algorithm that may be followed when assessing someone with ARF. This algorithm assumes patients are not on diuretics. If patients are on a diuretic, some clinicians substitute fractional excretion of urea for fractional excretion of sodium. A fractional excretion of urea <35% is indicative of prerenal azotemia.

The fractional excretion of Na is most useful in patients who have acute **oliguric** (urine output <500 cc/day) renal failure.

$$\% \, \text{FeNa} = 100 \times \frac{(\text{urine Na} \times \text{plasma creatinine})}{(\text{plasma Na} \times \text{urine creatinine})}$$

Remember that the creatinine in acute rapid onset renal failure may lag far behind its estimation of renal function. A creatinine that increases by 1 mg/dL/day is called an anephric rise, or roughly the amount that an average person's creatinine would

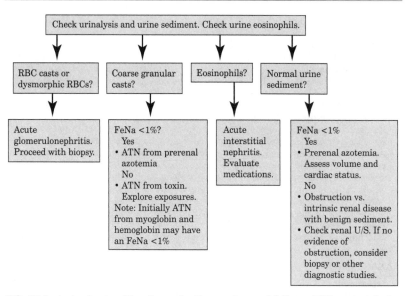

FIG. 17-1. A simple algorithm for evaluating acute renal failure. ATN, acute tubular necrosis.

increase in a noncatabolic state with a GFR of 0 mL/min. A patient whose creatinine rises from 2 mg/dL to 3 mg/dL may have a creatinine clearance of 0 mL/min.

ADDITIONAL CONSIDERATIONS IN POSTOPERATIVE RENAL FAILURE

1. Examine the intraoperative flow sheet carefully for episodes of hypotension during surgery. **Intraoperative renal hypoperfusion is the most common cause of postoperative renal failure.** Because of high vasopressin levels due to anesthesia and surgical stress, most patients will have a decreased urine output with concentrated urine for a few hours after surgery, despite adequate renal blood flow and renal function.
2. Patients with cardiopulmonary bypass are at high risk of renal failure proportional to the duration of cardiopulmonary bypass or cross clamping the aorta above the renal arteries.
3. Consider mechanical obstruction of the ureter or bladder by inadvertent ligation, hematomas, abscess, or (in the case of urologic surgery) ureteral edema.
4. In patients who are immobilized in awkward positions during surgery (e.g., urologic surgery, hip arthroplasty), consider rhabdomyolysis and myoglobinuric renal failure. Approximately one-third of patients with rhabdomyolysis develop ATN. Hyperphosphatemia, hyperkalemia, hyperuricemia, and hypocalcemia out of proportion to renal failure may be clues. Tea-colored urine that is dipstick positive for blood but without RBCs on microscopy is highly suggestive of the diagnosis. Evaluate with serum myoglobin or creatine kinase. Treat with fluids, mannitol, and urinary alkalinization.
5. Identify any history of IV dye administration in patients at high risk for dye-induced renal failure, who are those with poor renal perfusion (congestive heart failure, volume depletion), diabetes mellitus, chronic renal insufficiency, or multiple myeloma. **Contrast dye nephropathy** will have a UA and urine electrolyte changes that are usually indistinguishable from prerenal failure. Rarely, it may have a concomitant mild ATN. Initial rise in creatinine is within 48° of dye administration, peaking at approximately 3–4 days and then normalizing in 1 wk. The best "treatment" is prevention by ensuring that patients at risk are well hydrated

before contrast administration. The role of oral N-acetylcysteine (Mucomyst) in preventing dye nephropathy is not well established.

6. Patients who have had intravascular manipulation (e.g., aortic surgeries, cardiac catheterizations) may suffer from renal failure due to cholesterol emboli or atheroembolus. Cholesterol emboli may also occur spontaneously or with anticoagulation in patients with aortic atherosclerosis. Livedo reticularis, blue toes, and bright orange retinal arterioles may be evident. Blood eosinophil counts are often high, complements are usually low, and UA may resemble prerenal failure. Biopsy of skin lesions may be diagnostic. Classically, the loss of renal function is step-wise. Prognosis for renal recovery is dismal.

7. Recognize the abdominal compartment syndrome. This presents in patients with severe pelvic or abdominal trauma and in those who develop large intraabdominal fluid collections (ruptured abdominal aortic aneurysm, retroperitoneal bleed, pancreatitis, after reduction of a large hernia, massive ascites, etc.). Clinically, they develop distended, usually tense abdomens. Renal failure develops due to decreased cardiac output (from decreased blood return) and increased pressure on the renal parenchyma and vasculature. Respiratory compromise may also develop. Diagnosis is suggested by elevated intraabdominal pressures, usually measured through a Foley catheter. Normal intraabdominal pressure is <5 mm Hg (oliguria develops at >15 mm Hg, anuria at >30 mm Hg). Treatment involves surgical decompression.

MANAGEMENT

The treatment of ARF is determined by its etiology. Important aspects in the management of ARF include avoidance of nephrotoxic agents; the acute treatment of hyperphosphatemia, hyperkalemia, and metabolic acidosis; and maintaining a euvolemic state. Lasix to convert a patient to nonoliguric renal failure has not been shown to affect prognosis but may help with fluid management. Except in cases of hypotension or cardiogenic shock, dopamine has also not been shown to affect outcomes of renal function but may improve diuresis.

One should strive to **maximize renal perfusion** as well. Avoid hypotension, and keep the patient well hydrated. Remember to adjust medication doses for changing renal function.

As many of the causes of ARF are quite readily reversible, it is important to establish a prompt diagnosis and to treat the previously mentioned acute complications. Renal replacement therapy (e.g., hemodialysis) is indicated when

- Hyperkalemia or acidosis is refractory to medical management.
- There is evidence of volume overload (pulmonary edema).
- There are symptoms of uremia (encephalopathy, pericarditis, etc.).

Renal failure from ATN classically has a peak creatinine at 8–14 days, although there is wide variability. Most patients will recover adequate renal function within 6 wks.

KEY POINTS TO REMEMBER

- The UA is the single most important test in determining the etiology of renal failure.
- Determine the acuity of renal failure ideally by previous creatinine measurements. Small kidneys on renal U/S and anemia of renal failure both suggest that renal insufficiency has been chronic.
- In patients who develop renal failure while hospitalized, history should include "ins and outs," possible hypotensive episodes, medications, IV dye administration, and intravascular procedures.
- Always place a Foley catheter in men with ARF to rule out prostatic obstruction. Obstruction may be present even with normal urine output.
- Always remember to adjust medication doses for changing renal function.

REFERENCES AND SUGGESTED READINGS

Esson M. Diagnosis and treatment of acute tubular necrosis. *Ann Intern Med* 2002;137:744–752.

Thadhani R. Acute renal failure. *N Engl J Med* 1996;334(22):1448–1460.

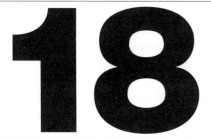

Approach to Hyperkalemia and Hypokalemia

Matthew J. Koch
and Evan D. Gross

APPROACH TO HYPERKALEMIA

Introduction

Hyperkalemia is defined as a plasma potassium level >5 mmol/L. Although this condition may be asymptomatic, with increasing levels of serum potassium, there is ultimately a decrease in cell membrane excitability, which can cause neuromuscular weakness and cardiac conduction defects.

Differential Diagnosis

Differential diagnoses are addressed in Tables 18-1 and 18-2.

History

Review of Medications
Particular attention should be paid to ACE inhibitors, angiotensin receptor blockers, beta blockers, NSAIDs, diuretics, potassium supplements, trimethoprim, pentamidine, and heparin. "Neutra-Phos" is an often unrecognized source of potassium.

Dietary History
Salt substitutes may contain large amounts of potassium salts. The presence or absence of diabetes may suggest hyporeninemic hypoaldosteronism/type IV renal tubular acidosis.

Physical Exam

The physical exam should focus on the **neurologic system** for generalized muscle weakness, which necessitates acute treatment for hyperkalemia.

Lab Evaluation

A rapid confirmation of K^+ level can be done on an ABG sample if the diagnosis is in doubt. Evaluation of renal function with serum creatinine should be performed.

Evaluating the **ECG** is paramount in determining treatment in hyperkalemia, although there may be a marked interpatient variability in the relationship between $[K^+]$ levels and ECG changes. Acute treatment is indicated in a patient with hyperkalemia and ECG changes, including peaked T waves and shortened QT interval (usually at $[K^+]$ levels >6 mmol/L), prolonged PR interval, loss of P wave, and QRS widening (usually at $[K^+]$ levels $\geq$ 7–8 mmol/L). This sine wave pattern can degenerate rapidly to ventricular fibrillation or asystole if untreated.

Evaluation of urinary potassium excretion may also be helpful. Unless the hyperkalemia is due to unreported massive ingestion, a spot urine potassium level is generally not of help. Calculation of the **transtubular potassium gradient (TTKG)** can be useful in evaluating hyperkalemia when the cause is not apparent by history and hypoaldosteronism is suspected [1].

TABLE 18-1. CAUSES OF HYPERKALEMIA

Increased potassium intake	PO (massive ingestion required)
	IV (including stored, nonwashed packed RBCs)
Decreased cellular uptake	Insulin deficiency
	Beta blockade (nonselective), digitalis toxicity
Extracellular shift of potassium	Hyperosmolar states
	Metabolic acidosis (nonorganic)
	Tumor lysis, rhabdomyolysis, extreme exercise, trauma
	Familial periodic paralysis, succinylcholine
Decreased renal excretion	Hypoaldosteronism (see Table 18-2)
	Chronic renal insufficiency
	Congestive heart failure, liver disease
	Hyperkalemic type I renal tubular acidosis
	Chloride shunt
	Selective potassium excretion defect
Pseudohyperkalemia	Variation in serum sample value
	Mechanical trauma during blood draw
	Increase in platelets or WBCs
	Repeated clinching of fist/tourniquet

- Before TTKG evaluation, any medication that can potentially affect the potassium level should be discontinued.
- The urine sodium should be >25 mmol/L (to ensure that potassium excretion is not limited by decreased sodium delivery).
- The urine osmolality should be greater than the plasma osmolality (to ensure that water is being reabsorbed in the collecting duct).

$$\text{TTKG} = \frac{(uK/pK)}{(uOSM/pOSM)}$$

uK, urine potassium; pK, plasma potassium; uOSM, urine osmolality; pOSM, plasma osmolality.

The normal value of a TTKG is approximately 8–9 but varies with potassium intake. The TTKG should be >11 in the presence of hyperkalemia and adequate aldosterone. **A TTKG <7** in the presence of hyperkalemia is suggestive of hypoaldosteronism or aldosterone receptor blockade.

TABLE 18-2. CAUSES OF HYPOALDOSTERONISM

Decreased renin	Hyporeninemic hypoaldosteronism/type IV renal tubular acidosis
	Medications: NSAIDs, cyclosporine, beta blockers
	HIV/AIDS
Decreased aldosterone	Primary adrenal failure, adrenal enzyme defects
	ACE inhibitors/angiotensin receptor blockers, heparin
	HIV/AIDS
Blockade of aldosterone receptor	Medications: amiloride, triamterene, trimethoprim

TABLE 18-3. RENIN AND ALDOSTERONE LEVELS WITH HYPERKALEMIA AND A LOW TRANSTUBULAR POTASSIUM GRADIENT

Disorder	Renin	Aldosterone
Primary or secondary hypoaldosteronism	↑	↓
Aldosterone receptor blockade, pseudohypoaldosteronism	↑	↑
Hyporeninemic hypoaldosteronism, chloride shunt	↓	↓

↑, increased; ↓, decreased.

Further workup in suspected hypoaldosteronism should include plasma renin, aldosterone, and cortisol levels (Table 18-3) obtained from a morning sample after the patient has been ambulating for at least 3 hrs or after the administration of furosemide the previous evening and again in the morning. The cortisol level is low in adrenal insufficiency. See Table 18-3 for renin/aldosterone interpretation.

Management

[K^+] levels ≥ 7 mmol/L require close clinical and cardiac monitoring and often indicate the need for acute treatment.

Calcium gluconate (1 g [10 cc of a 10% solution] given IV over 2 mins) should be given to stabilize the cell membrane in cases of hyperkalemia associated with severe weakness or marked ECG changes. The dose is repeated again in several minutes if there is no clinical improvement.

Insulin is usually given as a dose of 10 U regular insulin IV, along with 25–50 g of dextrose (1–2 amps of D_{50}). If the patient already has hyperglycemia, insulin can be given alone. The effect of insulin to lower the [K^+] is usually evident within 30 mins to 1 hr and lasts for several hours, with an expected decrease of 1–1.5 mmol/L.

Beta$_2$-adrenergic agents have a similar effect as insulin on intracellular transport of potassium. Albuterol is classically given in a dose of 10–20 mg by nebulizer or 0.5 mg IV.

Sodium bicarbonate, given as one ampule IV over several minutes, can be used to drive potassium intracellularly as well. The onset and duration of effect is approximately the same as with insulin. This may be more useful in patients with acidemia. In patients with end-stage renal disease, the effect is limited and also provides a significant sodium load.

Cation-exchange resins (Kayexalate) are used to eliminate excess potassium by exchanging potassium for sodium in the GI tract. The rectal preparation has a faster onset of action. Sorbitol is added to the preparations to reduce constipation and intestinal blockage. The normal dose is 15 g PO in 20% sorbitol given q6h prn. The rectal form is given as 50 g in 70% sorbitol and tap water, and should be kept in place for 2–3 hrs if possible. Repeat q4h prn. Colonic irrigation with tap water between each enema should be used to help reduce the risk of bowel injury. There is a significant risk of upper GI tract ulcers and bowel necrosis, especially in patients with decreased GI motility. Kayexalate should, therefore, be avoided in postoperative patients [2]. Each gram will remove up to 1 mmol of potassium.

Hemodialysis is used when hyperkalemia is not responsive to the usual measures, or when an extremely high [K^+] associated with significant ECG changes or severe weakness is present. Predialysis treatment should be limited to a dose of calcium gluconate, and a single agent, such as insulin, as further treatment (cellular shifts) can limit the amount of potassium removed during dialysis.

APPROACH TO HYPOKALEMIA

Introduction

Hypokalemia is defined as a plasma potassium level <3.5 mmol/L.

History

The clinical history, including the list of medications being taken, is often sufficient to diagnose the cause of hypokalemia. When the cause is not apparent, covert ingestion of diuretics or laxatives should be suspected, and specific tests to evaluate for their presence may be indicated.

Mild hypokalemia at levels of 3–3.5 mmol/L is generally asymptomatic. Weakness and muscle pain can develop as the $[K^+]$ drops <3 mmol/L.

Further decreases to <2.5 mmol/L can lead to paralysis, including involvement of the muscles of respiration. Some patients can present with an ileus due to the hypokalemic effects on smooth muscle.

Rhabdomyolysis can occur with severe hypokalemia. This elevates the $[K^+]$ and prevents further decrements, although it may also serve to mask the underlying etiology.

Increased BP and glucose intolerance may be a manifestation of chronic, mild hypokalemia. Renal manifestations can include nephrogenic diabetes insipidus.

Increased renal ammonia synthesis occurs in the presence of hypokalemia due to intracellular acidosis. In severe liver disease, this may trigger hepatic encephalopathy.

Causes of hypokalemia are listed in Table 18-4. Table 18-5 lists causes of primary or apparent excess aldosterone.

Lab Evaluation

ECG changes demonstrated in the presence of hypokalemia include: U waves, flat or inverted T waves, and S-T depression. The ECG changes do not correlate well with the degree of hypokalemia; however, with extremely low [K+] levels, the PR and QRS intervals can lengthen and lead to ventricular fibrillation.

Obtaining a **24-hr urine collection for potassium** is quite useful (Table 18-6), as the total urine excretion per day should be <15–25 mmol of potassium in the presence of hypokalemia.

The **TTKG** can be checked as well, and the value should be <4 if K+ is being conserved appropriately. The TTKG may be appropriately low in the presence of increased daily K+ excretion due to an osmotic diuresis, sodium wasting nephropathy, or diuresis.

Check a serum creatine phosphokinase in suspected hypokalemic-induced rhabdomyolysis. Further evaluation should include acid/base status and urine pH, as well as

TABLE 18-4. CAUSES OF HYPOKALEMIA

Decreased intake	
Increased cellular uptake	Insulin
	Sympathetic stimulation (beta$_2$-agonists, MI, arrhythmias)
	RBC or WBC production and transfusions
	Hypokalemic periodic paralysis (rare)
	Alkalosis
	Hyperthyroidism
Renal losses	Increased distal flow
	Nonabsorbed anions (e.g., glucosuria)
	Increased or apparent increased aldosterone (see Table 18-5)
	Type I and II renal tubular acidosis
	Amphotericin, cisplatinum, aminoglycosides
	Diuretics (thiazide, loop, acetazolamide)
	Hypomagnesemia
Nonrenal losses	GI (e.g., diarrhea), sweat

TABLE 18-5. PRIMARY OR APPARENT EXCESS ALDOSTERONE

Primary hyperaldosteronism (low renin–high aldosterone)	Adrenal adenoma, hyperplasia, carcinoma
	Glucocorticoid-remediable hyperaldosteronism
	Congenital adrenal hyperplasia
Secondary hyperaldosteronism (high renin–high aldosterone)	Renal artery stenosis, malignant HTN
	Renin secreting tumors, low effective circulating volume
Increased alternate mineralocorticoids (low renin–low aldosterone)	11-Beta-hydroxysteroid dehydrogenase deficiency (real licorice, chewing tobacco)
	Overwhelmed 11-beta-hydroxysteroid dehydrogenase (Cushing's)
Apparent mineralocorticoid excess (AME) (low renin–low aldosterone)	Liddle's syndrome (pseudohyperaldosteronism)
AME (high renin–high aldosterone)	Gitelman's syndrome (pseudothiazide)
	Bartter's syndrome (pseudofurosemide)

noting the presence of hypotension or HTN. Remote vomiting or diuretic use can present with the expected alkalosis and a low-potassium excretion.

Renin and aldosterone levels may also aid in the evaluation of possible apparent or true aldosterone excess.

Management

The approximate **potassium deficit** as the plasma potassium level decreases from 4 mmol/L to 3 mmol/L, is in the range of 200–400 mmol depending on the size of the patient. As the plasma level decreases to <3 mmol/L, the deficit can be >600 mmol but is unpredictable due to the potential release of potassium from cellular necrosis that maintains, and may even increase, the $[K^+]$.

These cellular shifts can mask a serious potassium deficit, and levels should be checked frequently to ensure adequacy of replacement.

Potassium replacement should be given orally whenever possible because of the potential cardiac risk of rapid IV K^+ administration, vein sclerosis, and cost.

Oral doses of 40 mEq of potassium are generally well tolerated and can be given q4h. Liquid potassium is generally unpalatable, and slow-release tablet forms should

TABLE 18-6. EVALUATION OF URINE POTASSIUM IN HYPOKALEMIA

Low daily urine potassium excretion	**Acidemia:** lower GI
	Alkalemia: prior upper GI, sweat, prior diuresis
Increased daily urine potassium	**Low transtubular potassium gradient excretion:** active diuresis (diuretics, salt wasting), osmotic diuresis
	High transtubular potassium gradient and acidemia: type I renal tubular acidosis, nonabsorbed anion
	High transtubular potassium gradient and alkalemia with increased BP
	Real or apparent hyperaldosterone **with decreased BP**
	Gitelman's, Bartter's syndrome

not be used because of the risk of gastric ulceration. **Potassium chloride** is usually administered as the chloride component helps to correct the often-coinciding alkalosis and bicarbonaturia. **Potassium citrate** can be given **if hypokalemia associated with acidemia is present.**

IV potassium can be administered in concentrations of 40 mmol/L via a peripheral line or 60 mmol/L via a central line. The rate of infusion should generally not be >20 mmol/hr unless the clinical situation dictates otherwise. The use of a femoral line has been recommended if rapid infusions are needed to avoid the administration of large concentrations of potassium directly into the cardiac chamber.

KEY POINTS TO REMEMBER

- The ECG is paramount in evaluating hyperkalemia. The presence of ECG changes, the earliest being peaked T waves, is an indication for rapid treatment of hyperkalemia.
- Therapy for hyperkalemia should start with IV calcium to stabilize the cardiac membrane. Albuterol, $NaHCO_3$, and insulin/glucose will cause rapid intracellular shifts as a temporizing measure, but potassium must be removed by Kayexalate or dialysis to prevent rebound hyperkalemia.
- Mild or moderate hypokalemia should preferably be repleted orally. There is a risk of vein sclerosis and cardiac arrhythmia with IV potassium replacement.

REFERENCES

1. West ML, Marsden PA, Richardson RM, et al. New clinical approach to evaluate disorders of potassium excretion. *Miner Electrolyte Metab* 1986;12:234–238.
2. Gardiner GW. Kayexalate (sodium polystyrene sulphonate) in sorbitol associated with intestinal necrosis in uremic patients. *Can J Gastroenterol* 1997;11:573–577.

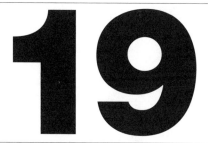

Hyponatremia and Hypernatremia

Matthew J. Koch and
Christopher H. Kwoh

APPROACH TO HYPONATREMIA

Introduction

Hyponatremia is defined by a serum sodium (Na^+) level <136 mmol/L. Serum Na^+ does not reflect total body Na^+ as much as it represents the ratio of Na to plasma volume.

History

Symptoms include CNS effects such as confusion, weakness, obtundation, or seizures and can progress to death from brainstem herniation [1]. Chronic hyponatremia (>48 hrs) is generally well tolerated, but symptoms may include cognitive defects as well as nausea and vomiting, weakness, and headache. SIADH may manifest years before the onset of an otherwise unapparent malignancy.

Physical Exam

Focus on assessing the **volume status** and mental status of the patient. Look for evidence of congestive heart failure or liver failure/cirrhosis.

Lab Evaluation

The first step is determining effective osmolality (eOSM) (Fig. 19-1):

- eOSM = measured plasma osmoles − (BUN/2.8 + ethanol/4.6)
- The normal eOSM is approximately 285 mOsm/kg. A low eOSM suggests true hypotonic hyponatremia, whereas a high and normal eOSM are hypertonic hyponatremia and pseudohyponatremia, respectively.

  Each of the categories is further discussed below.

Pseudohyponatremia

Pseudohyponatremia is due to a lab underestimation of Na^+ concentration from excess serum lipid and protein or WBCs. This is a benign lab artifact requiring only recognition.

Hypertonic Hyponatremia

Hypertonic hyponatremia is due to excess osmotically active substances drawing water into the **extracellular fluid (ECF)** and diluting serum Na^+. This increases risk of cellular dehydration. See Fig. 19-1 for specific etiologies.

The measured sodium must be corrected for hyperglycemia:

$$\text{Corrected } Na^+ = \text{Measured } Na^+ \left[2.4 \times \left(\frac{\text{glucose} - 150}{100} \right) \right]$$

Hypotonic Hyponatremia (True Hyponatremia)

True hyponatremia is further evaluated with measuring urinary Na (UNa):

- **Urine osmolality <100** identifies patients with decreased antidiuretic hormone (ADH).

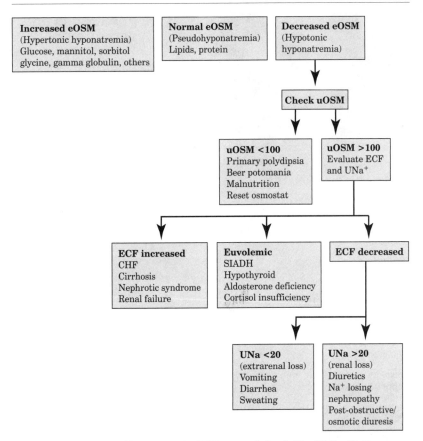

FIG. 19-1. Evaluation of hyponatremia. ECF, extracellular fluid; eOSM, effective osmolality; UNa, urinary sodium; uOSM, urinary osmolality.

- Reset osmostat is a variant of SIADH but with a stable Na^+. Etiologies are similar to SIADH and should be pursued in a similar fashion.
- **Extrarenal losses** will have a low UNa, with the exception of conditions that lead to alkalosis, as the bicarbonaturia may cause co-elimination of significant Na^+ in the urine. Ketonuria can have the same effect on UNa. The urine chloride, however, should still be low in both of these situations.
- **Urine osmolality >100** identifies patients with increased ADH activity and must be further defined depending on the **volume status** of the patient (see Fig. 19-1):
  - **Volume excess:** Congestive heart failure, cirrhosis, nephrotic syndrome; Na^+ tends to be stable at >125 mmol/L
  - **Euvolemic:** SIADH (see Table 19-1 for causes), hypothyroidism, Addison's, pregnancy. SIADH cannot be diagnosed in the setting of renal failure, and diagnosis must involve exclusion of adrenal insufficiency and thyroid disease.
- **Volume depletion:**
  - UNa >20: renal Na^+ loss (diuretics, salt-losing nephropathy). It is unusual for loop diuretics to produce significant hyopnatremia due to their effect on urine-concentrating ability. Thiazides more frequently cause hyponatremia.
  - UNa <20: extrarenal Na^+ loss (vomiting, diarrhea, sweating)

TABLE 19-1. COMMON CAUSES OF SIADH

CNS disorders	Hemorrhage, psychosis, infection, alcohol withdrawal
Malignancy (ectopic ADH)	Small-cell lung cancer (most commonly implicated), CNS, leukemia, Hodgkin's, duodenal, pancreatic, etc.
Pulmonary	Infection, acute respiratory failure, mechanical ventilation
Miscellaneous	Pain, nausea (powerful stimulator of ADH), HIV (multifactorial), general postoperative state, cortisol deficiency, hypothyroidism
Pharmacologic agents (either mimic or enhance ADH)	Cyclophosphamide, vincristine, vinblastine, NSAIDs, ecstasy (also polydipsia)
	Tricyclics and related agents, serotonin reuptake inhibitors, chlorpropamide, nicotine, bromocriptine, oxytocin, desmopressin (deamino-8-D-arginine vasopressin)

ADH, antidiuretic hormone.

Management

The correction of hyponatremia, either apparently acute or chronic in nature that presents **with significant symptoms**, requires hypertonic saline. Typically, 1 cc/kg/hr of 3% saline will raise the serum Na^+ by approximately 1 mmol/L/hr. A detailed approximation for the expected correction in serum Na^+ by giving 1 L of infusate is as follows [2]:

$$\frac{\text{Infusate } Na^+ \text{ (mmol/L)} + \text{infusate K (mmol/L)} - \text{serum } Na^+ \text{ (mmol/L)}}{\text{Estimated total body water (kg)} + 1}$$

- Normal saline = 154 mmol Na^+/L; 3% saline = 513 mmol Na^+/L
- Dividing the calculated volume by the desired time period gives the rate of infusion.
- The addition of potassium (K) to the solution is equivalent to adding additional Na^+ due to Na^+/K exchange and needs to be included in calculations as well.
- Loop diuretics are often also required either to prevent volume overload or to aid in free-water excretion by lowering the urine osmolality (uOSM).
- Calculations only provide a rough estimate to help initiate therapy and **do not replace frequent monitoring and adjustment**.

Acute, severe CNS symptoms can often be reversed with a 5% increase in the serum Na^+. Initially, aim to correct 1–2 mmol/L/hr unless continuing symptoms necessitate more rapid reversal.

Once symptoms are controlled, a maximum serum Na^+ increase in the first 24 hrs of 8 mmol/L is recommended (including initial correction). At this point, hypertonic saline is usually no longer necessary. The correction over the subsequent 24-hr periods should probably not exceed an additional 10 mmol Na^+/L [1,2].

Rapid correction may result in central pontine myelinolysis and osmotic demyelination. This is exceedingly rare with acute hyponatremia (<48 hrs duration).

The need to treat accidental overcorrection with free water or ADH analogs to decrease the serum Na^+ to the desired level of correction is possibly of benefit, especially if symptoms suggestive of osmotic demyelination appear [3].

Cognitive and movement disorders due to central pontine myelinolysis may not be apparent for days after correction of hyponatremia, and visible changes on MRI may take weeks to appear [4].

Chronic hyponatremia without acute neurologic events is best treated by fluid restriction.

For SIADH, free water restriction, loop diuretics, and high oral Na^+ and protein intake are the mainstay of treatment:

- The degree of free water restriction will depend on the uOSM present, as it will determine the amount of free water that can be excreted with the given osmotic load. For instance, a uOSM of 600 mOsm/kg would allow a daily dietary intake of

600 mOsm to be excreted in 1 L of urine, but decreasing the uOSM to 300 mOsm/kg with loop diuretics would allow the same intake to be excreted in 2 L of urine.
- Use hypertonic saline ± loop diuretics if severe symptoms or very high uOSM. Use of normal saline in SIADH may paradoxically worsen hyponatremia by allowing the kidney to extract the free water from the saline if uOSM are greater than the osmolarity of the infusate.
- **Oral urea** (30–60 g/day) is probably the safest current pharmacologic agent for the rare case in which standard management is unsuccessful [5].
- **Demeclocycline** (Declomycin) and **lithium** (Eskalith; Lithobid) have both been used to induce a nephrogenic diabetes insipidus. Lithium is unpredictable and has many side effects.
- Approximately one-third of cases are the reset osmostat variant and do not require therapy.

In hyponatremia from thiazides, complete resolution of the effect can sometimes take weeks after withdrawal. Patients who develop severe hyponatremia on a thiazide diuretic are at extreme risk of severe and rapid reoccurrence and should not receive these agents again [6].

APPROACH TO HYPERNATREMIA

Introduction

Hypernatremia is defined as serum Na^+ >145 mmol/L. All cases of hypernatremia are true hyperosmolar states.

Differential Diagnosis

The vast majority of hypernatremia is due to hypovolemia and dehydration.
   Hypervolemic hypernatremia is usually due to administration of hypertonic fluids (UNa >100) but may also be caused by primary hyperaldosteronism (reset osmostat hypernatremia).
   Hypernatremia of varying volume status may be caused by various mechanisms:

- Rapid ECF to intracellular fluid free water shift from rhabdomyolysis or prolonged seizures.
- Placental vasopressinase release during pregnancy (rare).

   Hypovolemic hypernatremia **etiologies** are included in Fig. 19-2:

- **Osmotic diuresis** may be caused by osmotic diuretics, glucosuria, high-protein diet, postacute tubular necrosis, or postobstructive diuresis (due to the urea load).

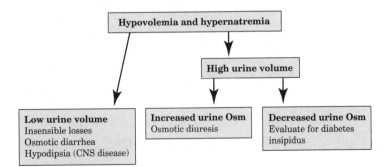

FIG. 19-2. Differential diagnosis and evaluation of hypernatremia with volume depletion. Osm, osmolality.

- **Central diabetes insipidus (DI)** is caused by disruption of the posterior pituitary by trauma, surgery, granulomatous diseases, meningitis, encephalitis, tumors, pituitary apoplexy, or, rarely, is hereditary.
- **Nephrogenic DI** is often due to drugs (lithium, foscarnet, cidofovir), electrolytes (K^+ <3.0, hypercalcemia), or kidney disease (obstructive uropathy, sickle cell, amyloidosis, Sjögren's).

History

Symptoms include lethargy, irritability, weakness, confusion, and progression to coma but are generally not apparent until the serum Na^+ has increased to 160 mmol/L [7].

Try to determine the amount of urine volume. Low urine volume is consistent with dehydration, but polyuria should raise suspicion for DI. Inquire about fluid intake as well.

Physical Exam

The physical exam should focus on assessing volume status. If DI is a consideration, then a neurologic exam, including visual fields, is indicated.

Lab Evaluation

History and physical exam will usually identify the cause of hypervolemic or euvolemic hypernatremia. Many patients with adequate thirst mechanisms may maintain volume status with DI.

Hypovolemic hypernatremia may be evaluated as per Fig. 19-2.

With hypovolemia due to free water loss, uOSM should be >700 mOsm/kg and the UNa should be <20 mmol/L.

Release of a total of >1000 urine osmoles/day (uOSM × 24-hr urine output) is consistent with an osmotic diuresis.

Patients with polyuria and hypernatremia may undergo a water deprivation test to differentiate central from nephrogenic DI:

- Water is withheld from the patient until three consecutive urine osmoles are stable (<30 mmol/kg increase). The patient is given desmopressin (deamino-8-D-arginine vasopressin, DDAVP), 1 μg SC with serum osmoles measured before injection and 45 mins later. In central DI, there is a >9% increase in uOSM with DDAVP. With nephrogenic DI, there is little change. Difficulty in diagnosis may arise in partial DI states.

Management

Correction of serum Na^+ at a **rate of 0.5 mmol/L per hr** has a low likelihood of causing complications.

The following formula calculates the approximate change with 1 L of infusate:

$$\frac{\text{Infusate } Na^+ \text{ (mmol/L)} + \text{infusate K (mmol/L)} - \text{serum } Na^+ \text{ (mmol/L)}}{\text{Total body water (L)} + 1}$$

Add 30–40 mL/hr for insensible losses and additional fluid prn continued losses.

The only indication for the use of normal saline in hypernatremia is in the patient with severe volume depletion requiring fluid resuscitation. Lesser degrees of clinical volume depletion can be treated with 0.2% or 0.45% saline solution (34 and 77 mmol/L Na^+, respectively).

Once volume status has been restored, 5% dextrose solution alone should be used to correct hypernatremia.

Total body water tends to be decreased by 10% in hypernatremic volume–depleted patients, and the estimated values most often used are 40% of body weight in women and 50% in men.

Calculations are valuable in initiating therapy, but repeated clinical and lab evaluation is necessary in the ultimate adjustment of fluid administration to ensure an appropriate correction rate.

Central DI may be treated with DDAVP SC titrated to effect.

Nephrogenic DI has several management options:

- Thiazide diuretics ± NSAIDs cause volume depletion and increase renal Na^+ retention.
- Amiloride may block access of lithium to the Na^+ channel of the collecting tubule and is useful in lithium-induced nephrogenic DI.

KEY POINTS TO REMEMBER

- The initial evaluation of hyponatremia is based on urine osmoles and volume status.
- Severe symptomatic hyponatremia may be treated with hypertonic saline. Do not exceed 2 mmol Na^+/L/hr correction. Calculations of free water excess are useful in initiating therapy, but one must still follow serial sodium measurements to assess appropriate response. Other cases are most safely treated with free water restriction.
- Normal saline may paradoxically decrease serum sodium in the case of SIADH. A trial of 1 L is safe and may be appropriate if volume depletion is suspected.
- Volume depletion is by far the most common cause of hypernatremia. Although calculation of free water deficit is important in determining initial IV infusion rates, they do not replace serial measurements of serum sodium. One of the most common mistakes in correcting hypernatremia is not accounting for the insensible free water loss of approximately 40 cc/hr.

SUGGESTED READING

Adrogue HJ, Madias NE. Hypernatremia. *N Engl J Med* 2000;342:1493–1499.

Adrogue HJ, Madias NE. Hyponatremia. *N Engl J Med* 2000;342:1581–1589.

Boton R, Gaviria M, Batlle DC. Prevalence, pathogenesis, and treatment of renal dysfunction associated with chronic lithium therapy. *Am J Kidney Dis* 1987;10:329.

Maraganore DM, Folger WN, Swanson JW, et al. Movement disorders as sequelae of central pontine myelinolysis: report of three cases. *Mov Disord* 1992;7:142.

Palevsky PM. Hypernatremia. *Semin Nephrology* 1998;18:20–30.

Sterns RH, Cappuccio JD, Silver SM, et al. Neurologic sequelae after treatment of severe hyponatremia: a multicenter perspective. *J Am Soc Nephrol* 1994;4:1522.

Verbalis JG. Adaptation to acute and chronic hyponatremia: implications for symptomatology, diagnosis, and therapy. *Semin Nephrol* 1998;1:3–19.

REFERENCES

1. Fraser CL, Arieff AI. Epidemiology, pathophysiology, and management of hyponatremic encephalopathy. *Am J Med* 1997;102:67.
2. Adrogue HJ, Madias NE. Aiding fluid prescription for the dysnatremias. *Intensive Care Med* 1997;23:309.
3. Soupart A, Ngassa M, Decaux G. Therapeutic relowering of the serum sodium in a patient after excessive correction of hyponatremia. *Clin Nephrol* 1999;51:383.
4. Brunner JE, Redmond JM, Harrar AM, et al. Central pontine myelinolysis and pontine lesions after rapid correction of hyponatremia: a prospective magnetic resonance imaging study. *Ann Neurol* 1990;27:61.
5. Decaux G, Genette F. Urea for long-term treatment of syndrome of inappropriate secretion of antidiuretic hormone. *BMJ (Clin Res Ed)* 1981;283:1081.
6. Friedman E, Shadel M, Halkin H, et al. Thiazide induced hyponatremia—reproduced by single dose challenge and analysis of pathogenesis. *Ann Intern Med* 1989;110:24.
7. Arieff AI, Guisado R. Effects on the central nervous system of hypernatremic and hyponatremic states. *Kidney Int* 1976;10:104.

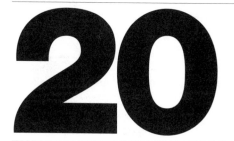

Approach to the Patient with Hematuria

Georges Saab

INTRODUCTION

The definition of microscopic hematuria by the American Urological Association is ≥ 3 RBCs per high-power field on microscopic evaluation of urinary sediment from two of three properly collected UA specimens.

In gross hematuria, urine appears red, cola-colored, or brown. In microscopic hematuria, urine appears grossly normal, and diagnosis is made by urine dipstick or microscopic exam of the sediment.

The prevalence of hematuria ranges from 2–16% by dipstick and 1–5% by microscopy. See Table 20-1 for differential diagnosis.

PRESENTATION

History

Hematuria clearing by the end of urination suggests a urethral source. If hematuria begins midway through, it suggests a bladder source. If hematuria is occurring throughout urination, it is probably from an upper urinary tract or kidney source. Ask about recent trauma, urinary catheters, and exercise habits. Make sure that the patient can urinate and is not obstructed by clots.

Aniline dye exposure, pelvic irradiation, and smoking all predispose to malignancy. Also inquire about weight loss.

A recent history of pharyngitis suggests a postinfectious glomerulonephritis, whereas a recent mucosal infection (upper respiratory infection, UTI, enteritis, etc.) may accompany IgA nephropathy. Bloody diarrhea may precede hemolytic uremic syndrome. Recurrent sinusitis/otitis may suggest Wegener's granulomatosis.

Dysuria, urinary frequency/urgency, and flank pain may be clues to cystitis/pyelonephritis. Urethral discharge occurs with urethritis. Nephrolithiasis may present with crampy abdominal pain radiating to the groin.

IV drug use is a risk factor for HIV, hepatitis, endocarditis, and (in those using IV heroin) focal segmental glomerular sclerosis. Blood transfusions increase the risk of HIV and hepatitis.

A detailed family history should include inquiries about deafness and kidney disease (Alport's), cerebral aneurysms and kidney disease (autosomal dominant polycystic kidney disease), and kidney stones.

A detailed sexual history may reveal risk factors for HIV, hepatitis, chlamydia, and gonorrhea. A menstrual history must also be obtained.

Physical Exam

A thorough skin exam may reveal rashes suggestive of a vasculitis or autoimmune disease (SLE). Palpable purpura occurs with Henoch-Schönlein purpura, especially if the distribution involves the abdomen and lower extremities. Also look for peripheral signs of endocarditis.

Examine for signs of arthritis and synovitis to suggest an autoimmune etiology.

A careful genitourinary exam is essential in the evaluation of hematuria. In men, examine for prostatitis, prostatic cancer, benign prostatic hypertrophy, testicular

TABLE 20-1. DIFFERENTIAL DIAGNOSIS OF HEMATURIA

Glomerular		
Proliferative GN	**Nonproliferative GN**	**Familial glomerular disease**
IgA nephropathy	Minimal change disease	Alport syndrome
Postinfectious GN	Focal glomerulo-sclerosis	Familial benign hematuria
Crescentic GN		Fabry disease
Membranoproliferative GN	Membranous nephropathy	Nail-patella syndrome
Fibrillary GN	Hemolytic uremic syndrome	
Henoch-Schönlein purpura		
SLE		
Anti-glomerular basement membrane nephritis		
Systemic vasculitides		
Chronic bacteremia		
Mixed cryoglobulinemia		

Nonglomerular			
Neoplasms	**Vascular**	**Infections**	**Other**
Renal cell carcinoma	Renal vein thrombosis	Acute cystitis	Cyclophosphamide
Transitional cell cancer	Renal infarction	Prostatitis	Trauma/exercise
Prostate carcinoma	Malignant HTN	Urethritis	
Squamous cell cancer of the urethra	A-V malformation	TB	
Wilms' tumor		Schistosomiasis	
Angiomyolipoma			
Multiple myeloma			

GN, glomerulonephritis.

masses, and signs of epididymitis. In women, a pelvic exam is essential to assess for masses or malignancy.

Lab and Imaging Evaluation

Initial lab data should include basic chemistries, CBC, PT, PTT, liver panel, UA, and urine sediment evaluation. Do not rely on the lab to discover casts; **examine the urine sediment yourself.**

A green color on the urine dipstick indicates presence of Hgb, with the degree of color change correlating with amount of Hgb. A speckled pattern indicates intact red cells, and a uniform pattern indicates free Hgb. False-positive dipstick results can be due to myoglobin, Hgb, contaminants (e.g., hypochlorite from container, menstrual blood, trauma, or bacterial peroxidase), or dehydration. Positive dipstick results for blood with no RBCs on microscopy should prompt an evaluation for myoglobinuria.

False-negative results can be due to ingestion of large amounts of ascorbic acid or other reducing agents, presence of low pH, or presence of formaldehyde.

If exam of the urine reveals dysmorphic RBCs (irregular cell membrane), red cell casts, and/or proteinuria, this suggests bleeding of glomerular origin. Additional testing includes the following serologies: ANA, ANCA, HIV, hepatitis panel, antiglomerular basement membrane, C3, C4, VDRL, and antistreptolysin O titer. A renal U/S and nephrology consultation may also be helpful. Consider a renal biopsy in patients with declining renal function.

Isomorphic RBCs in the presence of pyuria, dysuria, or bacteruria are likely related to a UTI. The presence of hematuria should be reevaluated after treatment of the UTI.

In the absence of a UTI, the presence of isomorphic RBCs warrants evaluation for tumors or calculi. Assess urine cytology for malignant cells. Begin the initial workup with a KUB as a "scout film" because 90% of renal calculi are radio-opaque. IV urography is the "gold standard" for evaluating for filling defects and/or obstruction along the urinary tract. However, its use is limited in patients with low GFR in which excretion of contrast is delayed. Alternatively, renal U/S has been used more frequently as a first-line investigation. Other diagnostic tests include CT, MRI, retrograde urography, and isotopic renography.

If the previously mentioned evaluations are nondiagnostic, then consider a urology consultation for possible cystoscopy.

Hematuria in the presence of supratherapeutic anticoagulation or bleeding diathesis still requires thorough evaluation.

MANAGEMENT

The management of patients with hematuria lies mainly in establishing the origin of the hematuria and rapid triage to the appropriate specialist. Any patient thought to have bleeding of glomerular origin should be seen promptly by a nephrologist, particularly those patients who have evidence of renal dysfunction. Patients with renal calculi or masses or positive urine cytology should be evaluated by a urologist.

KEY POINTS TO REMEMBER

- The most important first step in the evaluation of hematuria is to distinguish between hematuria from a glomerular source and a urinary tract source. Evaluation of the urine sediment is most critical. A glomerular source is indicated by the presence of dysmorphic RBCs or red cell casts on the UA. Isomorphic RBCs in the urine microscopy are more likely from the urinary tract.
- Hematuria in the presence of anticoagulation still requires evaluation, even with a supratherapeutic INR.

REFERENCES AND SUGGESTED READINGS

Culclasure TF, Bray VJ, Hasbargen JA. The significance of hematuria in the anticoagulated patient. *Arch Intern Med* 1994;154:649–652.

Fassett RG, Horgan BA, Mathew TH. Detection of glomerular bleeding by phase-contrast microscopy. *Lancet* 1982;1:1432–1434.

Fogazzi G, Ponticelli C. Microscopic hematuria diagnosis and management. *Nephron* 1996;72:125–134.

Grossfeld G, Wolf JS, Litwin M, et al. Asymptomatic microscopic hematuria in adults: summary of the AUA best practice policy recommendations. *Am Fam Physician* 2001;63(6):1145–1153.

Kohler H. Acanthocyturia. A characteristic marker for glomerular bleeding. *Kidney Int* 1991;40:115–120.

Webb JAW. Editorial imaging in haematuria. *Clin Radiol* 1997;52:167–171.

Woolhandler S, Pels R, Bor D, et al. Dipstick urinalysis screening of asymptomatic adults for urinary tract disorders. *JAMA* 1989;262:1215–1219.

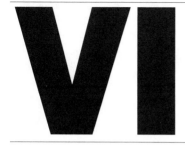

Infectious Disease

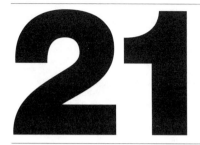

Pneumonia

Rebecca Chandler and
Christopher H. Kwoh

INTRODUCTION

There are approximately 2–3 million cases of community-acquired pneumonia (CAP) per year in the United States; approximately 0.5 million persons are hospitalized and approximately 10–15% of these persons die from their pneumonia [1,2].

Nosocomial pneumonia is defined as the acquisition of a pulmonary infiltrate within 48–72 hrs of hospitalization and ventilator-associated pneumonia developing after 48 hrs of mechanical ventilation. It has been documented to occur in 0.4–1% of hospitalized patients overall [3] and up to 25–58% of mechanically ventilated patients [4]. The overall mortality rate is calculated to be 20–50% [5].

DIFFERENTIAL DIAGNOSIS

CAP pathogens include bacteria (*Streptococcus pneumoniae* is most common, *Haemophilus influenzae, Moraxella catarrhalis, Chlamydia pneumoniae, Mycoplasma pneumoniae, Legionella*, and others), viruses (influenza and others), and fungi (e.g., histoplasma).

In nosocomial pneumonia, bacteria are implicated in >90% of cases. Distribution of pathogens varies with institution. Gram-negative rods account for up to 70% of cases, including *Pseudomonas aeruginosa, Klebsiella pneumoniae, Escherichia coli, Acinetobacter* species, *Serratia* species, and *Enterobacter* species. *Staphylococcus aureus* is the most important gram-positive cause, responsible for up to 30% of cases [6]. Viral pathogens, such as influenza and respiratory syncytial virus, have been implicated as well.

Congestive heart failure, malignancy, atelectasis, and pulmonary hemorrhage may all mimic pneumonia.

PRESENTATION

History

CAP has been historically divided into two categories:

- **"Typical" pneumonia** presents with the abrupt onset of fever, cough, purulent sputum, dyspnea, and pleuritic chest pain. Common etiologies are streptococcus pneumonia, *H. influenzae*, and oral anaerobes.
- **"Atypical" pneumonia** presents with the indolent onset of myalgias, headache, and nausea with cough productive of scant sputum. Common etiologies are legionella, mycoplasma, chlamydia pneumonia, and viral infections.

The diagnosis of nosocomial pneumonia is usually suggested by fever, cough, change in sputum, respiratory difficulty, or altered mental status.

Medical history should focus on comorbid conditions such as immune deficiency, cardiac, pulmonary, rheumatologic disease, history of tobacco and alcohol, and risk factors for pulmonary embolism. Recent antibiotic use may help in identifying likely resistance patterns in the eventually isolated pathogen.

In nosocomial pneumonia, inquire about risk factors, including mechanical ventilation, advanced age, severity of illness, depressed level of consciousness, nasogastric tubes, and use of stress ulcer prophylaxis (which may increase the bacterial density of aspirated gastric contents).

Physical Exam

Pulmonary exam may reveal evidence of consolidation or rales. Sputum should be examined, and any change in color is suggestive of infection. "Atypical" pneumonia may have an underwhelming pulmonary exam with a few rales or wheezes. Particular attention should be paid to the vital signs (fever, tachypnea, oxygenation), mental status, obvious sources of infection (catheters, wounds, purulent sinus drainage), signs of congestive heart failure, or deep venous thrombosis.

Lab Evaluation

In nosocomial pneumonia, it is most challenging to distinguish between colonization and infection in sputum results. Inpatients who are moderately to critically ill change their spectra of flora, becoming colonized with gram-negative rods within 4 days of hospitalization [7].

Sputum culture and blood culture (positive in <10%) should be obtained before administration of antibiotics. The use of sputum specimens from the upper respiratory tract is limited given the high rate of colonization of the oropharynx, trachea, and endotracheal tubes.

In the most critically ill patients, fiberoptic bronchoscopy and blind bronchial sampling are the means by which to obtain tissue by protected specimen brush and bronchoalveolar lavage:

- Gram staining of material from the distal airways, and in particular that obtained by bronchoalveolar lavage, has proven superior to that from proximal airways with a positive predictive value between 92–95% and a negative predictive value between 57–95% (8).
- Quantitative culture may be helpful. Nosocomial pneumonia is defined as a quantitative culture of 10^3 colony-forming units/mL by protected specimen brush and 10^4 colony-forming units/mL by bronchoalveolar lavage [9].

Consider a legionella urine antigen or pneumococcal or viral antigen testing.

Imaging Evaluation

A chest x-ray should be obtained in all patients for diagnosis, to rule out significant pleural effusion, and to follow progression. Radiographic abnormalities may persist for several weeks or progress for a couple of days despite appropriate therapy. Repeat the chest x-ray in 6–12 wks in older patients and smokers to document resolution and exclude an associated malignancy.

MANAGEMENT

Community-Acquired Pneumonia

Recommendations for inpatients include a regimen consisting of a beta lactam plus a macrolide [e.g., ceftriaxone (Rocephin), 1 g IV qd plus azithromycin (Zithromax), 250 mg PO qd] or a fluoroquinolone [e.g., moxifloxacin (Avelox), 400 mg PO/IV qd]. In those patients ill enough to require ICU placement, fluoroquinolone therapy should be combined with a beta lactam.

Nosocomial Pneumonia

The decision to treat positive sputum cultures should be based on the suspicion of pneumonia vs. colonization. Fever, leukocytosis, hypoxia, cough, increased tracheal secretions, or a change in the character of sputum/tracheal secretions all suggest pneumonia. New chest x-ray findings consistent with pneumonia are very specific for actual infection rather than colonization.

Mild to moderately ill patients (no comorbid conditions, no prior antibiotics) may be treated with monotherapy with a beta lactam + inhibitor [e.g., ticarcillin/clavulanate (Timentin), 3.1 g IV q4h], a second- or third-generation cephalosporin (e.g., ceftriaxone, 1–2 g IV qd), or a fluoroquinolone (e.g., gatifloxacin, 400 mg IV qd).

Moderately to critically ill patients (comorbid conditions, prolonged mechanical ventilation, previous antibiotics) may be treated with monotherapy with ciprofloxacin (Cipro) (400 mg IV qd), imipenem-cilastatin (Primaxin) (0.5 g IV q6h), or cefepime (Maxipime) (1–2 g IV q12h), but failure rate approaches 60%. Double coverage is therefore typically given with combinations of beta lactams and either an aminoglycoside (e.g., tobramycin [Tobrex], 5 mg/kg IV qd) or a fluoroquinolone.

In patients highly susceptible to pseudomonas (COPD, cystic fibrosis), an antipseudomonal beta lactam plus an aminoglycoside should be considered.

In patients at risk for aspiration (neurologic disease, alcoholics) or allergic to beta lactams, consider a fluoroquinolone plus clindamycin (Cleocin) (600 mg IV q8h).

Duration and Response to Treatment for Community-Acquired and Nosocomial Pneumonia

The Infectious Disease Society of America recommends that typical pneumonia should be treated until afebrile for 72 hrs, whereas atypical pneumonias should be treated for approximately 2 wks.

Duration of therapy for nosocomial pneumonias is uncertain, but 14–21 days is the general guideline. Necrotizing pneumonias may need treatment for up 28 days. Pulmonary toilet is a beneficial adjunct to antibiotics.

Defervescence is the most used measure of response to treatment; resolution of leukocytosis, hypoxia, and chest radiography are additional markers. Microbiologic studies reveal sterilization of distal airway secretion within 72 hrs of initiation of appropriate treatment.

If a pleural effusion is present, then consider a diagnostic thoracentesis to rule out an empyema, especially if there is >1 cm of fluid layers on a lateral decubitus. Chest tube placement may be necessary in some cases.

KEY POINTS TO REMEMBER

- Clinically, one must distinguish typical (abrupt onset of fever, cough with purulent sputum, dense consolidation on exam and imaging) from atypical pneumonia (often scant sputum, diffuse infiltrates). Also distinguish community acquired (onset before or within 48–72 hrs of admission) from nosocomial. Because of the differing pathogens in each syndrome, initial management and duration of therapy will differ. Know the pathogens for each syndrome, and learn the spectrum of nosocomial pathogens and their susceptibilities for your institution.
- In typical pneumonias, if 1 cm of pleural effusion layers out on a decubitus film, then consider thoracentesis to rule out empyema, which may necessitate a chest tube.

SUGGESTED READING

Bartlett JG. Practice guidelines for the management of community-acquired pneumonia in adults. *Clin Infect Dis* 2000;31:342–382.

Bartlett JG, Mundy L. Community-acquired pneumonia. *N Engl J Med* 1995;333:1618–1624.

Bassin AS, Niederman MS. Prevention of ventilator-associated pneumonia: an attainable goal? *Clin Chest Med* 1995;16:195.

Centers for Disease Control. CDC guideline for prevention of nosocomial pneumonia. *Infect Control Hosp Epidemiol* 1994;15:587.

Centers for Disease Control. CDC definitions of nosocomial infections, 1988. *Am Rev Respir Dis* 1989;139:1058.

Gross PA. Epidemiology of hospital acquired pneumonia. *Semin Respir Infect* 1987;2:2–7.

Kappstein I. Incidence of pneumonia in mechanically ventilated patients treated with sucralfate or cimetidine as prophylaxis for stress bleeding. *Am J Med* 1991;suppl 2A:S125–S131.

Pingleton SK, Fagon JY, Leeper KV Jr. Patient selection for clinical investigation of ventilator-associated pneumonia: criteria for evaluating diagnostic techniques. *Chest* 1992;102(suppl 1):553S.

REFERENCES

1. Centers for Disease Control and Prevention. Premature deaths, monthly mortality and monthly physician contacts: United States. *MMWR Morb Mortal Wkly Rep* 1997;46:556.
2. Marston BJ, Plouffe JF, File TM, et al. Incidence of community-acquired pneumonia requiring hospitalizations: results of a population based active surveillance study in Ohio. Community-Based Pneumonia Incidence Study Group. *Arch Intern Med* 1997;157:1709–1718.
3. Dal Nogare AR. Nosocomial pneumonia in the medical and surgical patient: risk factors and primary management. *Med Clin North Am* 1994;78:1081.
4. Jimenez P, Torres A, Rodriguez-Roisin R, et al. Incidence and etiology of pneumonia acquired during mechanical ventilation. *Crit Care Med* 1989;17:882.
5. George DL. Epidemiology of nosocomial pneumonia in intensive care unit patients. *Clin Chest Med* 1995;16:29.
6. Bartlett JG, O'Keefe P, Tally FP, et al. Bacteriology of hospital acquired pneumonia. *Arch Intern Med* 1986;146:868.
7. Johanson WG Jr, Pierce AK, Sanford JP, et al. Nosocomial respiratory infections with gram-negative bacilli: the significance of colonization of the respiratory tract. *Ann Intern Med* 1972;77:701.
8. Meduri GU, Beals DH, Maijub AG, et al. Protected bronchoalveolar lavage: a new bronchoscopic technique to retrieve uncontaminated distal airway secretions. *Am Rev Respir Dis* 1991;143:855.
9. Meduri GU, Chastre J. The standardization of bronchoscopic techniques for ventilator-associated pneumonia. *Chest* 1992;102:557S.

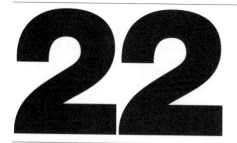

Urinary Tract Infections

Michelle Cabellon and
Christopher H. Kwoh

INTRODUCTION

Uncomplicated cystitis is common in women, with the vast majority caused by *Escherichia coli* and most of the remainder by *Staphylococcus saprophyticus* and enterococcus. Pyelonephritis—involvement of the upper urinary tract—typically involves *E. coli* and enterococcus. Common nosocomial UTI pathogens include *Pseudomonas, Klebsiella, Enterobacter*, and proteus.

It is critical to identify complicated UTIs (Table 22-1) for appropriate therapy. Patients with complicated UTIs frequently have polymicrobial infections, including *Pseudomonas*. Because of frequent infections and repeated therapy, they may have highly resistant organisms as well.

PRESENTATION

History

It is most important to distinguish simple cystitis from a complicated UTI and pyelonephritis. It may be difficult to differentiate cystitis from pyelonephritis in many patients because symptoms and signs may be nonspecific. Typical symptoms such as dysuria, urinary urgency, and frequency are common in all types of UTI. Fever, back pain, nausea, vomiting, and malaise suggest pyelonephritis, but these symptoms are neither sensitive nor specific.

Review the items listed in Table 22-1 to determine if the patient has a complicated UTI. Patients with complicated UTIs are more likely to have generalized symptoms such as fatigue, nausea and vomiting, or headache, often without urinary symptoms. A high suspicion must be maintained in patients with risk factors for complicated UTI.

Physical Exam

Patients with cystitis may have suprapubic tenderness. Fever and tenderness at the costovertebral angle indicates pyelonephritis. Men should have prostate exams to rule out prostatitis and genital exams to rule out orchitis or epididymitis.

Lab Evaluation

Many patients with a typical presentation of uncomplicated cystitis require only a UA and no culture or blood work.

UA is expected to show pyuria (>5–10 WBCs/high-power field) or positive leukocyte esterase. WBC casts are diagnostic of pyelonephritis. Hematuria and mild proteinuria are not uncommon in the setting of a UTI and do not necessarily indicate renal disease.

A pretreatment urine culture and Gram stain must be obtained in all patients with complicated UTI, as well as the elderly (age >65 yrs), those using a diaphragm, those with recurrent UTI, and those with long-standing symptoms (>7 days).

Obtain blood cultures in patients with systemic symptoms or pyelonephritis.

Repeated culture-negative pyuria should prompt evaluation for acid-fast bacilli and fastidious organisms, with the cultures held for an additional 14–21 days.

TABLE 22-1. DEFINITION OF COMPLICATED UTIs

Structural abnormalities: obstruction, prostatic infection, calculi, urinary diversion procedures, infected cysts, external drainage (urinary catheters, nephrostomy tubes), stents, vesicoureteral reflux, neurogenic bladder

Metabolic/hormonal abnormalities: diabetes mellitus, pregnancy, renal impairment, malakoplakia, primary biliary cirrhosis

Impaired host responses: transplant recipients, neutropenia, congenital or acquired immunodeficiency syndromes

Unusual pathogens: yeasts and fungi, *Mycoplasma* sp., resistant bacteria including *Pseudomonas aeruginosa*

MANAGEMENT

For **uncomplicated cystitis,** therapy with TMP-SMX (Bactrim; Septra) (160/800 mg PO bid × 3 days) is recommended by the Infectious Disease Society of America. Patients allergic to sulfa may have ciprofloxacin (Cipro), 250 mg PO bid, or trimethoprim (Proloprim; Trimpex), 100 mg PO bid, alone for 3 days or nitrofurantoin (Macrodantin), 50 mg PO qid, for 7 days. Elderly patients, men, patients with symptoms >7 days or with recurrent UTI, and those using a diaphragm should have 7 days of therapy. No follow-up UA is needed for first UTIs.

Patients with **pyelonephritis** may be treated as outpatients if they are able to take pills, not pregnant, aged <50 yrs, and only moderately ill:

- Outpatient therapy may be ciprofloxacin, 500 mg PO bid (or another quinolone), for 14 days.
- Inpatient therapy may be an IV fluoroquinolone, ampicillin + gentamicin (Garamycin), or an antipseudomonal penicillin given for 14 days. If enterococcus is highly suspected, then consider ampicillin, 1 g IV q6h, ± gentamicin, 1 mg/kg IV q8h.
- Patients who do not respond to appropriate antibiotics (based on culture and sensitivity results) in 72 hrs should have a urinary tract evaluation to look for structural disease, abscess, or calculi. Patients who are obstructed should undergo surgical decompression.
- A follow-up culture 1–2 wks posttherapy is recommended.

For **complicated UTI,** a 14-day course is recommended, with subsequent therapy tailored to the results of culture and sensitivities:

- Oral fluoroquinolones can be used as an outpatient.
- For hospitalized patients requiring IV antibiotics, ampicillin, 1 g IV q6h, + gentamicin, 1 mg/kg IV q8h; imipenem/cilastatin (Primaxin), 0.5–1 g IV q6-8h; piperacillin/tazobactam (Zosyn), 3.375 g IV q6h; or cefepime (Maxipime), 1 g IV q12h, are all appropriate to provide broad gram-negative coverage, including *Pseudomonas* species.
- If staphylococcal infection is also a concern, then vancomycin (Vancocin), 1 g IV q12h, may be added for empiric coverage until culture results are available.
- If *Enterococcus* species or *Pseudomonas* species are recovered from culture, longer courses of antibiotics (14 days) are preferred.
- Any foreign bodies, such as stents, that are in place must be removed for complete resolution of the infection.
- A follow-up urine culture 1–2 wks posttherapy is recommended.

KEY POINTS TO REMEMBER

- Antibiotics are *not* indicated for the presence of bacteriuria without urinary or systemic signs or symptoms except in selected high-risk populations: pregnant or neutropenic patients, transplant recipients, or patients undergoing genitourinary surgery.
- Remove all unnecessary urinary catheters as quickly as possible!

REFERENCES AND SUGGESTED READINGS

Ronald AR, Harding GKM. Complicated urinary tract infections. *Infect Dis Clin North Am* 1997;11(3):583–592.

Stamm WE, Hooton TM. Management of urinary tract infections in adults. *N Engl J Med* 1993;329(18):1328–1334.

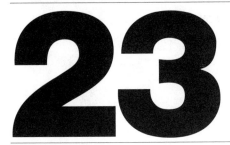

Cellulitis

Rick Starlin and
Christopher H. Kwoh

INTRODUCTION

The most common causes of cellulitis are group A streptococcus and *Staphylococcus aureus*. **Risk factors** for recurrent cellulitis include diabetes mellitus, chronic venous insufficiency, and lymphedema.

PRESENTATION

History

Inquire about immune deficiencies. An infection originating around a bite wound requires further imaging evaluation and different antibiotic regimens, depending on the source of the bite. Systemic symptoms such as fevers, rigors, and malaise may occur but are uncommon.

Physical Exam

The involved area is usually painful, warm, and erythematous. In contrast to erysipelas, the borders are not raised or sharply demarcated. Tender regional lymphadenopathy is frequent. Also look for evidence of an abscess. Patients who have crepitus or malodorous discharge likely have an anaerobic infection or necrotizing fasciitis.

Patients who appear toxic, have rapidly progressive involvement, have pain out of proportion to the exam findings, or have anesthesia of the infected area may have necrotizing fasciitis.

In lower extremity cellulitis, examine between the toes for tinea pedis as a potential source of entry.

Lab Evaluation

Blood cultures and CBC will almost always show left shift. Any fluid collection or abscess should be aspirated and evaluated for Gram stain and cultures. If a creatine phosphokinase is elevated, then consider the possibility of pyomyositis, necrotizing fasciitis, or some deeper infection.

Imaging Evaluation

Consider plain films of the involved areas to rule out osteomyelitis and gas within soft tissue (suggestive of necrotizing process).

If the lower extremity is involved, then consider a Doppler U/S to rule out deep venous thrombosis.

MANAGEMENT

Demarcation of the involved area should be outlined, and serial clinical assessments should be performed for rapidly advancing lesions and deeper tissue involvement that may need immediate surgical intervention. Get a surgical consult sooner rather than later! The discomfort from cellulitis may be severe, and appropriate pain medication should be provided.

Mild infections (localized, superficial, no constitutional symptoms) can be treated with oral antibiotics. Dicloxacillin (Dynapen), 500 mg PO q6h; cephalexin (Keflex), 500 mg PO q6h; or clindamycin (Cleocin), 450–600 mg PO q8h, are all reasonable choices.

Serious or rapidly progressing infections require hospitalization and IV antibiotics. Cefazolin (Ancef), 1 g IV q8h; nafcillin (Nallpen)/oxacillin (Bactocill), 1 g IV q6h; or clindamycin, 600 mg IV q8h is appropriate initial therapy.

KEY POINTS TO REMEMBER

- The typical pathogens are gram-positive cocci, most commonly *S. aureus* and streptococcus. Empiric therapy should be targeted at these bacteria.
- Demarcation of the involved area with a pen will allow the clinician to follow the progression or response of the cellulitis during therapy.
- Do not confuse cellulitis with a deeper soft tissue infection, such as necrotizing fasciitis, which may require surgical intervention.

REFERENCES AND SUGGESTED READINGS

Nichols RL, Florman S. Clinical presentations of soft-tissue infections and surgical site infections. *Clin Infect Dis* 2001;1(3 suppl 2):S84–S93.

Swartz MN. Skin and soft tissue infections. In: Mandell JL, Bennett JE, Dolin R, eds. *Mandell, Douglas, and Bennett's principles and practice of infectious diseases*, 5th ed. Philadelphia: Churchill Livingstone, 2000.

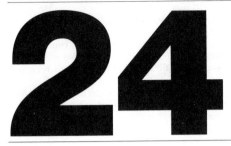

Osteomyelitis

Rick Starlin

INTRODUCTION

There are two general types of osteomyelitis: hematogenous osteomyelitis from bacteremia and contiguous-focus osteomyelitis through spread from an infected adjacent tissue. Osteomyelitis is most often caused by pyogenic bacteria but may also be due to other pathogens, such as mycobacteria and fungi. Osteomyelitis due to *Staphylococcus aureus, Staphylococcus epidermidis*, and *Pseudomonas aeruginosa* (vertebral) is common among IV drug users and hemodialysis patients.

Fungal osteomyelitis is rare and often the result of prolonged neutropenia or catheter-related fungemia. Tuberculosis often involves the thoracic vertebrae with compression deformities (Pott's disease).

Patients with sickle-cell disease are prone to *Salmonella* sp. and *Proteus* sp. osteomyelitis.

Diabetics with osteomyeleitis from a contiguous focus often have mixed microbial infections, including anaerobes.

PRESENTATION

History

Acute osteomyelitis presents with fever, chills, malaise, and bone pain. Chronic osteomyelitis has an indolent course with vague constitutional symptoms of 1–3 mos' duration. Patients with vertebral osteomyelitis typically present with neck/back pain and fever. Neurologic deficits, such as lower-extremity weakness, have been reported in approximately 50% of patients.

Physical Exam

Patients with chronic osteomyelitis often do not appear ill. If an ulcer can be probed to the bone, then it should be treated as osteomyelitis. A thorough neurologic exam should be performed in those with vertebral osteomyelitis to rule out impingement of nerve roots or spinal cord.

Lab Evaluation

Cultures of the ulcer do not necessarily reflect the pathogen unless they grow *S. aureus* and are not routinely obtained. Blood cultures should be drawn.

In chronic osteomyelitis, a bone biopsy for culture and sensitivities is ideally performed **before** starting therapy, unless there is evidence of cellulitis or sepsis (in which case antibiotics should be administered early).

The ESR is elevated and may be used to follow therapy.

Imaging Evaluation

Plain films of the involved bone may show soft tissue edema and periosteal elevation but are often normal.

Both CT and MRI have excellent resolution and help to identify the extent and severity of disease involvement, including soft tissue abscesses. MRI is particularly helpful in the diagnosis of vertebral disease.

Bone scan (technetium-99) is a sensitive test for the detection of early osteomyelitis.

MANAGEMENT

Generally a 6-wk course of parenteral antibiotic is recommended with the starting point as the last débridement or positive blood culture. Use the results of bone biopsy to guide therapy for chronic osteomyelitis.

Penicillin G (Pfizerpen) (4 million U IV q4h) or a first-generation cephalosporin (i.e., cefazolin (Ancef), 2 g IV q6h) is the drug of choice for beta-lactam–sensitive staphylococci and streptococci. Nafcillin (Nallpen) or oxacillin (Bactocill) (2 g IV q4–6h) is used for penicillin-resistant strains. Vancomycin (Vancocin) is reserved for documented methicillin-resistant or penicillin-allergic patients. Clindamycin (Cleocin) (600 mg PO/IV q6h) is the preferred drug if anaerobes are involved.

Fluoroquinolones (i.e., ciprofloxacin [Cipro], 750 mg PO q12h or 400 mg IV q12h) or third-generation cephalosporins (i.e., ceftriaxone [Rocephin], 2g IV q24h) may be used for gram-negative osteomyelitis. Consider high-dose ampicillin (1 g IV q6h) for patients with sickle cell anemia to cover for salmonella.

The ESR is usually measured serially to monitor response.

Patients with vascular insufficiency of the involved bone due to peripheral vascular disease should be considered for revascularization. Any associated foreign bodies should be removed.

CLINICAL PEARL

In diabetics, control of hyperglycemia speeds wound healing and limits infections. Also evaluate diabetics for arterial insufficiency. Prevention of foot infections is key and should involve daily inspection of the feet and gentle cleansing with soap and water, followed by the application of topical moisturizers.

KEY POINTS TO REMEMBER

- Maintain a high suspicion of osteomyelitis in soft tissue infections or you will miss the diagnosis. If an ulcer can be probed to bone, then it should be treated as osteomyelitis.
- Ideally, chronic osteomyelitis should have antibiotic therapy guided by bone biopsy. The bone biopsy will have the highest yield off of antibiotics. Revascularize if there is evidence of peripheral vascular disease of the involved area.

REFERENCES AND SUGGESTED READINGS

Caputo GM, Cavanagh PR, Ulbrecht JS, et al. Assessment and management of foot disease in patients with diabetes. *N Engl J Med* 1994;29;331(13):854–860.

Gillespie WJ. Prevention and management of infection after total joint replacement. *Clin Infect Dis* 1997;25(6):1310–1317.

Lew DP, Waldvogel FA. Osteomyelitis. *N Engl J Med* 1997;336(14):999–1007.

Lipsky BA. Osteomyelitis of the foot in diabetic patients. *Clin Infect Dis* 1997;25(6):1318–1326.

Swartz MN. Skin and soft tissue infections. In: Mandell JL, Bennett JE, Dolin R, eds. *Mandell, Douglas, and Bennett's principles and practice of infectious diseases*, 5th ed. Philadelphia: Churchill Livingstone, 2000.

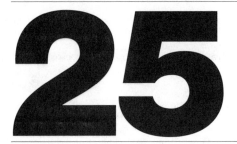

Approach to the Patient with Fever

Michelle Cabellon,
Erik R. Dubberke,
Erin K. Quirk, and
Christopher H. Kwoh

FEVER OF UNKNOWN ORIGIN

Introduction

Fever of unknown origin is defined as a temperature of ≥ 38.3°C for >3 wks with no identified etiology after 1 wk of inpatient evaluation. This evaluation should include CBC, chemistries, ESR, UA, HIV antibody, and ANA; purified protein derivative; chest radiograph; and three sets of blood cultures off antibiotics. Consider CT of the abdomen and pelvis and cultures of sputum, urine, and stool exam depending on the presenting symptoms.

Infection is implicated in one-third of all cases, neoplasm in 20–30%, collagen-vascular diseases in 10–20%, miscellaneous causes in 15–20%, and the undiagnosed in 5–15%. **Unusual presentations of common diseases are frequently seen.**

Causes

Differential Diagnosis

INFECTIOUS CAUSES. *CMV.* CMV can give a mononucleosis-like syndrome with low-grade fevers for >3 wks. Mildly elevated liver transaminases may be present. Send CMV IgM antibody or CMV polymerase chain reaction.

Disseminated TB. In patients with disseminated TB, increasing infiltrates, elevated ESR, and anemia may be seen. PPD is negative in one-half of patients, and sputum is positive for acid-fast bacilli in only one-fourth to one-half. Bone marrow biopsy may be revealing in up to 80% when anemia, leukopenia, and monocytosis are present. Culture from bronchoscopy may be helpful, but the bronchoalveolar lavage is rarely positive. Acid-fast bacilli stain and culture of sterile pyuria may also reveal the diagnosis.

Culture-Negative Endocarditis. If culture-negative endocarditis is suspected, blood cultures must be held for at least 2 wks to rule out the HACEK organisms. A TEE is positive for valvular vegetations in >90% of cases. Consider marantic endocarditis.

Abscesses. Abscesses may be identified with CT or radionuclide imaging.

MALIGNANT CAUSES. Look for lymphadenopathy and splenomegaly on exam, presence of B symptoms (weight loss, night sweats), thrombocytopenia, and anemia. A very high LDH may be a clue.

Other solid tumors causing fever are renal cell cancer, hepatocellular cancer, cerebellar tumors, atrial myxomas, and metastases to the liver.

COLLAGEN-VASCULAR DISEASE CAUSES. *Adult Still's Disease.* The classic triad in a young adult includes high fever, arthritis, and a macular or maculopapular rash on the trunk and peripheral extremities, which may appear in the evenings and may be exacerbated by skin irritation. Diffuse lymphadenopathy is common, and ESR and **ferritin** are almost always elevated.

Temporal Arteritis. Temporal arteritis comprises almost 15% of fever of unknown origin in patients older than 55. Ask about headache, jaw claudication, episodes of visual changes, and associated polymyalgia rheumatica symptoms. Fever is frequently the only symptom!

Polyarteritis Nodosa. Patient may have testicular tenderness, mononeuritis, or livedo reticularis on skin exam. Send ANCA if suspicious, and consider an angiogram.

NEWLY DISCOVERED CAUSES. *Hypergammaglobulinemia Immunoglobulin D Syndrome.* Hypergammaglobulinemia IgD syndrome presents with a large joint arthritis, rash, and very high levels of circulating IgD.

Kikuchi's Disease or Histiocytic Necrotizing Adenitis. Patients may have leukopenia, elevated hepatic transaminases, splenomegaly, and lymphadenopathy. Diagnose by lymph node biopsy.

OTHER CAUSES. Other often-overlooked causes include cirrhosis, alcoholic hepatitis, drug fever, hematoma, subacute thyroiditis, and sarcoidosis.

Presentation

History

A thorough history and physical is essential to obtaining the diagnosis. Inquire about medications, previous illnesses, alcohol ingestion, travel or occupational exposures, pets (birds, cats, farm animals, etc.), animal or insect bites, and familial disorders. Repeat the review of systems every couple of days to uncover new symptoms.

Physical Exam

The exam must be thorough. Pay special attention to the thyroid, teeth, skin, temporal arteries, lymph nodes, and eyes (funduscopy). This should also be thoroughly repeated every couple of days to uncover new clues.

Lab Evaluation

There are no good algorithms or pathways to follow. Clinical judgment based on the information in each case should guide what diagnostic tests are ordered next.

Review all lab and study results again. These facts should be pieced together with history and physical exam findings.

When you have a source to potentially obtain tissue diagnosis, pursue it quickly.

If the patient is stable, it is reasonable to just watch the patient until the fevers resolve or some other clue presents itself.

Very few tests have any value as screening tests. Some consider serum for cryoglobulins and temporal artery biopsy (if >55 yrs and ESR abnormal).

Imaging Evaluation

Gallium scans or indium scans may aid in finding an unsuspected source. Many clinicians obtain a CT of the chest, abdomen, and pelvis initially and often repeat the exam in 1 wk or more.

Management

Resist the temptation to administer empiric antibiotics or steroids if the patient is clinically stable. These therapies may decrease the yield of cultures or hide symptoms that would yield the diagnosis.

SPECIAL CONSIDERATIONS IN POSTOPERATIVE FEVER

History

It is important to consider the time period that has elapsed since the actual operation. See Table 25-1 for differential diagnosis of postoperative fever. A temperature >38.5°C is common in the postoperative patient—occurring in one-third—due to tissue injury from surgery. In general, a fever at <48 hrs postoperative is less worrisome unless severe symptoms are associated (mental status changes, etc.). A fever at >48 hrs is significant and should be thoroughly investigated.

<24 Hrs Postoperatively

Fever with onset <24 hrs after surgery is almost always due to atelectasis from shallow breathing and inadequate pain control. Encouraging deep breaths with respira-

TABLE 25-1. DIFFERENTIAL DIAGNOSIS OF POSTOPERATIVE FEVER

Onset time	Common etiologies to consider
<24 hrs	Atelectasis (by far the most common), pneumonia, wound infections from *Streptococcus* or *Clostridium* (necrotizing, bronze, weeping, painful wound), thyroid storm, transfusion reactions, postsurgical intestinal leaks, addisonian crisis
24–48 hrs	Any cause of fever <24 hrs, UTI from Foley, bacteremia from lines
3–5 days	Any cause of fever <48 hrs, wound infections or leakage (most common), hematomas, inserted hardware, drug fever, pneumonia, DVT (consider pelvic also), acalculous cholecystitis, pancreatitis, candidiasis (with TPN)
>5 days	Any cause of fever <6 days, anastomosis leaks, abscesses (intraabdominal sources may involve both gram-negative aerobes and anaerobes), infected hematomas and deep wound, *Clostridium difficile* colitis, parotitis (with a nasogastric tube, usually *Staphylococcus*)

DVT, deep venous thrombosis.

tory therapy can resolve the problem. If the patient is having a lot of secretions, a chest x-ray may be helpful to rule out pneumonia. It is rare to have a wound infection at this stage, but if present, the likely organisms are *Streptococcus* and *Clostridium* (necrotizing, bronze, weeping, painful wound). Other things to consider are thyroid storm, Addisonian crisis, transfusion reactions if the patient received blood products, and intestinal leaks, depending on the type of surgery involved.

Postoperative Days 1–2

One must consider the same etiologies as in the first 24 hrs, in addition to other infections related to instrumentation such as UTI if a Foley catheter was inserted and bacteremia from central lines. A CBC, UA and urine culture, blood cultures, and chest x-ray are part of the initial workup.

Postoperative Days 3–5

Postoperative days 3–5 are when more serious causes of fever appear. Again, consider the above sources, along with some that are not as obvious. Pneumonia may develop in this period, especially if the patient is on a ventilator. Deep venous thrombosis can occur in both the lower extremities and the pelvic veins. Acalculous cholecystitis, especially in immobile patients or those who received large amounts of blood products, may present with fever as well as pancreatitis. Candidiasis in patients on total parenteral nutrition must be considered. Wound infections and leakage are most common, along with hematomas.

Postoperative Days >6

Again, etiology of fever tends to be more serious in this period. Anastomosis leaks, abscesses (intraabdominal sources may involve both gram-negative aerobes and anaerobes), infected hematomas, and deep wound infections must be ruled out. New problems to consider are *Clostridium difficile* colitis for those patients who received antibiotics and parotitis in those who have or had an NG tube. Usually, the causative organism in parotitis is *Staphylococcus*. Patients at higher risk for this are those with poor oral hygiene initially, those who are NPO, and those with dehydration.

Physical Exam

Perform a wound inspection and exam of all lines inserted, respiratory exam, and inspection for thrombosis.

Culture any possible existing fluid collections if no other source is apparent, but there is suspicion for infection: pleural effusions, ascites, percutaneous drains, sputum, CSF, blisters, catheter tips. Culture of wounds is generally not helpful.

If loculated collections or undrained pus is suspected, do not hesitate to obtain further imaging to help pinpoint the diagnosis.

Management

Treatment should be directed at the underlying cause. Use antipyretics for symptomatic relief.

Atelectasis should be treated with pulmonary toilet and adequate pain control.

SPECIAL CONSIDERATIONS FOR FEVER IN THE ICU

Introduction

Infections are the most common cause of fever in the ICU patient, but many noninfectious, inflammatory conditions can cause fever.

Conversely, not every patient in the ICU with an infectious process will mount a febrile response. 10% of septic patients are hypothermic at presentation, and 35% are normothermic. See Table 25-2 for differential diagnosis of common causes of fever in ICU patients.

Differential Diagnosis

Ventilator-associated pneumonia can be difficult to diagnose, and no single method is ideal. 25% of patients who are mechanically ventilated will develop pneumonia with a subsequent 27% attributable mortality. Ventilator-associated pneumonia should be suspected in patients with changes in the lung exam such as the development of crackles, consolidation, an effusion, or a change in respiratory secretions. Purulent sputum may precede radiographic evidence of pneumonia.

TABLE 25-2. COMMON CAUSES IN THE DIFFERENTIAL DIAGNOSIS OF ICU FEVER

Infectious etiologies	Noninfectious etiologies
Ventilator-associated pneumonia	Drug fever
UTI	Thyroid storm
Clostridium difficile colitis	Addisonian crisis
Infected decubitus ulcer	Acalculous cholecystitis
Line infections	Pancreatitis
Sinusitis	Fat emboli
Wound infection	Withdrawal from alcohol, benzodiazepines, or opiates
	Transfusion reaction
	DVT or pulmonary embolus
	Subarachnoid hemorrhage
	Malignant hyperthermia

DVT, deep venous thrombosis.

C. difficile should be suspected if patients have stool that conforms to the container in which it is placed, prior exposure to antibiotics (particularly cephalosporins, ampicillin, or clindamycin), systemic inflammatory response syndrome, positive fecal leukocytes, and evidence of colitis on CT scan or endoscopy. Some patients with *C. difficile* may have ileus or toxic megacolon and produce little, if any, stool.

Central venous catheter infection should be suspected with bacteremia/fungemia in an immunocompetent patient without underlying disease, no underlying local infection, the presence of an intravascular device at the onset of fever, inflammation or purulence at the catheter insertion site or along the tunnel, abrupt onset of infection that is associated with fulminant shock, and multiple blood cultures positive for organisms that might otherwise be disregarded as contaminants. 25% of central venous catheters will become colonized with bacteria, and 20–30% of these will result in bloodstream infection (5% of central venous catheter infections).

Sinusitis develops in up to 85% of nasally intubated patients within 1 wk. Purulent nasal discharge is present in only 25% of ICU patients with proven sinusitis.

Most noninfectious etiologies of fever in the ICU do not lead to a temperature >38.9°C. The main exceptions include fever secondary to drugs and transfusion reactions.

Fever complicates blood transfusions 0.5% of the time and is more common with platelet transfusions. Febrile reactions often start 30 mins to 2 hrs after the transfusion has begun.

Drug fever may be associated with leukocytosis, eosinophilia, or relative bradycardia. The fevers in drug fever are usually asymptomatic but can result in significant systemic toxicity. A drug fever may begin months after the drug was initiated! Commonly implicated drugs include antibiotics, procainamide, quinidine, and phenytoin.

Physical Exam

The exam should focus on the sinuses, lungs, abdomen, urinary tract, and skin, as well as any sites of prior invasive procedures or prosthetic material.

Lab Evaluation

Evaluation should focus on ruling out dangerous causes of fever.

At least two blood cultures should be taken from two different sites, as well as cultures from other suspicious sites. UA to assess for pyuria, as well as urine culture and sensitivities, should be performed.

If *C. difficile* colitis is suspected, then enzyme-linked immunoassay for the toxin (sensitivity 72%) and fecal leukocytes should be sent to the lab. If the enzyme-linked immunoassay is negative, a second sample should be sent (sensitivity 84% for two assays).

Imaging Evaluation

Upright chest x-ray should be performed to rule out pneumonia. Keep in mind that early in the course there may be no radiographic findings, and a repeat film at a later time may reveal a pneumonia.

A CT of the sinuses should be performed on patients with suspected sinusitis. If the CT is consistent, the definitive diagnosis may be obtained by sterile aspiration of the sinuses for Gram stain and culture.

Management

The take home note for fever in the ICU patient is if infection is suspected, empiric broad-spectrum antibiotics should be initiated promptly after appropriate specimens have been obtained for Gram stain and culture. Mortality is 10–15% lower in septic patients who are initially treated with effective antibiotics. If patients are suspected to have severe *C. difficile* colitis, then it is reasonable to start empiric metronidazole (Flagyl) while awaiting the results of stool enzyme-linked immunoassay.

KEY POINTS TO REMEMBER

- Fever of unknown origin is a strict definition based on fever for 3 wks and 1 wk of inpatient evaluation. Cultures should be obtained after antibiotics have had time to leave the system. The highest diagnostic yield is from a very thorough history, review of systems, and physical exam. Remember that the most common etiologies in fever of unknown origin are infections, neoplasms, and collagen vascular diseases.
- Repeat a thorough physical exam and review of systems every day. Often, the most valuable clues are not there when the fever first begins!
- Patients with fever and sepsis in the ICU should be treated empirically as soon as they are cultured. Mortality in sepsis is highly dependent on time elapsed until effective antibiotic therapy is administered.

REFERENCES AND SUGGESTED READINGS

Arnow PM, Flaherty JP. Fever of unknown origin. *Lancet* 1997;350:575–580.

Clarke DE. The evaluation of fever in the intensive care unit. *Chest* 1991;100:213–230.

Cunha BA. Fever of unknown origin. *Infect Dis Clin North Am* 1996;10(1):111–127.

De Kleijn EM. Fever of unknown origin: diagnostic procedures in a prospective multicenter study of 167 patients. *Medicine* 1997;76:401–414.

Hirschmann JV. Fever of unknown origin in adults. *Clin Infect Dis* 1997;24:291–302.

Marik PE. Fever in the ICU. *Chest* 2000;177(3);855–869.

O'Grady NP, Barie PS, Bartlett JG, et al. Practice guidelines for evaluating new fever in critically ill adult patients. *Clin Infect Dis* 1998;26:1042–1045.

Schwartz SI, ed. *Principles of surgery*, 7th ed. New York: McGraw-Hill, 1999:447–448.

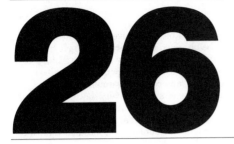

Bacteremia

Erik R. Dubberke and
Christopher H. Kwoh

Gram-positive cocci are now the most common cause of nosocomial bloodstream infections (64%), followed by gram-negative bacilli (GNB) (27%) and *Candida* sp. (8%).

GRAM-POSITIVE COCCI BACTEREMIA

Introduction

In one study involving 49 hospitals over a 3-yr period, coagulase-negative *Staphylococcus* accounted for 32% of nosocomial bloodstream infections, *Staphylococcus aureus* 16%, and *Enterococcus* 11% (80–90% *Enterococcus faecalis*, 5–10% *Enterococcus faecium*).

Risk factors for *Staphylococcus epidermitis* bacteremia include neutropenia and abnormal heart valves, as well as having prosthetic devices and indwelling central venous catheters.

Risk factors for *S. aureus* bacteremia include diabetes requiring insulin injections, chronic hemodialysis, chronic ambulatory peritoneal dialysis, dermatologic conditions, IV drug abuse, HIV infection, poor leukocyte function, and the postoperative state.

Risk factors for *Enterococcus* bacteremia include prior GI colonization, serious underlying disease, prolonged hospital stay, neutropenia, transplantation, HIV, IV drug abuse, urinary or vascular catheters, and recent ICU stay.

S. aureus bacteremia is associated with mortality rates of 11–43%.

Presentation

History

Most patients with gram-positive cocci bacteremia present with fevers and chills. Only *S. aureus* commonly presents with shock.

S. aureus has a high incidence of metastatic infections, and bacteremic patients may present with osteomyelitis, septic arthritis, or endocarditis.

Origins of enterococcal bacteremia (in descending order) include the urinary tract, intraabdominal/pelvic infections, wounds (burns, decubitus ulcers, diabetic foot ulcers), indwelling central lines, and the hepatobiliary tract.

Physical Exam

Review vital signs for episodes of fever. Tachycardia and hypotension may indicate sepsis. All patients should have central lines thoroughly examined.

S. aureus commonly causes folliculitis, carbuncles, impetigo, hidradenitis, cellulitis, wound infections, and abscesses. Also look for bone or joint infections and endocarditis findings.

Lab Evaluation

Up to 85% of solitary positive blood cultures for coagulase-negative *Staphylococcus* and many for enterococcus represent contamination rather than infection. A single positive culture for *Enterococcus* or coagulase-negative *Staphylococcus* suggests contamination. If a patient has risk factors for bacteremia, repeat cultures should be drawn. Multiple positive cultures of the same organism suggest infection. The presence of fever or signs of sepsis also indicates true infection.

Antibioticograms can be compared to see if multiple positive cultures represent the same or different strains (matching antibiotic resistance patterns).

Imaging Evaluation

Hospitalized patients with *S. aureus* should be evaluated for pneumonia.

Transthoracic echocardiogram or TEE should be considered in *S. aureus* infections (0–26% incidence of endocarditis) and with repeatedly positive coagulase-negative staphylococcus cultures. Only 1:50 of enterococcus bacteremias are associated with endocarditis, but it is likely if clinical presentation is suggestive.

Maintain a high suspicion for deep wound infection, osteomyelitis, or abscess with *S. aureus*.

Management

Repeat blood cultures before initiating therapy, but it is not necessary to await the repeat culture results before administering antibiotics.

Staphylococcus

Initial empiric therapy with vancomycin (Vancocin), 1 g IV q12h, should be initiated promptly while awaiting sensitivities. Regimens can then be adjusted, preferably involving semisynthetic beta-lactams (e.g., oxacillin, 2 g IV q4–6h). Vancomycin may be continued, but it is actually less effective against beta-lactam–sensitive *Staphylococcus* than beta-lactam antibiotics. Duration of therapy for *S. aureus* is 2 wks with a negative TEE or 4 wks if TEE cannot be performed.

In patients with a single positive culture for coagulase-negative *Staphylococcus* who are stable and asymptomatic, repeat cultures and consider observation rather than empiric therapy.

Enterococcus

Penicillin and ampicillin are the initial antibiotics of choice, even if the susceptibility report shows moderate resistance to penicillin (which is "standard" for enterococci) and sensitivity to vancomycin. Penicillin/ampicillin alone is fine if bactericidal therapy is not needed:

- If bactericidal therapy is needed (e.g., endocarditis, meningitis), then an aminoglycoside should be added.
- Resistance to aminoglycosides can be overcome by addition of appropriate cell wall–active agents, although some strains have acquired true resistance to aminoglycosides.
- Treatment of vancomycin-resistant enterococcus requires susceptibility testing. Chloramphenicol (Chloromycetin) and high-dose ampicillin-sulbactam (3 g IV q6h adjusted for renal failure) have been used with some success. Dalfopristin-quinupristin (Synercid) is effective against some strains of *E. faecium*, but not *E. faecalis*. Linezolid (Zyvox; 600 mg IV q12h) is a new option that has also had modest success.

All abscesses/infected devices should be drained/removed.

GRAM-NEGATIVE BACILLI BACTEREMIA

Introduction

GNB remains the most common cause of **community-acquired** bacteremia. The most common gram-negative isolates are *Escherichia coli*, *Klebsiella pneumoniae*, *Proteus mirabilis*, *Haemophilus influenzae*, and *Bacteroides* sp. The most common nosocomial isolates include *E. coli*, *Klebsiella* sp., *Enterobacter* sp., *Serratia* sp., and *Pseudomonas aeruginosa*. Approximately 15% of GNB bacteremias are polymicrobial.

Risk factors include neutropenia (most significant), advanced age, prolonged hospitalization, prior antimicrobial use, and severe underlying comorbid conditions and skin lesions (decubitus ulcers, burns). GNB bacteremia is also associated with urinary tract manipulation, corticosteroid use, respiratory tract manipulation, and surgical procedures.

GNB bacteremia is associated with a 20–25% mortality rate.

Presentation

History
Fevers, chills, and signs of sepsis may predominate the clinical picture.

Physical Exam
Indwelling lines and skin should be evaluated for infection or as a source of entry or infection. Skin lesions can be seen with *E. coli*, *Klebsiella*, *Enterobacter*, and *Serratia* bacteremia, including colorful vesicular/bullous lesions, cellulitis, diffuse erythema, and petechiae. Ecthyma gangrenosum is associated with *P. aeruginosa* bacteremia. Skin lesions may be aspirated for Gram stain and culture.

Lab Evaluation
The bacteremia should be confirmed with two to three sets of blood cultures from separate sites over 15–30 mins. Thorough evaluation of known common sources of GNB bacteremia is warranted (urinary tract, hepatobiliary tract, and pelvis).

The bacterial species isolated suggests a source. 80% of *E. coli* bacteremias originate in the genitourinary or GI tracts. 50% of *Pseudomonas* bacteremias have a urinary or lung source. *Klebsiella* is twice as likely to originate in the urine than the lung. *Bacteroides* bacteremias almost exclusively originate in the abdomen.

Management

Community hepatobiliary tract infections with bacteremia can empirically be treated with ampicillin-sulbactam (Unasyn; 3 g IV q6h adjusted for renal function), clindamycin (Cleocin) plus gentamicin (Garamycin), aztreonam (Azactam), ciprofloxacin (Cipro; 400 mg IV q12h adjusted for renal function), cefoxitin/cefotetan, or a third-generation cephalosporin (e.g., ceftriaxone) plus metronidazole (Flagyl). **Community UTI** can be empirically treated with ampicillin and gentamicin, ciprofloxacin, aztreonam, or a third-generation cephalosporin. **Nosocomial GNB bacteremias** and **granulocytopenic** patients can be empirically treated with antipseudomonal penicillin/cephalosporin, aztreonam (2 g IV q8–12h adjusted for renal function), or imipenem (Primaxin; 500 mg IV q6–8h adjusted for renal function) ± aminoglycoside. Therapy should be for 14 days depending on response.

Any obstruction should be mechanically relieved.

KEY POINTS TO REMEMBER

- Patients with *S. aureus* bacteremia should be clinically evaluated for septic arthritis, osteomyelitis, and endocarditis.
- Gram-negative bacteremia is a serious illness with high mortality. Empiric therapy should be based on the suspected source of the pathogen and local resistance patterns.

REFERENCES AND SUGGESTED READINGS

Bhavnani SM, Drake JA, Forrest A, et al. A nationwide, multicenter, case-control study comparing risk factors, treatment, and outcome for vancomycin-resistant and -susceptible enterococcal bacteremia. *Diagn Microbiol Infect Dis* 2000;36:145–158.

Edmond MB, Wallace SE, McClish DK, et al. Nosocomial bloodstream infections in United States hospitals: a three-year analysis. *Clin Infect Dis* 1999;29:239–244.

Kreger BE, Craven DE, Carling PC, et al. Gram-negative bacteremia III. Reassessment of etiology, epidemiology and ecology in 612 patients. *Am J Med* 1980;68:332–343.

Kreger BE, Craven DE, McCabe WR. Gram-negative bacteremia IV. Re-evaluation of clinical features and treatment in 612 patients. *Am J Med* 1980;68:344–355.

Lowy FD. *Staphylococcus aureus* infections. *N Engl J Med* 1998;339(8):520–532.

Young LS, Stevens P, Kaijser B. Gram-negative pathogens in *Septicaemic* infection. *Scand J Infect Dis* 1982;31:78–94.

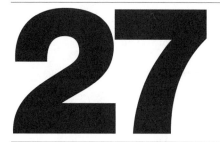

Central Venous Catheter Infections

Erik R. Dubberke and
Christopher H. Kwoh

INTRODUCTION

The most common causative organism in central venous catheter (CVC) infections is coagulase-negative *Staphylococcus* (CNS), followed by *Staphylococcus aureus*, *Enterococcus*, gram-negative bacilli (GNB), and fungi (typically *Candida*).

Risk factors for CVC infections include the type of catheter, location of CVC (likelihood of infection is greatest if femoral, then internal jugular, followed by subclavian), duration of catheter placement, number of lumens, and number of manipulations.

PRESENTATION
Physical Exam

The most sensitive sign is fever. Inflammation and purulence of the catheter site are more specific but less sensitive. Also look for tenderness and milk the pocket to extrude pus. Look for evidence of metastatic infection, including signs of endocarditis or osteomyelitis. Other sources of infection may secondarily infect the catheter.

Lab Evaluation

Blood cultures should be drawn, at least one peripheral and one central.

Two catheter-culturing techniques are commonly used: semiquantitative (roll plate) and quantitative (vortex, sonification):

- CVC infections occurring <1 wk after insertion suggest skin organisms, and roll plate culturing (semiquantitative) is most sensitive (≥ 15 colonies is positive).
- If the CVC has been in place for >1 wk, then intraluminal sources are more likely, and quantitative methods (sonification or vortex) are more appropriate (≥ 100 colony-forming units is positive).
- If the catheter culture is positive and clinical scenario is appropriate, then sensitivity is 60% for semiquantitative and 80% for quantitative.

Consider quantitative blood cultures if the CVC cannot be removed: If a colony count of the culture drawn from the CVC is 5–10 times greater than the peripheral colony count, then a CVC source is likely.

Gram stain may be helpful, but it is not as sensitive as quantitative methods. Cultures should be sent of extruded purulent material if there is an exit site infection.

MANAGEMENT

Vancomycin (Vancocin), 1 g IV q12h, is the antibiotic usually recommended for empiric therapy. Additional coverage for GNB should be considered in patients who are severely ill, recently hospitalized, or immunocompromised. See Chap. 26, Bacteremia, for possible regimens. Results of bacterial culture sensitivities should guide specific further therapy.

Nontunneled CVCs infected with *S. aureus* or *Enterococcus*, GNB, or *Candida* should be removed and treated with 14 days of antibiotics (including antipseudomonals if GNB). If the patient remains febrile and/or has bacteremia >3 days after catheter removal and/or initiation of antibiotics, then a longer course of antibiotics is needed (4–6 wks), and evidence of metastatic infection should be investigated.

Nontunneled catheters infected with CNS without symptoms or persistent bacteremia may undergo attempted salvage therapy (see later):

- Persistent fevers, persistent bacteremia, or relapse after antibiotics are discontinued are clear indications for CVC removal.
- If the CVC with CNS bacteremia is removed, systemic antibiotics should be administered for 5–7 days.

Tunneled catheters should be removed if there is a tunnel site or pocket infection or port abscess and should be treated with 14 days of parenteral antibiotic therapy. Tunneled catheters should also be removed if there is evidence of a complicated CVC infection (septic thrombosis, endocarditis, or osteomyelitis) and then treated with 4–6 wks of IV antibiotics.

Salvage therapy may be attempted on selected tunneled CVCs or CNS infections. There is an 80% salvage rate with 10 days of vancomycin for lines infected by CNS. Parenteral antibiotics may be given with 14 days of therapy and antibiotic lock therapy. Cultures should be redrawn after completion of therapy. Persistently positive cultures or fevers should prompt removal of the CVC.

Due to poor response to salvage therapy, all CVC infections associated with *Candida* sp., *Pseudomonas* sp. (other than *P. aeruginosa*), *Burkholderia* sp., *Stenotrophomonas* sp., *Agrobacterium* sp., *Actinobacteria baumanii*, *Bacillus* sp., or *Corynebacterium* sp. should prompt removal of the device.

If a tunneled CVC is present during an episode of candidemia, then the likelihood of catheter-related candidemia must be determined. Predictors of tunneled CVC–related candidemia include isolation of *Candida parapsilosis* from the blood, neutropenia with a CVC and no other apparent source for bloodstream infection, receiving hyperalimentation through the catheter, and persistent candidemia in a patient who is not responding to systemic antifungal therapy.

Removal of the catheter and amphotericin B [Amphocin (0.5 mg/kg/day IV for total 250–500 mg), Fungizone] is recommended for suspected catheter-related candidemia in patients who are hemodynamically unstable or who have received prolonged fluconazole (Diflucan) therapy or fungal isolates resistant to fluconazole. In other cases, fluconazole may be used. Therapy should be continued for 14 days after the last positive blood culture and when signs and symptoms of infection have resolved.

The risk of CVC infections can be decreased by good aseptic insertion technique; avoiding femoral catheters (should be removed within 72 hrs), antimicrobial impregnated catheters, and cuffs; tunnelled catheters; and clean catheter care.

KEY POINT TO REMEMBER

- Removal of the catheter provides the best opportunity to clear the infection. Salvage therapy may be attempted with tunneled catheters unless infected with certain bacteria or candida, which cannot be cleared with antibiotics. Make sure there is no evidence of seeding of infection to other sites. Also consider the possibility that another primary infection may have seeded the catheter.

REFERENCES AND SUGGESTED READINGS

Mermel LA, Farr BM, Sherertz RJ, et al. Guidelines for the management of intravascular catheter-related infections. *Clin Infect Dis* 2001;32:1249–1272.

Mundy L. Treatment of infectious diseases. In: Ahya, Flood, Paranjothi, eds. *The Washington manual of medical therapeutics*, 30th ed. Philadelphia: Lippincott Williams & Wilkins, 2001:297–298.

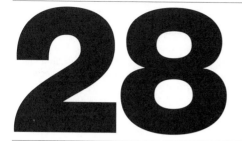

Infective Endocarditis

Rick Starlin and
Christopher H. Kwoh

INTRODUCTION

The annual incidence of infective endocarditis (IE) is 10–20 per million with a mortality rate of 16–27%.

PRESENTATION

History

Fever (in 90%) and new murmur are the most common presentations. Congestive heart failure develops in 25%. Weight loss and diaphoresis may occur. **10% are afebrile!**

Pulmonary symptoms are important in IV drug abuse because septic emboli may occur from a right-sided endocarditis.

Presentation and etiologies vary with clinical subtypes:

- Acute bacterial endocarditis rapidly progresses over 1–2 days, and the infecting organism is highly pathogenic (e.g., *Staphylococcus aureus*).
- Subacute bacterial endocarditis symptoms evolve for weeks to months, and the infecting organism is less virulent (e.g., *Streptococcus viridans*).
- Native valve endocarditis in adults ages 15–60, excluding IV drug users and nosocomial infection, most commonly occurs (7–30%) in the setting of mitral valve prolapse with an associated murmur. Congenital heart disease accounts for 6–24% of cases. The most common cause is strep (usually viridans). *Staphylococcus* is the second most common isolated.
- IV drug users have a high risk for IE, typically tricuspid. *S. aureus* accounts for >60% of the cases.
- Early prosthetic valve IE occurring within 2 mos (peak at 3–9 wks) of surgery is most commonly caused by coagulase-negative *Staphylococcus*.
- Late prosthetic valve IE is most commonly caused by *S. viridans*. It is believed to be related to incidental bacteremias and not associated with surgery.
- Nosocomial endocarditis is probably more common than suspected. The most common offending organisms are *Staphylococcus*, *Enterococci*, *Candida* species, and gram-negative bacilli.

Physical Exam

Cardiac exam should focus on new or changing murmurs and congestive heart failure findings. In addition to conjunctival petechiae, a fundoscopic exam should be done to look for retinal hemorrhages, Roth spots, and evidence of ophthalmitis. Roth spots are retinal lesions with a pale center surrounded by a red halo.

Neurologic findings are present in 30–50% of patients and include confusional states, focal neurologic findings from emboli, hemorrhages from mycotic aneurysms, and cerebritis symptoms.

Osler's nodes are painful erythematous nodules, usually on the hands, that may have pale central areas without necrosis. Janeway lesions are painless, flat, red spots found on the palms and soles of some patients that blanch with pressure.

TABLE 28-1. DUKE CRITERIA*a*

Major criteria

Positive blood cultures (two cultures >12 hrs apart, all of 3 or most ≥ 4 with first and last at least 1 hr apart) for *S. viridans*, *S. bovis*, HACEK organisms, *Staphylococcus aureus*, or *Enterococcus*. There must be no primary focus for *Staphylococcus* or *Enterococcus*.

Echocardiogram showing vegetations, abscess, new valvular regurgitation, or prosthetic valve dehiscence.

Minor criteria

Predisposing heart disease or IV drug abuse

Fever (>38C)

Immunologic: Osler's nodes, Roth spots, rheumatoid factor, glomerulonephritis

Vascular: Janeway lesions, conjunctival or intracranial hemorrhages, mycotic aneurysm, septic pulmonary infarcts, major arterial emboli.

Blood cultures positive for bacteria known to cause infective endocarditis but not meeting major criteria.

Echocardiogram consistent with infective endocarditis but not meeting major criteria.

*a*Requires 2 major, 1 major and 3 minor, or 5 minor to be positive.
From Durack DT, Lukes AS, Bright DK. New criteria for diagnosis of infective endocarditis: utilization of specific echocardiographic findings: Duke endocarditis service. *Am J Med* 1994;96:200–209, with permission.

Splinter hemorrhages (subungual hemorrhages) can be detected on the fingernails with the background of a penlight.

Splenomegaly is common and is found in 15–55% of cases.

Look for evidence of IV drug use.

Lab Evaluation

Evaluation should follow the requirements of the Duke criteria (Table 28-1), which have a specificity of 98–99% for the diagnosis of IE. Only rarely is therapy for IE emergent, and it is usually appropriate to obtain all the necessary cultures before administering antibiotics. Save the cultures for 2–3 wks to isolate fastidious organisms.

UA may reveal a microscopic hematuria and proteinuria. Immune complex glomerulonephritis is associated with RBC casts, gross proteinuria, and decreased total complement levels. Renal infarction from embolic disease may manifest as gross hematuria.

Imaging Evaluation

A chest x-ray should be obtained.

ECG should be obtained to look for evidence of embolic disease to coronary arteries and to assess for conduction delays suggestive of abscess formation.

When IE is suspected, patients should initially undergo transthoracic echocardiogram (TTE), which has a sensitivity of 60–75%. If patients have a negative or nondiagnostic TTE, then they should undergo TEE, which has a sensitivity of up to 95%. Some clinicians prefer to do a TEE as the initial test if suspicion for IE is sufficiently high. If both the TTE and the TEE are negative, this provides a negative predictive value of 95%. If the suspicion is still high despite negative echocardiography, then repeat the evaluation in 7–10 days.

Follow-up echocardiograms after therapy are usually not helpful because vegetations will remain for years, even with resolution of the infection.

TABLE 28-2. CARDIAC CONDITIONS REQUIRING PROPHYLAXIS

High risk

 Prosthetic valves

 Previous infective endocarditis

 Surgical pulmonic-systemic shunts

 Complex cyanotic congenital heart disease (tetralogy of Fallot, transposition of the
  great vessels, etc.)

Moderate risk

 Mitral valve prolapse only with regurgitation

 Hypertrophic obstructive cardiomyopathy

 Acquired valvular disease

 Other congenital heart disease

Low risk (no prophylaxis)

 Atrial septal defect

 Repaired ventriculoseptal defect

 Cardiac pacemakers

 Automatic implantable cardiovascular defibrillators

MANAGEMENT

It is easier to prevent endocarditis than it is to treat it. See Table 28-2 for indications
for prophylaxis and Table 28-3 for suggested regimens.

 In general, an infectious diseases consult should be obtained in patients being
treated for endocarditis.

 Bactericidal antibiotics should be used whenever possible. Empiric therapy should
be instituted while the etiologic organism and antibiotic sensitivities are being determined. For acute IE, initial coverage includes oxacillin (Bactocill), 2 g IV q4h, plus gentamicin (Garamycin), 1.5 mg/kg IV q8h. If methicillin-resistant *S. aureus* is likely,
vancomycin, 1 g IV q12h, should be substituted for ofacillin until sensitivities return.

 Obtain **daily blood cultures** until they become sterile. Patients should defervesce
within 7 days of appropriate therapy. If they are still spiking fevers, then assess them for
potential complications, such as abscess, and reassess the sensitivity of the pathogen.

 The combination of heparin and penicillin has been shown to increase the risk of
intracerebral hemorrhage. In general, avoid heparin unless there is an urgent indication. Warfarin should also be avoided unless there is a necessary indication, such as a
mechanical prosthetic valve.

 Patients with *Streptococcus bovis* endocarditis require a GI evaluation to rule out
associated colon cancer.

 Surgery is ultimately required in approximately one-third of patients. The major
indications for surgery are moderate to severe heart failure not responding to medical
therapy, valvular obstruction, periannular or myocardial abscess, prosthetic valve
dehiscence, uncontrollable infection despite antibiotics, and fungal infections. The relative indications for surgery include recurrent emboli, *Staphylococcus* and gram-negative bacilli infection especially with prosthetic valve endocarditis, persistent fever
despite treatment, and vegetations that enlarge despite treatment.

 Surgery performed too early subjects the patient to unnecessary risks from the surgery itself, combined with an inadequately controlled infection. Surgery postponed too
long could result in patients deteriorating rapidly to the point that surgery is of no
benefit. As a result, patients with IE in whom surgery might be indicated must be
evaluated closely both clinically and with serial echocardiograms. This is a situation
in which experienced specialists should be involved.

TABLE 28-3. PROCEDURES AND REGIMENS FOR ENDOCARDITIS PROPHYLAXIS

Dental procedures requiring prophylaxis: procedures likely to cause gingival bleeding, professional tooth cleaning, tonsillectomy.

Respiratory procedures requiring prophylaxis: rigid bronchoscopy, surgery on respiratory mucosa. Consider for high-risk cardiac conditions with flexible bronchoscopy or biopsy. Not for simple endotracheal intubation.

Esophageal procedures requiring prophylaxis: sclerotherapy for esophageal varices, dilatation. Esophagogastroduodenoscopy or biopsy only for high-risk patients.

Regimens for oral, respiratory, or esophageal prophylaxis: amoxicillin (Amoxil), 2 g PO 1 hr prior (or ampicillin, IV/IM 30 mins prior).

Penicillin allergic: clindamycin (Cleocin), 600 mg PO 1 hr prior (or IV/IM 30 mins prior), **or** azithromycin (Zithromax), 500 mg PO 1 hr prior, **or** cephalexin (Keflex), 2 g PO 1 hr prior.

GI procedures requiring prophylaxis: endoscopic retrograde cholangiopancreatography, surgery involving the GI mucosa or biliary tree or gallbladder. For routine endoscopy or biopsy, one can consider prophylaxis for high-risk patients.

Genitourinary procedures requiring prophylaxis: cystoscopy, prostate surgery, catheterization or surgery with a UTI, vaginal delivery in the setting of an infection, vaginal hysterectomy, urethral dilatation. High-risk patients may have prophylaxis for vaginal delivery. Prophylaxis is **not** needed with cesarean section.

Regimens for GI and genitourinary prophylaxis

High risk: ampicillin (2 g IV/IM) and gentamicin (Garamycin) (1.5 mg/kg up to 120 mg) 30 mins prior, then amoxicillin, 1 g PO 6 hr after (or ampicillin IV/IM).

PCN-allergic high risk: vancomycin (Vancocin), 1 g IV and gentamicin (1.5 mg/kg up to 120 mg) completed 30 mins prior.

Moderate risk: amoxicillin, 2 g PO 1 hr prior (or ampicillin IV/IM 30 mins prior).

PCN-allergic moderate risk: vancomycin, 1 g IV completed 30 mins prior.

From Dajani AS, Taubert KA, Wilson W, et al. Prevention of bacterial endocarditis. Recommendations by the American Heart Association. *JAMA* 1997;277:1794, with permission.

KEY POINTS TO REMEMBER

- Symptoms of endocarditis may be vague, and 10% of cases present without fever, so maintain a high level of suspicion. Consider endocarditis in any patient with *S. aureus* bacteremia.
- If the patient is stable, withhold antibiotics until adequate cultures are obtained separated by sufficient time to meet major requirements for Duke's criteria. TEE remains the most sensitive test for endocarditis.
- Long-term IV antibiotic therapy should be guided by the susceptibilities of the pathogen. Consider a formal infectious disease consult to establish appropriate therapy.

REFERENCES AND SUGGESTED READINGS

Bayer AS. Diagnosis and management of infective endocarditis and its complications: AHA scientific statement. *Circulation* 1998;98:2936–2948.

Dajani AS, Taubert KA, Wilson W, et al. Prevention of bacterial endocarditis. Recommendations by the American Heart Association. *JAMA* 1997;277:1794.

Durack DT, Lukes AS, Bright DK. New criteria for diagnosis of infective endocarditis: utilization of specific echocardiographic findings: Duke endocarditis service. *Am J Med* 1994;96:200–209.

Kamath NV, Warner MR, Camisa C. Infective endocarditis: cutaneous cues to the diagnosis. *Consultant* 1999:3085–3097.

Meningitis

David Anand Rengachary
and Christopher H. Kwoh

INTRODUCTION

Meningitis has an annual incidence of approximately 3–5 per 100,000 people. Risk factors include immunocompromised states, traumatic or surgical breakdown of the blood-brain barrier, and exposure. Bacterial endocarditis may seed the meninges, as well as cause abscesses.

Bacterial meningitis still has a high mortality rate (up to 25% without appropriate treatment), and early diagnosis and therapy are critical for improving outcomes.

PRESENTATION

History

Symptoms of meningitis (headache, meningismus, malaise, fever, photophobia) present in hours to days with bacterial causes and days to weeks with fungal or tuberculous causes. Decreased alertness and seizures may also be present.

One must determine whether a patient is immunocompromised. Initial history should establish HIV risk factors, presence of immunosuppressive agents, history of alcohol abuse/cirrhosis, malnutrition, diabetes, or splenectomy. Upper respiratory symptoms strongly suggest a viral cause. Skull fracture with nasopharyngeal communication resulting in meningitis is classically *Streptococcus pneumoniae*.

A history of cancer should create a high suspicion of carcinomatous meningitis. Neurologic symptoms predominate, and leg weakness or numbness, ataxia, or cranial nerve symptoms may be the only clue.

See Table 29-1 for a differential diagnosis of aseptic meningitis and Table 29-3 for the most common causes of bacterial meningitis.

Physical Exam

Meningismus and photophobia are common.

Kernig's sign can be performed as follows: flex thigh on abdomen with knee also in flexed position, then extend the knee. It is positive if it elicits pain or resistance.

Brudzinski's sign can be performed as follows: Flexion of the neck leads to flexion of the hips and/or knees.

Cranial nerve palsies can be seen in 10–15% of bacterial infections (3, 4, 6, and 7 most commonly affected).

Papilledema or absent retinal venous pulsations, obtundation, bilateral cranial nerve III palsies and Cushing's response (bradycardia, HTN, erratic respirations) suggest severe increased intracranial pressure.

Cerebellar ataxia is relatively common in VZV encephalitis.

Petechial rash suggests meningococcus, but this can also be seen in pneumococcal disease and others. Maculopapular rashes are common with viral infections.

Lab Evaluation

Lumbar puncture (LP) is imperative. It should be performed as soon as possible. Patients who have suspected bacterial meningitis should receive antimicrobial therapy immediately if the LP is delayed. See Table 29-2 for CSF interpretation.

141

TABLE 29-1. ETIOLOGIC DIFFERENTIAL DIAGNOSIS OF ASEPTIC MENINGITIS

Partially treated bacterial (most common)	Drugs
Carcinomatous meningitis	Azathioprine
Kawasaki's	Penicillin
Wegener's granulomatosis	IV immune globulin
Spirochetes	TMP-SMX
Vaccines (MMR, polio)	Isoniazid
Sarcoidosis	Carbamazepine
Lupus and Sjögren's syndrome	NSAIDs and COX2 inhibitors
Brucella	Muronomab-CD3
Mollaret's meningitis	
Behçet's	
Toxins	

TABLE 29-2. COMMON CSF PATTERNS IN NORMAL AND DISEASE STATES

Condition	Color	Pressure (mm H$_2$O)	Cells/mL	Protein (mg/dL)	Glucose (mg/dL)
Normal	Clear	10–180	0–5 mononuclear	15–45	2/3 serum value (range 45–80)
Viral meningitis	Clear or opalescent	Normal	>5–2000, >50% lymphs, may be PMNs early in course	20–200	Normal or slightly decreased
Bacterial meningitis	Opalescent	Increased (may be normal)	Increased with PMNs	50–1500	Decreased
Tuberculous meningitis	Clear or opalescent	Usually increased	50–500 lymphocytes	45–500	Decreased
Fungal meningitis	Clear or opalescent	Normal or increased	5–800 lymphocytes	Normal or increased	Decreased
Carcinomatous meningitis	Clear or opalescent	Normal or increased	5–1000 mononuclear	Up to 500	Decreased
Subarachnoid hemorrhage	Bloody or xanthochromic	Normal or increased	Many RBCs, with WBC:RBC same as blood	Up to 2000	Decreased

PMNs, polymorphonuclear neutrophils.

Gram stain of the CSF has a sensitivity of 66–90% for bacterial meningitis, depending on the pathogen, severity, and immune status.

Herpes simplex virus (HSV) frequently has hemorrhagic CSF. Approximately 4% of bacterial meningitis presents with no CSF pleocytosis. Approximately 30% of *Listeria* meningitis has lymphocyte predominance in the CSF. Viral meningitis may have neutrophil CSF predominance for up to 48 hrs of illness and then become lymphocyte predominant.

CBC (will usually show leukocytosis), complete metabolic profile, PT/PTT, and U/A should be performed. Obtain blood, urine, and sputum cultures. Also consider HIV testing and throat and stool cultures for a viral source.

CSF Tests to Consider in Chronic, Aseptic, Fungal, and HIV-Related Meningitis

- Cytology (fresh bedside cytology to rule out HSV in Mollaret's) and flow cytometry.
- Acid fast and India ink stains, VDRL/FTA-ABS
- Fungal tests: Cryptococcal antigen, histoplasma antigen, *Blastomyces*, *Coccidioides* complement fixation antibody.
- PCR for HSV, CMV, VZV, human herpesvirus 6, JC virus, Epstein-Barr virus.
- Latex agglutination for *S. pneumoniae*, *Neisseria meningitidis*, *Haemophilus influenzae*, *Escherichia coli*, and group B strep can often identify the pathogen in partially treated bacterial meningitis.

Imaging Evaluation

CT of the head for evidence of abscess or other focal disease should be undertaken for patients with focal neurologic signs, evidence of increased intracranial pressure, or marked obtundation. Also consider a head CT for persistent neurologic dysfunction, endocarditis with meningitis, and lack of CSF response despite several days of apparently appropriate antibacterial therapy.

MANAGEMENT

Initial therapy is empiric and may be based on clinical characteristics of the patient, especially age and immune status. See Table 29-3 for likely bacterial pathogens and empiric therapies. See Table 29-4 for treatment based on Gram stain. Subsequent therapy should be tailored toward the specific identified organism and results of sensitivities.

Duration of therapy is 10–14 days; most physicians treat for 14 days. Gram-negative and *Listeria* infections may require 21–28 days of therapy.

Consider acyclovir (Zovirax), 10 mg/kg IV q8h, × 10–21 days if the history and CSF are consistent with HSV viral meningitis (viral, often with increased RBCs as well). This decreases mortality in HSV encephalitis, and most physicians would discontinue therapy if the HSV polymerase chain reaction result is negative (80–98% sensitive) or another diagnosis is established.

All patients with meningitis should initially be placed on respiratory isolation for at least 24 hrs of effective therapy (especially *H. influenzae* and *N. meningitides*). Enterovirus cases should have contact isolation. Measles, mumps, and influenza should have respiratory isolation through the duration of illness.

The role of corticosteroids is not clear. A recent trial of dexamethasone (10 mg IV q6h × 4 days) in bacterial meningitis demonstrated a reduction in disability and mortality [1].

TUBERCULOUS MENINGITIS TREATMENT

Begin with isoniazid, 300 mg PO per day; pyridoxine (Nestrex), 50 mg PO per day; rifampin (Rifadin, Rimactane), 10 mg/kg PO per day; ethambutol (Myambutol), 15–25 mg/kg PO per day; and pyrazinamide, 30 mg/kg/day. If the patient is clinically

TABLE 29-3. LIKELY BACTERIAL PATHOGENS AND EMPIRIC THERAPY BASED ON CLINICAL CHARACTERISTICS

Age or risk factor	Bacterial pathogens	Empiric IV therapy
3 mos to 18 yrs	*Streptococcus pneumoniae, Neisseria meningitides, Haemophilus influenzae.*	Ceftriaxone, 2 g q12h, ± vancomycin, 1 q12h if in an area of >5% *S. pneumoniae* PCN resistance
18–50 yrs	*N. meningitides, S. pneumoniae, H. influenzae.*	Ceftriaxone, 2 g q12h, ± vancomycin, 1 g q12h if in an area of >5% *S. pneumoniae* PCN resistance
>50 yrs	*S. pneumoniae, Listeria monocytogenes*, gram-negative bacilli.	Ceftriaxone, 2 g q12h, + ampicillin, 2 g q4h, ± vancomycin, 1 g q12h, if in an area of >5% *S. pneumoniae* PCN resistance
Immunocompromised	Varied but includes *Listeria, Pseudomonas*. With AIDS, *Cryptococcus* is very likely.	Ceftazidime, 2 g q8h, + ampicillin, 2 g q4h
Recent neurosurgery, CSF shunts, penetrating head trauma	*S. aureus*, diphtheroids, gram-negative bacilli (including *Pseudomonas*).	Ceftazidime, 2 g q8h, + vancomycin, 1–2 g q12h

responding after 8 wks, then pyrazinamide and ethambutol may be stopped, and the remaining agents are continued for 6–12 mos [2].

KEY POINTS TO REMEMBER

- Administer empiric antibiotics in suspected meningitis if the LP cannot be performed immediately.
- Recognize the CSF characteristics of bacterial, viral, and mycobacterial/fungal meningitis. Empiric therapy may be adjusted based on Gram stain. If CSF is consistent with HSV meningitis, then empiric acyclovir therapy is indicated until HSV can be ruled out. Remember to place patients on respiratory isolation if the CSF is consistent with a highly contagious meningitis.

TABLE 29-4. EMPIRIC THERAPY BASED ON CSF GRAM STAIN RESULTS

Gram-positive cocci	Ceftriaxone, 2 g q12h, + vancomycin, 1–2 g q12h
Gram-negative cocci	Penicillin G, 4 million units q4h
Gram-positive bacilli	Ampicillin, 2 g q4h, + gentamicin, 1 mg/kg q8h
Gram-negative bacilli	Ceftazidime, 2 g q8h, + gentamicin, 1 mg/kg q8h

SUGGESTED READING

Coyle PK. Overview of acute and chronic meningitis. *Neurol Clin* 1999;17:691–670.

Marra CM. Bacterial and fungal brain infections in AIDS. *Semin Neurol* 1999;19:177–184.

Roos KL. Acute bacterial meningitis. *Semin Neurol* 2000;20:293–306.

Rotbart HA. Viral meningitis. *Semin Neurol* 2000;20:277–292.

Spach DH, Jackson LA. Bacterial meningitis. *Neurol Clin* 1999;17:711–735.

Thwaites G, Chau TT, Mai NT, et al. Tuberculous meningitis. *J Neurol Neurosurg Psychiatry* 2000;68:619–636.

Zunt JR, Marrra CM. Cerebrospinal fluid testing for the diagnosis of central nervous system infections. *Neurol Clin* 1999;17:675–689.

REFERENCES

1. de Gans J. Dexamethasone in adults with bacterial meningitis. *N Engl J Med* 2002;347:1549–1556.
2. Roos KL. Mycobacterium tuberculosis meningitis and other etiologies of the aseptic meningitis syndrome. *Semin Neurol* 2000;28:329–335.

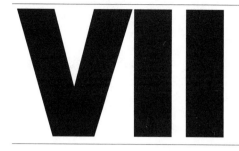

VII

Neurology

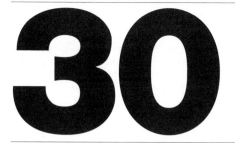

Approach to Altered Mental Status

Kyle C. Moylan and
Christopher H. Kwoh

INTRODUCTION

Delirium is a common medical syndrome affecting up to 30% of hospitalized inpatients, with the elderly being at greatest risk. Postoperatively, the incidence may approach 60% of the elderly. These patients are at risk for complications of their hospitalization such as dehydration, malnutrition, aspiration, skin ulcers, deconditioning, falls, institutionalization, and increased length of stay. The mortality rate is also high (approximately 8%), which is in part related to the severity of the underlying medical conditions. Table 30-1 provides a differential diagnosis of altered mental status.

PRESENTATION

History

The DSM-IV criteria define delirium as an impaired level of consciousness (either alertness or attention) and impaired cognition (memory, orientation, or language), with onset over hours to days and fluctuation over the course of the day.

Collateral history is imperative. History should be elicited from family members or other caregivers and should focus on several items (Table 30-2).

Try to elicit a history of subtle signs of a prior cerebrovascular accident. In the face of acute medical illness, findings of an old stroke, which have been compensated for at baseline, may become evident again.

Physical Exam

The purpose of the physical exam in delirious patients is to **identify possible precipitating causes or evidence of a focal neurologic process.**

In a complete physical exam, look for evidence of infections, dehydration, and head trauma. Evaluate for fecal or urinary retention.

The **Mini-Mental Status Exam** is a useful screen for cognitive dysfunction. A score <24 on the Folstein Mini-Mental Status Exam is abnormal, but false-positives can occur with advanced age and poor education. The Short Blessed Test (Table 30-3) is much more time efficient and of nearly equal accuracy to the Folstein Mini-Mental. A score of <9 on the Short Blessed is considered normal. A **single** normal exam **does not exclude** the diagnosis because it does not take into account fluctuations. Serial exams are likely to be more useful for identifying and following delirious patients. **A baseline exam on admission on all admitted patients with the diagnosis or at high risk for developing delirium is useful.**

A **Delirium Writing Test** (with evaluation of reluctance to write, motor impairment, and spatial understanding) is rapid and can be useful perioperatively (preoperatively and then the third day postoperative and as needed) for identifying patients with early delirium [1].

Passive exams of patient behaviors are important to observe and document:

- **Motor activity:** Is there psychomotor agitation or retardation?
- **Alertness:** What level of stimulus is required to arouse the patient?

TABLE 30-1. DIFFERENTIAL DIAGNOSIS

Infections: UTI, pneumonia, surgical wound or site, line infection.

Medications: anticholinergics (antihistamines, clonidine, tricyclic antidepressants), **narcotics, benzodiazepines, H$_2$-blockers,** steroids, theophylline, digoxin, antiparkinsonian agents, neuroleptic malignant syndrome, sulfonylureas, NSAIDs, anticonvulsants, antihypertensives.

Cardiac: myocardial ischemia or MI.

Withdrawal: ethanol, narcotics, benzodiazepines.

Electrolyte abnormalities: hyper- or hyponatremia, hypercalcemia.

Postoperatively: uncontrolled pain, postanesthetic.

Metabolic derangements: uremia, hepatic encephalopathy, vitamin B$_{12}$ deficiency, Wernicke-Korsakoff syndrome, hyper- or hypoglycemia, hyper- or hypothyroidism, hypoxia, hypercapnia, acidosis or alkalosis.

CNS disorders: cerebrovascular accident sleep deprivation, previously unrecognized dementia, vasculitis, neoplasia (primary or metastatic), meningitis, encephalitis, neurosyphilis, relative hypotension, postictal state, nonconvulsive status epilepticus.

Psychiatric disorders: depression/pseudodementia, psychosis.

Environmental: hyperthermia, hypothermia, trauma, burns, fractures.

- **Attentiveness**: Can the patient maintain focus during a conversation, or are they easily distracted? Can the patient shift attention appropriately?
- **Speech:** Pay attention to content and flow of thought.

Lab Evaluation

Lab evaluation includes UA with microscopic analysis (culture if abnormal), pulse oximetry, electrolytes (including calcium and BUN/Cr), glucose (bedside stick), liver panel, and CBC. Most patients should have an ECG as well; the elderly may have delerium as the only symptom of myocardial ischemia or infarction.

Consider further testing, when appropriate, with ABGs, ethanol level, toxicology screens, thyroid function tests, VDRL, and HIV.

Lumbar puncture to exclude meningoencephalitis can be considered for patients with unexplained mental status changes, especially in the face of fever, leukocytosis, or other evidence of sepsis that is not readily attributable to another source of infection.

Electroencephalogram is not routinely indicated but can be useful in cases in which the diagnosis remains in doubt or there is concern for seizure activity.

Imaging

Most patients should have a **chest x-ray** to rule out pneumonia.

TABLE 30-2. KEY HISTORICAL FEATURES

Baseline mental status (has there been evidence of progressive cognitive decline suggesting dementia)

Previous history of delirium

History of falls or head injury

Medications (prescription and over-the-counter), especially recent changes

Ethanol use

TABLE 30-3. SHORT BLESSED TEST

1. What year is it? Maximum error: 1; weight × 4.
2. What month is it? Maximum error: 1; weight × 3.

   Repeat this address (three attempts): John Brown, 42 Market Street, Chicago.

3. Without looking at a watch or clock, what time is it? (Within 1 hour.) Maximum error: 1; weight × 3.
4. Count backwards from 20 to 1. Maximum error: 2; weight × 2.
5. Say the months in reverse order. Maximum error: 2; weight × 2
6. Repeat the address as above. Maximum error: 5; weight × 2.

Note: Sum of scores (up to maximum error multiplied by weight); 0–8: normal to mild impairment; 9–19: moderate; >19: severe.
From Thompson P, Blessed G. Correlation between the 37-item mental test score and abbreviated 10-item mental test score by psychogeriatric day patients. *Br J Psychiatry* 1987;151:206–209, with permission.

In **neuroimaging studies,** a noncontrast head CT should be performed if there are new focal neurologic deficits (to evaluate for old CVA or other structural abnormality) or if there is a history of falls (to exclude a subdural hematoma). MRI may further identify causes of encephalopathy.

MANAGEMENT

Preoperative and admission assessment of mental status is critical in applying appropriate interventions and assessing their response.

Prevention and early intervention with **increasing mobility and activity, preventing sleep deprivation/interruption, full hydration,** and **reversing hearing and visual impairment** is effective in decreasing delirium in hospitalized patients [2].

Treatment is primarily supportive until the underlying precipitants are identified and treated.

Review medications and give a therapeutic and diagnostic trial of stopping suspect medications. Avoid starting new medications that could worsen the problem.

Maximize the safety of the surrounding environment: institute "fall precautions." Avoid physical restraints, which can result in iatrogenic injuries.

Evaluate sensory input:

- **Avoid sensory extremes**.
- Avoid placing two delirious patients in the same room.
- Use sitters (especially **familiar faces**—ask family members to stay with the patient).
- Use windows and a visible clock to orient the patient to the day/night cycle.

Treat pain adequately.
Medications are indicated for specific disruptive or harmful behaviors:

- **Neuroleptic agents** may be useful in treating hyperactive patients who represent a danger to themselves or the staff. **Haloperidol (Haldol) is the drug of choice.** Initially administered IM/IV for prompt control, the starting dose should be low (0.5–2 mg) and given parenterally; it can be doubled every hour until control is achieved. Repeated doses can then be given q4–8h and then switched to oral administration if continued maintenance is needed. For conversion, give 50–100% of the parenteral dose required in 24 hrs, divided up bid or tid. Newer, atypical antipsychotics do not appear to be any more effective at this time.
- **Benzodiazepines** can be useful adjuncts to antipsychotic agents for severe agitation, insomnia, and withdrawal syndromes. Medium-acting agents are preferable

[lorazepam (Ativan), 0.5–2 mg PO], as short-acting agents risk a paradoxic agitation after drug withdrawal.

KEY POINTS TO REMEMBER

- Baseline mental status is critical in assessing the severity and response to patients with delirium. All patients at risk for delirium (e.g., an elderly patient undergoing a preoperative evaluation) should have a mental status exam. History provided by other (less delirious) family members may be extremely helpful.
- Use nonpharmacologic methods initially to control delirium. Optimize patient safety, but try to avoid using restraints if possible. If behavioral management requires medications, then use antipsychotics before using sedatives.

SUGGESTED READING

Katzman R. Validation of a short orientation-memory-concentration test of cognitive impariment. *Am J Psychiatry* 1983;140:734–739.
Meagher D. Delirium: optimising management. *BMJ* 2001;322:144–149.
Tune L, Hazzard WR, ed. *Principles of geriatric medicine and gerontology*. New York: McGraw-Hill, 1999:1229–1237.

REFERENCES

1. Aakerlund LP. Writing disturbances: an indicator for postoperative delirium. *Int J Psychiatry Med* 1994;24:245–257.
2. Inouye SK, Bogardus ST Jr, Charpentier PA, et al. A multicomponent intervention to prevent delirium in hospitalized older patient. *N Engl J Med* 1999;340;669–676.

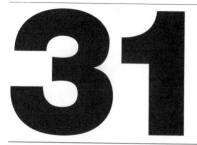

Approach to the Patient with Vertigo

David Anand Rengachary
and Christopher H. Kwoh

INTRODUCTION

Vertigo is defined as the sensation of movement or rotation in space. Patients may describe a sensation of the room spinning around them or impulsion—the sensation that they are being hurled through space. It is distinct from dizziness or lightheadedness.

PRESENTATION

History

History should include head trauma, strokes, neoplasms, ear infections, antiepileptic medication use, ethanol abuse, diving/air flights, or sinusitis.

Important associated symptoms include hearing loss and tinnitus, which isolates the pathology to the auditory nerve or inner ear.

Benign paroxysmal positional vertigo, the most common cause of vertigo, presents with brief (5–90 secs) attacks brought on by position changes and is reproducible. **Attacks lasting seconds** are **rarely** another diagnosis.

Ménière's disease has the classic triad of hearing loss, tinnitus, and vertigo lasting several minutes to several hours. The presentation may also be syncopal (Tumarkin drop attacks preceded by the sensation of being spun around) or with fullness in the ear. An increase with Valsalva or increase with loud noises (Tullio's phenomenon) suggests a **perilymphatic fistula.** Tullio's can also be found in Ménière's.

Vestibular labyrinthitis or neuronitis is preceded by a viral infection in approximately 50% of cases and presents with constant symptoms for days (although worsening with movement).

Acoustic neuroma presents with progressive symptoms of vertigo, hearing loss, or tinnitus and may be accompanied by ataxia and cranial nerve VII deficits.

Isolated attacks of vertigo may be a sign of vertebrobasilar ischemia (TIAs). (For differential diagnoses, see Tables 31-1 and 31-2.)

Physical Exam

A detailed neurologic exam, focusing on cranial nerves, helps to identify focal neurologic findings and further localization (Table 31-3). Other CNS deficits should raise suspicion for a central lesion.

An external ear exam may reveal signs of infection or vesicles of Ramsay-Hunt syndrome (VZV of cranial nerve VII).

The **Dix-Hallpike** maneuver helps to identify benign paroxysmal positional vertigo: With the patient seated, have him or her turn the head 45 degrees to the right. In one firm motion, allow the patient to fall back with the head around 20 degrees below vertical. Observe for vertigo and rotational nystagmus. Repeat the procedure to the left. Patients may also develop nystagmus and vertigo when returned to the seated position.

Calorics may aid in the diagnosis. **Always** establish the integrity of the tympanic membrane before performing calorics. Elevate the head of the bed to 30 degrees. Use cold water only if warm water is unable to elicit responses:

TABLE 31-1. DIFFERENTIAL DIAGNOSIS OF PERIPHERAL VERTIGO

Benign paroxysmal positional vertigo

Ménière's disease

Vestibular labyrinthitis/neuronitis

Perilymphatic fistula

Ramsay Hunt syndrome

Ototoxic medications: aminoglycosides, furosemide (Lasix)

Acoustic neuroma

Otitis media

Cholesteatoma

Mastoiditis

Barotrauma

Otosclerosis

Otogenic syphilis

- **Normal:** warm water produces nystagmus with the fast phase **toward** the irrigated ear. Cold water–induced nystagmus directs the phase **away.**
- **Vestibular disease:** diminished or absent responses.

Imaging Evaluation

Straightforward diagnoses by history and physical may not require further evaluation.

Electrooculography and audiometry may be useful in unclear cases.

Perform MRI for suspected central vertigo or acoustic neuroma. MRI should also be performed when symptoms are accompanied by a headache or in a patient at high risk for cerebrovascular accident. Also consider imaging in cases of acute peripheral vertigo that progress after 48 hrs.

Magnetic resonance angiography or traditional angiography may identify vertebrobasilar vascular disease.

MANAGEMENT

Pharmacologic therapeutic options include meclizine (Antivert), 25–50 mg q6h × 3 days; diazepam (Valium), 2–5 mg PO tid; promethazine (Phenergan), 25 mg PO q12h; or prochlorperazine (Compazine), 5–10 mg PO or IV q4–6h.

For patients with benign positional vertigo:

- A bedside Epley maneuver is >70% effective on first attempt and >90% after two attempts.

TABLE 31-2. DIFFERENTIAL DIAGNOSIS OF CENTRAL VERTIGO

Brainstem infarctions and other lesions	Basilar migraines
Vertebrobasilar transient ischemic attacks	Meningitis
Cerebellopontine angle tumors	Trauma
Multiple sclerosis	Cerebellar lesions
	Seizures

TABLE 31-3. HISTORY AND EXAM FEATURES SUGGESTING PERIPHERAL VS CENTRAL VERTIGO

Suggests peripheral	Suggests central
Nausea and vertigo tend to be more disabling	Imbalance and ataxia tend to be more prominent symptoms
Sudden onset, episodic	Gradual onset, constant
Associated hearing loss or tinnitus	Associated diplopia or dysarthria
Positional	Severe oscillopsia
Ear pain or fullness, facial weakness	Neighboring brainstem symptoms
Increased with Valsalva or loud noises	Direction changing disconjugate nystagmus
Unilateral horizontal jerk nystagmus	Isolated vertical/down-beating nystagmus
Fatigable nystagmus	Nonfatigable nystagmus
Nystagmus suppressible with fixation	Gaze-evoked nystagmus

- Brandt-Daroff habituation exercises involve head and trunk tilts and may be effective for decreasing symptoms when Epley maneuvers fail.
- Symptomatic pharmacologic therapy can be applied as needed.

Ménière's disease can be managed with 2-g salt restriction or diuretic therapy (acetazolamide or hydrochlorothiazide). Additional symptomatic medications may be given. Surgery may be useful for refractory cases of Ménière's.

Vestibular neuronitis may be improved with steroid pulse therapy and symptomatic therapy.

The course of Ramsay-Hunt syndrome may be shortened with acyclovir (Zovirax).

Acoustic neuroma or cerebellar hemorrhage should be handled surgically.

KEY POINTS TO REMEMBER

- The most important initial step is clearly identifying the patient's sensation as vertigo, the sensation that they are spinning or being hurled through space. Vertigo is not equivalent to lightheadedness or dizziness.
- Key findings that suggest peripheral rather than central vertigo include horizontal rather than vertical nystagmus, associated auditory symptoms, and fatigability. A careful neurologic exam may reveal other deficits that may suggest a significant CNS pathology.

REFERENCES AND SUGGESTED READINGS

Baloh RW. Vertigo. *Lancet* 1998;352:1841–1846.

El-Kashan HK, Telian SA. Diagnosis and initiating treatment for peripheral system disorders: imbalance and dizziness with normal hearing. *Otolaryngol Clin North Am* 2000;33:563–577.

Simon RP, Aminoff MJ, Greenberg DA, eds. Disorders of equilibrium. In: *Clinical neurology*, 4th ed. New York: McGraw-Hill, 1999:102–132.

Strupp M, Arbusow V. Acute vestibulopathy. *Curr Opin Neurol* 2001;14:11–20.

Tusa RK. Vertigo. *Neurol Clin* 2001;19:23–55.

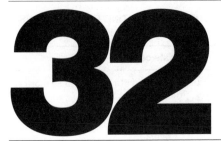

Approach to the Carotid Bruit

Christopher H. Kwoh

INTRODUCTION

The prevalence of a carotid bruit is estimated at 4% of those older than 40 and 8% of those older than 75. Not all bruits indicate significant carotid stenosis. Studies of patients with carotid bruits reveal positive predictive values of moderate stenosis of approximately 75%. Carotid bruits also do not correlate well with intracranial disease [1]. A 25% stenosis appears to be significant enough to cause a bruit. **Severe occlusion may not cause a bruit** because of limited blood flow.

PRESENTATION

History

Most patients with carotid bruits are asymptomatic, with the bruit discovered on routine physical exam. Symptoms of carotid stenosis include transient monocular blindness (amaurosis fugax) or cerebrovascular events with aphasia, dysarthria, or contralateral weakness or numbness.

Physical Exam

Other signs of atherosclerotic disease are often present, including diminished lower extremity pulses and subclavian bruits.

A thorough neurologic exam is critical because management for asymptomatic patients is different from management of those with prior cerebrovascular accidents.

Imaging Evaluation

Duplex U/S is commonly used with accuracy estimated at 85–95% but with wide operator variability. Most operators will **underestimate** stenosis, especially in high-grade lesions. **Magnetic resonance angiography** is widely used, with cost somewhere between U/S and angiography. Most MRI readings will **overestimate** the degree of stenosis. **Angiography** is the gold standard for diagnosis but with a complication rate around 5%, most of which are transient neurologic events.

MANAGEMENT

Approaches differ for symptomatic vs. asymptomatic stenosis.

Management of Symptomatic Carotid Stenosis

Carotid Endarterectomy
Carotid endarterectomy (CEA) has shown benefit in patients with **>70% stenosis** in two large randomized controlled trials vs. medical therapy [2,3]. (See Appendix A for details of NASCET.) **CEA should therefore be performed on symptomatic patients with >70% stenosis** unless another contraindication exists.

In patients with **50–69% stenosis,** a CEA resulted in an absolute risk reduction of 6.5% for ipsilateral stroke at 5 yrs in one trial [2]. **American Heart Association recommendations for 50–69% stenosis** are to consider endarterectomy if operating risk is <3% for high-risk patients: males, age ≥ 75 yrs, hemispheric symptoms, stroke within 90 days, intracranial stenosis, lack of microvascular ischemia, or more severe stenosis [4,5].

Patients with **<50% stenosis** received **no benefit from CEA** in most large trials of medical management vs. CEA.

Medical Therapy

Medical management should be offered regardless of whether the patient is a candidate for CEA. Medical therapy should focus on modifying the risk factors of smoking, HTN, hyperlipidemia (see Appendix A for details of the 4S Study), diabetes, alcohol use, obesity, and sedentary lifestyle.

Antiplatelet therapy should be prescribed [ASA, 325 mg PO qd; clopidogrel (Plavix), 75 mg PO qd; ticlopidine (Ticlid), 250 mg PO bid; or combined ASA and dipyridamole (Persantine)].

In the Warfarin-Aspirin Recurrent Stroke Study (WARSS), warfarin did not demonstrate additional benefit over ASA for carotid stenosis and is not recommended by the American Heart Association committee.

There may be additional benefit from ACE inhibitors vs. other antihypertensives in reducing stroke [6]. See Appendix A for details of the HOPE trial.

Management of Asymptomatic Carotid Stenosis

Carotid Endarterectomy

In large studies of CEA vs. medical therapy for asymptomatic patients [7,8], benefit was seen only with low operative risk.

The **American Heart Association** recommends that **asymptomatic** patients with **>60% stenosis** be considered for CEA if they are <80 yrs old with surgical risk <3% (based on Asymptomatic Carotid Atherosclerosis Study trial; see Appendix A for details) [7].

A **Cochrane database metaanalysis** states, however, that there is insufficient evidence to recommend CEA in asymptomatic patients [9].

Medical Management

Medical management is identical to that for symptomatic carotid stenosis.

KEY POINTS TO REMEMBER

- The history should focus on determining whether the patient has had any symptoms attributable to carotid stenosis, as this greatly affects management. A thorough neurologic exam may reveal an unrecognized neurologic deficit.
- Symptomatic carotid stenosis >70% should be surgically managed with CEA. Patients with asymptomatic bruits >60% or symptomatic bruits >50% may benefit from CEA depending on surgical risk.

SUGGESTED READING

Grubb RL. Risks of stroke and current indications for cerebral revascularization in patients with carotid occlusion. *Neurosurg Clin North Am* 2001;36:473–487.

Hobson RW. Efficacy of carotid endarterectomy for asymptomatic carotid stenosis. *N Engl J Med* 1993;328:221–227.

Mayo Asymptomatic Carotid Endarterectomy Study Group. Results of a randomized controlled trial of carotid endarterectomy for asymptomatic carotid stenosis. *Mayo Clin Proc* 1992;67:513–518.

NASCET Collaborators. Beneficial effect of carotid endarterectomy in symptomatic patients with high-grade carotid stenosis. *N Engl J Med* 1991;325:445–453.

Sacco RL. Extracranial carotid stenosis: clinical practice. *N Engl J Med* 2001;345: 1113–1118.

REFERENCES

1. Ingall TJ. Predictive value of carotid bruit for carotid atherosclerosis. *Arch Neurol* 1989;46(4):418–422.
2. Barnett HJ. NASCET: benefit of carotid endarterectomy in patients with symptomatic moderate or severe stenosis. *N Engl J Med* 1998;339(20):1415–1425.
3. The European Carotid Surgery Trialist's Collaborative Group. Randomized trial of endarterectomy for recently symptomatic carotid stenosis: final results of the MRC European Carotid Surgery Trial. *Lancet* 1998;351:1379–1387.
4. Albers GW. Supplement to the guidelines for the management of transient ischemic attacks: a statement from the Ad Hoc Committee on Guidelines for the Management of Transient Ischemic Attacks, Stroke Council, American Heart Association. *Stroke* 1999;30:2502–2511.
5. Moore WS. Guidelines for carotid endarterectomy: a multidisciplinary consensus statement from the Ad Hoc Committee, American Heart Association. *Circulation* 1995;91:566–579.
6. Heart Outcomes Prevention Evaluation Study Investigators. Effects of an angiotensin-converting-enzyme inhibitor, ramipril, on death from cardiovascular causes, myocardial infarction, and stroke in high-risk patients. *N Engl J Med* 2000;342:145–153.
7. Executive Committee for the Asymptomatic Carotid Atherosclerosis Study. Endarterectomy for asymptomatic carotid stenosis. *JAMA* 1995;273:1421–1428.
8. The CASANOVA Study Group. Carotid surgery vs medical therapy in asymptomatic carotid stenosis. *Stroke* 1991;22:1229–1235.
9. Cochrane Database, 1999.

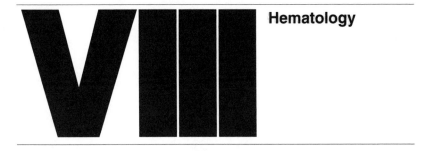

VIII Hematology

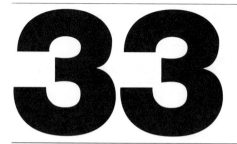

Approach to Anemia

Jennifer M. Quartarolo
and Stephen J. Wen

INTRODUCTION

Anemia is frequently seen in hospitalized patients. An orderly approach to diagnosis is needed because a "shotgun" approach can lead to dramatic increases in cost of care.

DIFFERENTIAL DIAGNOSIS

Causes of anemia can be divided into three broad categories: blood loss, increased destruction of RBCs (e.g., hemolytic anemia), or decreased production of RBCs (hypoproliferative anemia).

Anemia may also be classified by RBC size (mean corpuscular volume or MCV): microcytic, normocytic, macrocytic.

Microcytic Anemia

See Table 33-1 for the differential diagnosis of microcytic anemia.

- Iron (Fe) deficiency is the most common cause of microcytic anemia in adults, usually due to chronic blood loss but may be due to malabsorption or excessive phlebotomy.
- Anemia of chronic disease is commonly seen in the hospitalized patient as a result of abnormal ferrokinetics.
- Sideroblastic anemia may be hereditary; idiopathic; or caused by alcohol, lead, INH, chloramphenicol, malignancy, myelodysplasia, or chronic inflammation.
- Also consider lead poisoning in microcytic, hypochromic anemia.

Normocytic Anemias

Normocytic anemias can be divided into two groups based on the reticulocyte count.

- Increased reticulocyte count: hemolytic anemia or bleeding.
- Decreased reticulocyte count: hypoproliferative disorder.
- Anemia of chronic renal failure generally starts to occur when CrCl <45 mL/min and worsens with increasing renal failure. Classically, this is a hypochromic normocytic anemia.

Macrocytic Anemias

Macrocytic anemias are divided into megaloblastic or nonmegaloblastic based on peripheral smear. **Megaloblastic anemia** may be caused by vitamin B_{12} deficiency or folate deficiency, or may be drug induced [phenytoin (Dilantin), hydroxyurea, TMP-SMX (Bactrim), azidothymidine (Retrovir), and methotrexate (Folex) have been implicated]. **Nonmegaloblastic macrocytic anemia** may be caused by reticulocytosis, hemolysis, alcohol, liver disease, hypothyroidism, or various bone marrow disorders.

Hemolytic Anemia

See Table 33-2 for the differential diagnosis of hemolytic anemia.

TABLE 33-1. DIFFERENTIAL DIAGNOSIS FOR MICROCYTIC ANEMIA

	Fe deficiency	Anemia of chronic disease	Thalassemia	Sideroblastic
Serum Fe	Decreased or normal	Decreased	Normal	Increased
Total iron-binding capacity	Increased	Normal or decreased	Normal	Increased
Transferrin saturation	Decreased	Normal or decreased	Normal	Normal or increased
Serum ferritin	Decreased	Increased or normal	Normal	Increased
Bone marrow iron stores	Absent	Normal or decreased	Increased	Increased
RBC morphology	Microcytic, hypochromic, anisocytosis	Microcytic or normocytic, normochromic	Microcytic, hypochromic	Microcytic, hypochromic, dimorphic

Fe, iron.

PRESENTATION

History

General symptoms of anemia may include dyspnea, fatigue, or palpitations.

Vitamin B_{12} deficiency may present with a burning sensation of the tongue, vague abdominal pain, diarrhea, numbness, or paresthesias.

Weight loss, night sweats, and fever may all point to an underlying malignancy.

TABLE 33-2. DIFFERENTIAL DIAGNOSIS OF HEMOLYTIC ANEMIA

Autoimmune hemolytic anemia	Nonimmune hemolytic anemia
IgG autoantibody	Microangiopathic/traumatic
IgM autoantibody	DIC, TTP, HUS
Drug induced	Enzyme defects (e.g., G-6-PD deficiency)
Cold agglutinin	Drug induced
Malignancy associated	Paroxysmal nocturnal hemoglobinuria
Systemic lupus	Hemoglobinopathy (e.g., sickle cell)
	Malignant HTN
	RBC membrane diseases
	Infections (e.g., malaria)
	Eclampsia
	Transfusion reactions (immune)

DIC, disseminated intravascular coagulation; G-6-PD, glucose-6-phosphate dehydrogenase; HUS, hemolytic uremic syndrome; TTP, thrombotic thrombocytopenic purpura.

A careful history concerning blood loss (especially perioperatively or in the stool or menses), frequency of Hgb and Hct evaluations, and family history of anemia should be sought. Dark urine may be due to indirect bilirubin in the urine and a hemolytic anemia. Early cholecystectomy in a family member may be a clue to familial hemolytic anemia.

A good dietary history should be obtained, including Fe intake, B_{12} (deficient in vegans), and folate (from uncooked leafy vegetables), as well as pica symptoms (seen in Fe deficiency).

Physical Exam

Anemia may result in pallor, tachycardia, or signs of high output heart failure. In Fe deficiency, one may see alopecia, atrophic glossitis, angular cheilosis, koilonychias (spoon nails), or brittle nails. B_{12}-deficient patients often have glossitis/smooth tongue, dorsal column findings (decreased vibration and proprioception), or corticospinal tract findings.

Assess for jaundice or splenomegaly, sometimes present in hemolytic anemias. Lymph nodes may be enlarged in hematologic malignancies. **All** patients need a stool guaiac to look for GI blood loss.

Lab Evaluation

Review the full CBC. The presence of leukopenia or thrombocytopenia should raise suspicion for bone marrow failure, infiltration, or severe nutritional deficiency.

The **peripheral smear** is the single most important test to obtain. Some pertinent findings include the following:

- Target cells in Fe deficiency, hemoglobinopathies, liver disease, asplenia, and lecithin-cholesterol acyltransferase deficiency.
- Megaloblastic changes in macrocytic anemia include hypersegmentation of neutrophils, anisocytosis, large ovalocytes, and often pancytopenia.
- Hemolysis is suggested by acanthocytes, spherocytes, or reticulocytes.
- Look for evidence of malignant blood cells.

The **reticulocyte count** (normal 0.5–1.5%) should be corrected for anemia using the following formula:

$$\text{Corrected reticulocyte count} = \text{uncorrected reticulocyte count} \times (\text{patient's Hct/45})$$

RBC indices (MCV, mean corpuscular hemoglobin concentration, and RBC distribution width) should be noted to aid in the diagnosis.

Normocytic anemia should be evaluated with a reticulocyte count after looking at the peripheral smear:

- A high reticulocyte count suggests bleeding or hemolysis, and the patient should be evaluated for both of these possibilities.
- An inappropriately low reticulocyte count indicates poor bone marrow function. Rule out renal failure as the cause. Evaluate further based on the peripheral smear. Consider hypothyroidism, adrenal insufficiency, or gonadal insufficiency. Anemia of chronic disease will be a common cause.
- Always rule out blood loss.

Macrocytic anemia should first be evaluated by determining whether it is megaloblastic or nonmegaloblastic based on the peripheral smear:

- **Megaloblastic:** Obtain serum folate and vitamin B_{12}. In cases of borderline low B_{12} values, one can measure serum methylmalonic acid and homocysteine levels, which are elevated in vitamin B_{12} deficiency. When B_{12} and folate deficiency are excluded, then consider one of the drug-induced causes (see Macrocytic Anemias).
- **Nonmegaloblastic:** Check the reticulocyte count. If it is elevated, then it is most likely a hemolytic cause (see earlier). If the reticulocyte count is inappropriately

low, then consider one of the other causes of nonmegaloblastic macrocytic anemia (see Macrocytic Anemias).

Obtaining a serum ferritin is the most cost-effective way to diagnose Fe deficiency. A ferritin of ≤30 μg/L almost always indicates iron deficiency. Levels of 30–100 μg/L require more interpretation. In the presence of malignancy, infection, and inflammation, the ferritin value may be elevated and should be interpreted cautiously. In these settings, total Fe binding capacity, transferrin saturation, and serum Fe are helpful additional labs.

Thalassemia may be diagnosed by Hgb electrophoresis. Alpha-thalassemia trait, the most commonly diagnosed thalassemia, will have a normal Hgb electrophoresis but an MCV that is low out of proportion to the anemia and a chronically low Hct on review of previous lab data.

In hemolytic anemias, one often sees signs of increased RBC destruction, such as an increased LDH, decreased haptoglobin, increased unconjugated bilirubin, or hemoglobinuria (in intravascular hemolysis or severe extravascular hemolysis). Reticulocytosis should also be seen. If there is evidence of hemolysis, then evaluation with an indirect and direct Coomb's test is indicated. Direct Coomb's test will be positive in autoimmune hemolytic anemias, detecting IgG and C3 antibodies. A false-negative direct Coomb's may occur with IgM-mediated or cold agglutinin hemolysis.

Consider a bone marrow evaluation in difficult cases.

SPECIAL CONSIDERATIONS IN POSTOPERATIVE ANEMIA

1. Patients who experience hypothermia or cold cardioplegia with cardiac surgery may have a shortened RBC life span due to membrane damage. RBCs recovered with the "cell-saver" also experience significant membrane damage and early hemolysis.
2. Patients with valvular surgery may have a valve-induced hemolytic anemia. Also consider evaluation of the mooring, which, if loosened, can cause significant hemolysis.
3. Bone marrow suppression may occur owing to surgical inflammation and may continue for 1 wk or more.
4. Perioperative hemodilution is common due to aggressive intravenous hydration. Review the ins and outs and anesthesiology flow sheets.
5. Consider drug-induced hemolysis and glucose-6-phosphate dehydrogenase due to anesthetics or pain medications.
6. Stress gastritis is common perioperatively and can be the source of significant blood loss. This is easier to prevent (with prophylactic H_2-blockers, proton pump inhibitors, or sucralfate) than it is to treat.
7. Consider postoperative bleeding at the site of the surgery.

MANAGEMENT

Iron-Deficiency Anemia

Discover and treat the underlying source of blood loss. $FeSO_4$, 325 mg PO bid to tid, may be initiated. Parenteral Fe (500–1000 mg + 1 mg/mL of blood deficit) may be administered in cases of intolerance or failure to take PO Fe, malabsorption, or severe renal failure. The risk of anaphylaxis is significant but somewhat lower with newer preparations (e.g., ferrous gluconate).

Expect an increase in the reticulocyte count within 7–10 days of therapy. Correction of anemia usually occurs within 6–8 wks, but treatment should continue for approximately 6 mos (if on oral Fe) to fully restore tissue stores.

Nonmenstruating adults should have endoscopy to evaluate for a potential gastrointestinal source of chronic blood loss.

Vitamin B₁₂ Deficiency

Vitamin B_{12} deficiency should be treated with vitamin B_{12}, 1 mg IM daily for 7 days, then weekly for 1 mo, followed by monthly doses thereafter. An evaluation for the underlying mechanism should be undertaken. Failure to correct or identify the underlying cause of deficiency should result in lifetime therapy.

Folate Deficiency

Folate deficiency should be treated with folate, 1 mg PO qd with resolution of hematologic abnormalities within 2 mos.

Chronic Renal Failure

Anemia of chronic renal failure may respond to erythropoietin, 50–100 U/kg IV or SC 3×/wk with readjustments based on response. Ensure adequate Fe stores. Transfuse as needed.

KEY POINTS TO REMEMBER

- The peripheral smear should always be examined. It is your most powerful diagnostic tool!
- Always rule out blood loss in an acute anemia.
- Renal failure as a cause of anemia is often overlooked. Calculate the glomerular filtration rate.

REFERENCES AND SUGGESTED READINGS

Berkow R, ed. Anemias. In: *The Merck manual*, 16th ed. Rahway, NJ: Merck Research Laboratories, 1992:1136–1174.

Eckman JR. Orderly approach to the evaluation and treatment of anemia. *Emory Univ J Med* 1991;5(2):80–90.

Goroll AH. Evaluation of anemia. In: Goroll AH, ed. *Primary care medicine: office evaluation and management of the adult patient*, 3rd ed. Philadelphia: Lippincott, 1995:447–455.

Rosse W, Bunn HF. Hemolytic anemias. In: Isselbacher KJ, ed. *Harrison's principles of internal medicine*, 13th ed. New York: McGraw-Hill, 1994:1743–1754.

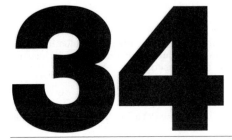

Thrombocytopenia

Jennifer M. Quartarolo and
Christopher H. Kwoh

INTRODUCTION

The normal platelet number is 150–450 × 1000/mL blood. At any given time, approximately one-third of mature platelets are sequestered in the spleen, whereas two-thirds circulate in blood. The lifespan of circulating platelets is 7–10 days. In general, thrombocytopenia is caused by decreased production, increased splenic sequestration, or increased destruction of platelets. See Table 34-1 for differential diagnosis of thrombocytopenia.

PRESENTATION

History

Symptoms of low platelets vary depending on the platelet count:

- Platelets >100,000/μL should have normal hemostasis.
- Platelets <50,000/μL may have a history of prolonged bleeding after a procedure, mucosal bleeding (gingival, GI), menorrhagia, easy bruising.
- Platelets <20,000/μL may have a petechial rash or spontaneous bleeding.
- Platelets <10,000/μL are at risk for spontaneous intracerebral hemorrhage.

In addition, look for symptoms and risk factors associated with etiologies of decreased platelets (Tables 34-1 and 34-2).

- Fatigue, weight loss, or night sweats may be associated with infection or malignancy.
- A medication history and an accurate alcohol history are critical.
- Try to elicit a history of symptoms suggesting an autoimmune disease.
- The classic pentad of thrombotic thrombocytopenic purpura (TTP) is fever, altered sensorium, renal failure, microangiopathic hemolytic anemia, and thrombocytopenia. Only rarely are all elements present.

Obtain a transfusion history. **Posttransfusion purpura** is a rare disorder caused by an overwhelming platelet antibody response in patients who are PLA1 antibody negative. Consider this in the postsurgical patient who has a precipitous drop in platelets 7–10 days after platelet transfusions.

Physical Exam

Vital signs may reveal evidence of sepsis (hypotension, tachycardia, fever). A fever is also frequently present in TTP.

Look for petechiae. Be certain to thoroughly examine skin as well as the oropharynx, subconjunctiva, and retina.

The spleen size helps to narrow the differential and rule out splenic sequestration. Look for stigmata of liver disease or autoimmune disease.

Lab Evaluation

The most important test to do is the **peripheral blood smear:**

TABLE 34-1. DIFFERENTIAL DIAGNOSIS OF THROMBOCYTOPENIA

Decreased production	Splenic sequestration	Increased destruction
Marrow infiltration	Splenic enlargement	Nonimmune
Malignancy	Tumor infiltration	Vascular prostheses
Myelofibrosis	Infection	Disseminated intravascular coagulation
Granulomatous disease	Splenic congestion	
Marrow failure	Portal HTN or liver disease	Sepsis
Medication		Vasculitis
Chemotherapy		Thrombotic thrombocytopenic purpura
Aplastic anemia		
Severe iron deficiency		Immune
Infection (HIV, Epstein-Barr virus, TB)		Autoantibody (idiopathic thrombocytopenic purpura)
Alcohol use		Drug-associated[a]
Nutritional deficiency		Circulating immune complexes (systemic lupus erythematosus, viral, bacterial sepsis)
Iron, folate, vitamin B_{12}		
		Posttransfusion ab (PLA1)

[a]One of most common causes of thrombocytopenia in inpatients.

- Look for platelet clumping (spurious thrombocytopenia/pseudothrombocytopenia) in which platelet numbers are normal but clumped by the ethylenediaminetetraacetic acid and missed by the automated counter.
- Look for schistocytes [TTP, disseminated intravascular coagulation (DIC)].
- Look for evidence of malignancy, myelofibrosis, blasts.
- Look for micro- or macrocytosis (associated with vitamin deficiency).

Identify whether this is a pancytopenia (all cell lines decreased, which suggests marrow failure) or isolated thrombocytopenia.

Bleeding time (BT) is an estimate of platelet function (normal is 2–9 min):

- >100 K platelets, the BT is generally normal.
- 50–100 K platelets, the BT is mildly prolonged.
- <50 K platelets, the BT is significantly prolonged.

HIV should be checked in any patient suspected of having idiopathic thrombocytopenic purpura. Also consider checking an ANA because ITP may be the first manifestation of SLE.

TABLE 34-2. MEDICATIONS COMMONLY ASSOCIATED WITH THROMBOCYTOPENIA

Quinidine	Heparin
H_2-blockers	Vancomycin
Digoxin	Danazol
TMP-SMX	Amiodarone
Quinine	Methyldopa
Rifampin	Valproic acid

Consider bone marrow biopsy if the etiology is uncertain or to rule out marrow failure or infiltration.

Other labs may be associated with underlying etiology:

- Evaluating PT/PTT and fibrin degradation products may help identify DIC and distinguish a hemolytic anemia from TTP.
- TTP may present with hemolytic anemia (decreasing Hgb and Hct, elevated LDH) and renal failure. Hemolytic uremic syndrome may also present with renal failure and thrombocytopenia.

A severely decreased ferritin, folate, or vitamin B_{12} level suggests nutritional deficiency. When other causes are ruled out, then ITP is the most likely diagnosis.

MANAGEMENT

Platelet transfusion is generally contraindicated in cases of TTP and posttransfusion purpura. Otherwise, in cases of platelet number $<20,000/\mu L$ or spontaneous bleeding, platelet transfusion is appropriate. A single donor unit of platelets is equivalent to six random donor platelets and should increase the platelet count by 30 K. In sequestration- or destruction-mediated thrombocytopenia, the platelets may not last long, and administration shortly before procedures is warranted. Otherwise, repeated checks of platelet counts can be done on a daily basis.

Avoid anticoagulants such as NSAIDs and ASA.

Plasmapheresis is the initial therapy for TTP and should be initiated promptly.

A diagnosis of **drug-induced** thrombocytopenia should prompt withdrawal of medication (resolution of thrombocytopenia postwithdrawal also confirms diagnosis).

For **heparin induced thrombocytopenia,** stop heparin, including heparin flushes. Low-molecular-weight heparins still have cross-reactivity. Hirudin may be used in cases in which anticoagulation is necessary.

Posttransfusion purpura may be treated with IV immunoglobulin.

Most cases of **ITP** can be controlled with glucocorticoids. Initial dosage is prednisone (Deltasone), 1 mg/kg/day, and slowly tapered. Refractory and chronic cases may require IV immunoglobulin or splenectomy. Management guidelines are published on the American Hematology Association Web site (http://www.hematology.org).

In cases of infection, malignancy, liver disease, and autoimmune disease, treatment involves supportive care and treatment of underlying disorder.

Synthetic thrombopoietin is becoming available for use in patients with decreased production due to malignancy, toxins, or marrow failure.

KEY POINTS TO REMEMBER

- The most critical first step in the evaluation of thrombocytopenia is to look at the peripheral smear. Many patients with spurious thrombocytopenia have undergone unnecessary, expensive evaluations for thrombocytopenia. It is also important to identify those with isolated thrombocytopenia and those with more cell lines affected, suggesting bone marrow failure or infiltration. Also look for schistocytes, suggesting TTP or DIC.
- Have a low threshold for considering heparin-induced thrombocytopenia.

REFERENCES AND SUGGESTED READINGS

Elalamy I, Lecrubier C, Horellou MH, et al. Heparin-induced thrombocytopenia: laboratory diagnosis and management. *Ann Intern Med* 2000;32(Suppl 1):60–67.

Elliott M, Nichols W. Thrombotic thrombocytopenic purpura and hemolytic uremic syndrome. *Mayo Clin Proc* 2001;76:1154–1162.

George J, Raskob GE, Shah SR, et al. Drug-induced thrombocytopenia: a systematic review of published case reports. *Ann Intern Med* 1998;129:886–890.

Handin R. Disorders of the platelet and vessel wall. In: Braunwald E, Longo DL, Jameson JL. *Harrison's principles of internal medicine*, 15th ed. New York: McGraw-Hill, 2001.

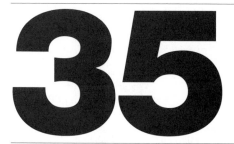

Approach to a Prolonged Prothrombin Time/ Partial Thromboplastin Time

Jennifer M. Quartarolo
and Christopher H. Kwoh

INTRODUCTION

Prolongation of the PT and PTT are common findings in hospitalized patients. Often, the internist is called preoperatively to assess these abnormalities.

PT screens the extrinsic or tissue-factor–dependent coagulation pathway (including most of the vitamin K–dependent factors). PTT screens the intrinsic pathway (factors 8, 9, 11, 12, high-molecular-weight kininogen, prekallikrein). **Both** PT and PTT evaluate the common coagulation pathway.

PRESENTATION

History

History should include medications, nutritional status, and any personal or family history of severe bleeding. Specifically inquire about prior excessive surgical bleeding or bleeding during childhood tooth extraction, which may be a clue to a long-standing factor deficiency. Many "coagulation abnormalities" are lab artifacts without clinical bleeding. Antibiotics with the MTT side chain (some cephalosporins) inhibit synthesis of the vitamin K–dependent proteins.

The patient should also be assessed for associated conditions, including liver or autoimmune disease.

Physical Exam

Look for evidence of bleeding, bruising, hemarthroses, and hematomas. Also look for stigmata of liver disease or autoimmune disease.

Differential Diagnosis

There are several points at which the coagulation cascade can be interrupted. See Table 35-1 for some common etiologies and Table 35-2 for differential diagnosis by lab abnormality.

Lab Evaluation

In patients who have an elevated PTT as well as an elevated INR while on warfarin (Coumadin), the approximate expected PTT should be approximately $(5 \times \text{INR}) + 25$. Elevations several points or more higher than expected may point to an etiology other than excessive warfarin dosing alone.

Elevations of the PT/PTT without an obvious cause should be evaluated by a 50:50 mix of the patient's blood to normal blood:

- If correction is achieved on a 50:50 mix, then there is a factor deficiency.
- If no correction is achieved, then an inhibitor is likely present.

If a factor deficiency is present, then further evaluation may be performed by assaying specific factors based on the differential listed in Table 35-2.

TABLE 35-1. DIFFERENTIAL DIAGNOSIS OF PROLONGED PT/PTT

	Etiology	Diagnosis
Liver disease	Decreased production of clotting factors	Signs and symptoms of liver failure
		Reverses with FFP
Vitamin K deficiency	May be secondary to fat malabsorption, nutritional deficiency, or loss of vitamin storage with liver disease	Reverses with vitamin K supplementation (within 24–48 hrs)
Medications	Warfarin and cephalosporin antibiotics (primarily leads to elevated PT)	Medication history/resolution with discontinuation of medication
	Heparin	
Circulating coagulation inhibitor	IgG antibodies	Failure of 50:50 mix with plasma to correct elevated PT/PTT
	Nonspecific examples include lupus anticoagulant and anticardiolipin Ab (associated with thrombosis rather than bleeding)	
	Increased risk in postpartum patients, patients with history of frequent plasma transfusions, autoimmune diseases, and reaction to penicillin or streptomycin	
DIC	Accelerated coagulation reactions diminish factor levels	Clinical presentation
	Associated with malignancy, bacterial sepsis, trauma	Thrombocytopenia, decreased fibrinogen, elevated fibrin degradation products
Inherited factor deficiency	Factor VIII and IX, hemophilia A and B	Bleeding history
	Factor VII deficiency: rare autosomal recessive	Assays for factor levels

DIC, disseminated intravascular coagulation.

MANAGEMENT

Generally, therapy depends on the underlying disorder.

First repeat the PT/PTT and ensure that enough blood is placed in the tube.

Patients without prolonged PTT due to deficiency of factor XII, high-molecular-weight kininogen, or PK are not at risk of bleeding. The bleeding risk in factor XI deficiency is very mild. These patients do not need specific preoperative therapy.

Vitamin K (5–20 mg PO or 5–10 mg SC) can be administered to patients with vitamin K deficiency or liver disease. Patients who are supratherapeutic on warfarin respond well to oral vitamin K, 2–5 mg. The response takes days, and patients with liver disease often see very little response. After a few days of vitamin K, the body's stores are replenished, and additional administration will have little or no effect.

FFP contains all of the coagulation factors at normal serum levels. Administer 2 U before procedures if the PT/PTT is prohibitively prolonged. Patients with severe elevations or who are having life-threatening bleeding should receive 3–4 U to start. Frequent monitoring should be done to ensure that the PT and PTT correct to the appropriate range.

Cryoprecipitate contains high levels of fibrinogen (factor I), factor VIII (80 U), and von Willebrand factor. This may be used in bleeding for the volume-overloaded patient

TABLE 35-2. DIFFERENTIAL DIAGNOSIS OF PROLONGED PT/PTT BY COAGULATION ABNORMALITY

Abnormal lab result	Causes
Prolonged PT only	Deficiency of factor VII
	Vitamin K deficiency or warfarin therapy
	Liver disease
Prolonged PTT only	Deficiency of factor 8, 9, 11, 12; high-molecular-weight kininogen; or prekallikrein
	von Willebrand disease
	Antiphospholipid syndrome
Prolonged PT and PTT	Deficiency of factor 1 (afibrinogenemia), 2, 5, 10
	Disseminated intravascular coagulation
	Severe vitamin K deficiency or excessive warfarin
	Severe liver disease
	Heparin

and when factor VIII is not available for hemophiliacs. It has also been used topically to stop bleeding from wounds.

Specific **coagulation inhibitors** may resolve in 6–12 mos. In cases of severe hemorrhage, plasma transfusion or plasmapheresis to lower antibody titer may be necessary.

There is no proven benefit to treating the coagulation defects associated with **disseminated intravascular coagulation**. Focus should be on treating the underlying disorder.

KEY POINTS TO REMEMBER

- Always confirm any abnormal coagulation test. A small amount of saline or insufficient quantities of blood collected in the tube may result in alterations of the PT and PTT. The next step is to repeat the test using a mixing study, which determines whether there is a factor deficiency of an inhibitor of coagulation.
- Try to obtain old PT/PTT results. Normal prior coagulation studies will essentially rule out any hereditary deficiency.

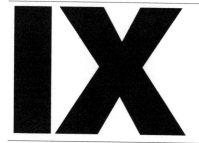

IX

Oncology

Pain Control in the Cancer Patient

Ron Lubelchek

INTRODUCTION

In a study of 200 patients being treated at a cancer pain clinic, pain caused by tumor growth was found in 158 (79%) of the patients. The level of pain should be assessed frequently and systematically using a verbal numerical scale (0–10) or visual scale such as the "faces of pain" scale. In patients with cognitive impairment, autonomic signs such as tachycardia, HTN, and diaphoresis may suggest inadequate analgesia.

MANAGEMENT

Analgesia is often best accomplished by antitumor therapy using radiation, chemotherapy, or palliative surgery to debulk the tumor when appropriate.

The World Health Organization (WHO) has proposed a three-step approach for the pharmacologic treatment of cancer pain:

Step 1	Use nonopioids and adjuvant drugs.
Step 2	For increasing pain, add an opioid analgesic.
Step 3	If inadequate control, add a more potent opioid [1].

Nonopioid Analgesics

NSAIDs and acetaminophen are commonly used for the treatment of cancer pain, as part of step 1 of the WHO guidelines. When given on a scheduled basis, they are also useful for limiting opioid doses and their side effects.

Opioid Analgesics

Opioids predictably induce tolerance and physical dependence. Disease progression (rather than tolerance) is more often the cause of increasing analgesic requirements.

Opioid addiction (psychological dependence) is rare in cancer patients [2,3].

Opioid Dosing

When starting therapy, a short-acting drug should be given q2–3h. After five or six half-lives (1 day for morphine), the daily requirement is determined, and a scheduled long-acting preparation should be used.

Short-acting agents, at 5–15% of the daily dose, may be used q2–4h for breakthrough pain.

If the short-acting opioid is used more than 3× /day, the dose of the long-acting drug should be increased at intervals of one-third to one-half of the previous dose.

With treatment of underlying cancer, narcotics may be withdrawn. Reducing the dose gradually, by <75% daily, prevents symptomatic withdrawal.

Patient-controlled analgesia provides a rapid, efficient means by which to titrate the analgesic dose to individual needs.

TABLE 36-1. EQUIPOTENT ANALGESIC DOSES (MORPHINE, 10 MG IV/IM = 1 U)

Drug	Onset (mins)	Dose interval (hrs)	PO equivalent dose (mg)	IM/IV equivalent dose (mg)
Codeine	10–30	4	200	130
Hydrocodone	15–30	4	30	—
Hydromorphone (Dilaudid)	15–30 (PO)	2–4 (IV) 4–6 (PO)	7.5	1.5
Meperidine (Demerol)	10–45 (PO)	4–6 (PO) 4 (IV)	300	75
Morphine sulfate	15–60 (PO)	4 (PO) 2–4 (IV)	30	10
Morphine sulfate, sustained release	60	12	90	—
Oxycodone	15–30	6	30	—
Oxycodone, sustained release	15–30	12	30	—
Methadone[a]	30–60	6	20	10

[a]A dose ratio of 1:4 of oral methadone to oral morphine is used for oral morphine doses <90 mg/day. For doses of 90–300 mg, a ratio of 1:8 and >300 mg should use a ratio of 1:12 of oral methadone to oral morphine.

Incomplete cross-resistance may lead to unanticipated potency with a new agent. When converting large opioid doses, the initial dose should be halved to account for this reduced cross-resistance. If inadequate analgesia has led to the change in agents, then the new drug may be started at a nearly equivalent dose (Table 36-1).

Some medications will accumulate in renal insufficiency. These include codeine, tramadol (Ultram), and the active metabolites of meperidine (normeperidine) and morphine (morphine-6-glucoronide). Tramadol and normeperidine lower seizure threshold.

The **fentanyl** transdermal patch at 25 μg/hr is equivalent to 45–134 mg of controlled-release morphine/day. It takes 24 hrs to reach maximal activity, so previous pain medications must be continued through this period.

MANAGEMENT OF OPIOID-RELATED SIDE EFFECTS

General approaches to limit side effects include reducing doses by adding NSAIDs, changing opioids, changing route of administration, and providing symptomatic therapy.

Nausea/vomiting is usually caused by a direct effect on chemoreceptor trigger zone. However, it may be related to delayed gastric emptying, refractory constipation, or stool impaction.

• Various antiemetics include **phenothiazines, antihistamines, serotonin antagonists,** or **steroids. Metoclopramide (Reglan; 5–10 mg PO qAC)** is useful for postprandial nausea. **Meclizine (Antivert; 12.5–25 mg PO bid to tid)** helps with movement-associated nausea.
• Constipation and stool impaction must be diagnosed and treated if present.

Constipation

A bowel regimen containing a stool softener such as docusate (100 mg PO bid) and cathartic agent, such as bisacodyl (10 mg PO qd), should routinely accompany the analgesic regimen. Senokot (start at 2–4 tablets PO qd to bid) is often used prophylactically.

TABLE 36-2. COMMONLY USED ANALGESIC ADJUVANTS

Drug	Use
Tricyclic antidepressants	Neuropathic pain
Anticonvulsants	Neuropathic pain
Local anesthetics	Mucositis, postherpetic neuralgia
Capsaicin	Postherpetic neuralgia
Bisphosphonates	Osteolytic metastases
Corticosteroids	Mass effect, bony/parenchymal infiltration, neural compression

Patients may benefit from disimpaction. This may involve mineral oil, glycerin suppositories, or saline enemas.

After impaction is ruled out, osmotic laxatives, such as lactulose (15–30 mL PO q2–6h prn) or magnesium citrate (120 mL PO q4–6h prn), may be used.

Oral naloxone (Narcan) may be helpful in refractory cases.

Respiratory Depression

Respiratory depression may occur to an equal extent with equipotent doses of any pure opioid agonists when given systemically. Tolerance often develops rapidly, and most patients can tolerate mild respiratory depression (respiratory rate of 8–12). **Naloxone** (20–80 μg IV) may be given in repeated doses, as needed. The half-life of naloxone is shorter than most opioid analgesics.

See Chap. 48, Opioid Overdose and Withdrawal, for further information.

PAIN CONTROL ADJUVANTS

Adjuvants may be used for neuropathic pain to reduce opioid doses (Table 36-2).

Anticonvulsants commonly used for neuropathic pain include carbamazepine (Tegretol), phenytoin (Dilantin), valproate (Depacon), and gabapentin (Neurontin). Gabapentin has the fewest serious side effects and drug interactions.

Further information on cancer-related pain may be found at http://www.cancer-pain.org.

KEY POINTS TO REMEMBER

- The WHO guidelines recommend starting with acetaminophen and NSAIDs for pain control. Do not hesitate to control pain with opioids for fear of addiction, which is exceedingly rare among cancer patients.
- When initiating therapy with opioids, start with frequent dosing of short-acting agents to determine the daily amount of opioid needed to control pain, then change to longer-acting formulations.

REFERENCES

1. World Health Organization. Cancer pain relief and palliative care. (WHO Technical Report Series, 804). Geneva: WHO, 1990.
2. Kanner RM, Foley KM. Patterns of narcotic drug use in a cancer pain clinic. *Ann N Y Acad Sci* 1981;362:161.
3. Joranson DE, Ryan KM, Gilson AM, et al. Trends in medical use and abuse of opioid analgesics. *JAMA* 2000;283:1710.

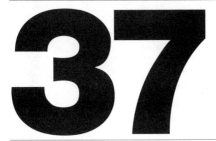

Perioperative Care of the Cancer Patient

Michael E. Lazarus

INTRODUCTION

Patients with cancer may present for surgery several times for a variety of procedures from major surgical resection to gastric or venous line placement. The patient's health stability at preoperative evaluation may be in a variable range from wellness to significant immunosuppression or cachexia.

CLINICAL PEARLS FOR SPECIFIC CANCERS

Breast Cancer

Tamoxifen, often used preoperatively, can result in preoperative nausea, emesis, dehydration, and rarely skin rash.

Patient anxiety associated with altered body image can be significant. Preoperative evaluation should focus on providing the patient and family with education to aid their understanding of the disease and reduce anxiety and fears.

Colorectal Cancer

Preoperative intravascular fluid deficits may have occurred secondary to bowel preparation and should be corrected to prevent hypotension. Patients with abdominal distention may have perioperative respiratory compromise and an increased incidence of aspiration.

Esophageal Cancer

Dehydration preoperatively, as well as cachexia, reflux esophagitis, and an increased incidence of aspiration, are all concerns. Patients should be evaluated for any evidence of tracheal compression whenever mediastinal lymphadenopathy is present.

Gastric Cancer

Anemia secondary to GI bleeding should be corrected. Pulmonary complications occur in 15% of patients, with a decrease in functional residual capacity, respiratory muscle weakness, and aspiration being the principal culprits.

Head and Neck Cancer

Associated cigarette smoking with underlying pulmonary disease should be evaluated. Perioperative morbidity includes cardiovascular events, cranial nerve injury, pneumothorax, chylothorax, vascular injury, and air embolus.

Intracranial Tumors

Evaluate for the presence of raised intracranial pressure, which usually presents with nausea, emesis, altered mental status, visual disturbance, and seizures.

Leukemia

Associated immunosuppression will increase the risk of infection, sepsis, interstitial pneumonia, and encephalopathy. Coagulation disorders and electrolyte disorders may also be present.

Lung Cancer

Management of associated COPD and cardiovascular disease is important.

Endobronchial obstruction with active pneumonia should be identified and treated. Atelectasis should also be minimized.

Pericardial effusion and superior vena cava syndrome should be considered in patients with distended neck veins, hypotension, and facial swelling.

In advanced disease, patients may have malnutrition and coagulopathies.

Electrolyte disorders could indicate underlying ectopic hormone secretion and other paraneoplastic disorders.

Pancreatic Cancer

Pancreatic cancer involves gastric outlet obstruction with abdominal pain and dehydration secondary to anorexia, nausea, and emesis. Bile duct obstruction may result in sepsis and liver dysfunction with associated coagulopathy.

Prostate Cancer

Prostate cancer occurs in a predominantly elderly population, with an increased likelihood of associated medical conditions. Patients who are receiving hormonal therapy may have an abnormally high liver metabolism, requiring adjustments in anesthesia management.

Renal Cancer

On occasion, a lesion or thrombus extends into the inferior vena cava. Portal vein obstruction can occur, causing coagulopathy, GI bleeding, and hepatic encephalopathy.

Thyroid Cancer

Tracheal obstruction may cause dyspnea, wheezing, and stridor. The esophagus may be compressed and partially obstructed. Assess the size of any mediastinal mass and potential tracheal compression.

KEY POINTS TO REMEMBER

- Recognize the location and size of tumors preoperatively, and be on the lookout for any evidence of adjacent mechanical complications postoperatively.
- Patients who have a history of heavy smoking (a common carcinogen) are also at risk for COPD.

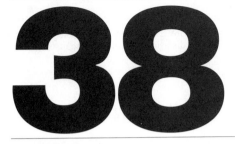

Neutropenic Fever

Erik R. Dubberke and
Christopher H. Kwoh

INTRODUCTION

Neutropenic fever is defined as a single temperature $\geq 38.3°C$ or a temperature $\geq 38°C$ over at least 1 hr in a patient with an absolute neutrophil count (ANC) $<500/mm^3$ or $<1000/mm^3$ with a predicted decline to $\leq 500/mm^3$. The onset of fever should be dated from the first day of the last cycle of chemotherapy, which allows estimation of the duration of neutropenia.

50–60% of febrile neutropenic patients have an established or occult infection, and >20% of patients with an ANC $<100/mm^3$ have bacteremia.

Common etiologic agents include various *Staphylococcus*, *Streptococcus*, *Enterococcus*, *Escherichia coli*, *Klebsiella*, *Pseudomonas*, and anaerobes.

Risk factors include a rapid decrease in the neutrophil count and protracted neutropenia (ANC <500 for >10 days). Chemotherapy-induced mucosal damage facilitates bacterial translocation from the gastrointestinal tract.

PRESENTATION

History

History should focus on subtle symptoms of infection. Even with severe bacterial infection, a neutropenic patient may be asymptomatic.

Exposure and recent hospitalization may aid in recognizing exposure to nosocomial infections.

Retrosternal burning pain suggests esophagitis (herpes simplex virus or *Candida*).

Physical Exam

Exam should focus on signs of infection at commonly affected sites, including the periodontium, pharynx, lower esophagus, lung, perineum and anus, skin lesions, bone marrow aspiration sites, the eye, vascular access sites, and tissue around the nails. Inflammation may be subtle to nonexistent because of the neutropenia.

Many physicians would recommend against performing a digital rectal exam, as it may induce more mucosal damage and allow further bacterial translocation.

Consider mucormycosis or aspergillus if there is sinus tenderness or ulcers.

If there is right lower quadrant tenderness, then suspect typhlitis, which may prompt anaerobic therapy.

Lab Evaluation

Perform CBC, liver function tests, serum chemistries, electrolytes, and renal function tests every 3 days.

Blood cultures ×2 from different sites, UA (and culture if pyuria, Foley catheter, or symptoms), and Gram stain and culture should be taken from any suspicious site. If the lesions are chronic, samples should be sent for fungal and atypical mycobacteria cultures.

If the patient has diarrhea, stool should be tested for *Clostridium difficile* toxin, stool culture, ova and parasites, bacterial pathogens, viruses, and protozoa.

CSF should be obtained only if there are signs or symptoms of CNS infection.

Imaging Evaluation

A chest x-ray should be obtained. Further imaging should be guided by clinical judgment. Many physicians have low thresholds for obtaining CT scans of the sinuses and noncontrast CT scans of the chest.

MANAGEMENT

Initial antibiotics should be given promptly in neutropenic patients because overwhelming sepsis can occur in a short period of time. The type, frequency, and antibiotic susceptibilities of the bacterial isolates found in similar patients at a particular institution should guide the initial antibiotic regimen.

- Only broad-spectrum, bactericidal, gram-negative coverage (antipseudomonal) has influenced mortality.
- Monotherapy regimens include carbapenems, ceftazidime (Fortaz; 1 g IV q8h adjusted for renal function), and cefepime (Maxipime; 1 g IV q12h adjusted for renal function). Quinolone monotherapy is not recommended.
- Duotherapy regimens include an aminoglycoside with an antipseudomonal penicillin or cephalosporin.
- No study has demonstrated striking differences in efficacy between monotherapy and multidrug combinations.
- Vancomycin (Vancocin) is indicated for initial therapy, along with appropriate gram-negative coverage, in patients with severe mucositis, prior quinolone prophylaxis, known colonization with oxacillin-resistant *Staphylococcus aureus* or cephalosporin-resistant *Pneumococcus*, obvious catheter-related infection, or hypotension. Empiric vancomycin should be discontinued if initial cultures are negative for gram-positive organisms after 3–4 days.

After three days, further treatment is determined by culture results, fever resolution, the ANC, the patient's risk stratification, and whether the patient's condition has deteriorated:

If a **pathogen** or site of infection is **identified,** then therapy is directed appropriately.

If **no pathogen** is identified, but the patient is **afebrile within 3 days,** then management depends on their level of risk:

- **Low risk:** if the patient is low risk ("clinically well" and ANC ≥ 100), then change to oral antibiotics. If ANC ≥ 500/mm^3 by day 7 and the patient remains stable and afebrile, then antibiotics can be discontinued. If the ANC <500/mm^3 by day 7 but the patient remains clinically well, then antibiotics should be continued until the patient is afebrile for 5–7 days.
- **High risk:** (ANC <100/mm^3, severe mucositis, or unstable vital signs). Continue antibiotics until leukocyte recovery has been present for at least 5 days.

If **no pathogen** is identified and **persistent fever** for first 3 days:

- Suggests a nonbacterial infection, a resistant bacterial infection, emergence of a secondary infection, inadequate tissue levels of antibiotic, drug fever, or infection at an avascular site.
- Reassess on day 4 and every 4–5 days if fever is persistent. This involves a thorough physical exam, chest and sinus radiographs, vascular catheter inspection, reculture of blood and specific sites of infection, and imaging of any organ suspected of infection. Special studies may be done for *Toxoplasma gondii,* herpes simplex virus, CMV, Epstein-Barr virus, enterovirus, enteric protozoa, *Mycobacterium tuberculosis,* nontuberculous mycobacteria, and *Chlamydia pneumoniae* if clinical features suggest any of these disease processes.

If reassessment does not reveal a cause of fever, then any of four management options can be pursued:

1. Stopping antibiotics if the ANC is >500/mm³ for 4–5 days and patient has no mucositis.
2. Continue current antibiotics if patient has no clinical deterioration and neutrophil recovery is expected in the next 5 days.
3. Change or add antibiotics if there is evidence of disease progression. Consider vancomycin if not already given.
4. Add amphotericin B (Amphocin, Fungizone). Perhaps one-third of neutropenic fevers not responsive in 1 wk have a fungal infection (*Candida* or aspergillus). Fluconazole (Diflucan) may be considered if in an institution with low candidal fluconazole resistance, low rates of mold infections, and no sinus or pulmonary disease. Consider a CT of the chest prior to therapy. Discontinue antifungal therapy after 2 wks if there are no lesions on exam, chest radiography, and CT of the abdomen.

Routine use of **antivirals** is not indicated. If skin or mucous membrane lesions are suggestive of herpes simplex virus or VZV, treatment with acyclovir (Zovirax; 5 mg/kg IV q8h) is indicated even if the patients are afebrile.

The routine use of granulocyte colony-stimulating factors (G-CSF) is not indicated because it does not affect mortality. It may decrease hospitalization time and decrease duration of neutropenia. Consider G-CSF with severe deterioration or expected prolonged neutropenia, or if no bone marrow recovery after 5 days.

Neutropenic patients should be on reverse isolation.

Consider rotating antibiotics through each lumen of multilumen catheters.

KEY POINTS TO REMEMBER

- Prompt empiric therapy is indicated in febrile neutropenic patients. Overwhelming sepsis may ensue in a matter of hours. The range of pathogens is quite wide, and initial therapy should also be broad, covering gram-positives, gram-negatives, and anaerobes.
- Consider empiric antifungals if febrile neutropenia persists after the first week or so.

REFERENCES AND SUGGESTED READINGS

Hughes WT, Armstrong D, Bodey GP, et al. 1997 guideline for the use of antimicrobial agents in neutropenic patients with unexplained fever. *Clin Infect Dis* 1997;25: 551–573.

Pizzo P. Management of fever in patients with cancer and treatment induced neutropenia. *N Engl J Med* 1993;328:1323–1332.

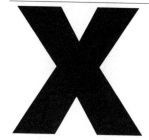

Endocrinology

Inpatient Diabetes Management

Christopher H. Kwoh and
Michael E. Lazarus

INTRODUCTION

Appropriate management of blood glucose levels in inpatient diabetics decreases infections, improves wound healing, and avoids diabetic ketoacidosis and hyperosmolar hyperglycemia. Importantly, appropriate management minimizes the risk of hypoglycemia.

The physician must anticipate difficulties with hyperglycemia from stress, as well as risk of hypoglycemia from bed rest, interrupted meal schedules, and inpatient dietary differences. It should be recognized that most of these changes are temporary, and discharge regimens should reflect anticipated outpatient conditions rather than being based on inpatient control.

Blood glucose goals as an inpatient are not well defined, and few studies are available to support various glucose targets.

- Many physicians set blood sugar goals to <180–200, which minimizes glycosuria and also seems to be the level at which wound healing and leukocyte function decline.
- The low end of blood sugar goal is typically set at approximately 100 with the belief by many physicians that the dangers of inpatient hypoglycemia outweigh the benefits of short-term strict treatment of hyperglycemia.
- One recent study suggests that glucose levels <120 instead of <200 may further reduce mortality in hyperglycemic (not necessarily diabetic) patients in surgical ICUs with prolonged hospitalizations.
- Many diabetologists argue for strict control of diabetes as an inpatient because it is an opportunity to fine tune medical management and stresses to the patient the importance of optimum control.

One important principle is that diabetics require both glucose (dietary or IV) and insulin to prevent catabolism and achieve a balance between hypo- and hyperglycemia.

Recognize the effect that diabetic gastroparesis or narcotics may have on decreasing oral bioavailability of inpatient medications (especially sulfonylureas for which timing is critical), and consider IV administration of the most important treatments.

MANAGEMENT OF INPATIENTS WHO ARE EATING

Provide a diet that resembles the patient's outpatient eating habits unless the patient is expected to make significant changes in the diet at discharge. Include late-night snacks if typically eaten by the patient.

For inpatients with **insulin-dependent diabetes** who are **eating:**

- Continue their outpatient regimens with anticipated supplements owing to stress response and inactivity.
- Plan procedures requiring the patient to be NPO for the early morning.

For inpatients with **non–insulin-dependent diabetes** who are **eating:**

- Continue outpatient regimens and supplement short-acting insulin as needed. Reassess the response of non–insulin-dependent diabetes patients to insulin because many of them will require very large amounts to control hyperglycemia.

- If patients are not well controlled on PO agents, recognize the possibility that they have achieved secondary failure of PO diabetic agents and may require a change to full insulin therapy.

For algorithmic short-acting insulin supplements:

- Frequently, "sliding-scale" regimens are ordered to supplement regular insulin based on blood glucose values. Most endocrinologists frown on this practice because it frequently results in poor blood sugar control and is not physiologic.
- Many diabetologists prefer adjustments based on premeal values by adding more regular insulin with the meal and, if blood sugars are very high, administering the insulin with a greater lead time (30–45 mins before meal instead of 15 mins). This requires premeal and bedtime blood glucose assessments.

PREOPERATIVE DIABETES EVALUATION AND MANAGEMENT

The preoperative evaluation of the diabetic patient should focus on the long-term complications of diabetes (microvascular, macrovascular, and neuropathic), which may potentiate risk.

Particular attention should be given to assessment of cardiovascular and renal function abnormalities, which may be undiagnosed.

Diabetic autonomic neuropathy may further complicate and prolong the postoperative recovery phase and has been associated with excess nonsurgical mortality.

It is important to note that the effects of antecedent metabolic control independent of the extent of the chronic complications of diabetes are not well established, and few recommendations can be made regarding the outcome of surgical patients with chronically poor diabetes control and/or those whose glucose levels have been rapidly normalized preoperatively.

Little evidence exists to substantiate obtaining near optimal blood glucose control preoperatively, but it **is** important to optimize the patient's nutritional status preoperatively.

Management of diabetes for the patient who is NPO for a short procedure or test is summarized in Table 39-1. **Consider treating patients with insulin-dependent diabe-**

TABLE 39-1. MANAGEMENT OF DIABETES MELLITUS FOR SHORT PROCEDURES

Timing of procedure	Diabetic regimen	Recommended management strategy
Early morning	Any	Delay diabetic agent dosing.
Late morning	Oral agents	Hold oral agent on day of surgery. Supplemental insulin (short acting) may be used to achieve tighter control.
Late morning	Single-dose insulin (Ultralente/Lantus)	Give two-thirds of total daily dose preoperatively.
Late morning	2–3 doses of insulin daily	Give one-half of the total morning dose of long-acting insulin.
Late morning	Multiple doses of short-acting insulin	Give one-third of morning dose.
Afternoon	Oral agents	Hold oral agent.
Afternoon	Single-dose insulin	Give one-half of daily dose.
Afternoon	2–3 doses of insulin daily	One-third of total morning dose.
Afternoon	Multiple doses of short-acting insulin	Give one-third of the morning and lunch time doses.
Any	Insulin pump	Continue basal rate only.

tes who will be NPO from midnight to mid- or late afternoon as if they are undergoing major surgery (see later).

Diabetics who are undergoing major surgery or who will be NPO for >24 hrs require both calories and insulin to minimize ketosis and catabolism.

- Many physicians recommend 5–10 g glucose/hr (500–1000 kcals/day), which will, on average, require about 0.5–1 U insulin/hr. D_{10} (one-fourth NS) at 75 cc/hr provides 7.5 g glucose/hr.
- 5 g glucose/hr often results in ketosis 12-hr postprocedure, whereas 10 g/hr appears protective.
- Consider increasing glucose rates if ketonuria develops (do urine dipstick for ketones q24h).
- Adjust insulin administration based on glucose levels. IV drips are easiest to manage. Check hourly blood glucose levels for several hours until stable and slowly taper off glucose checks to every few hours.
- Anticipate that type II diabetics will typically require much higher doses of insulin than type I diabetics. Select the initial rate based on daily insulin injections.
- Beware of resultant hypokalemia with insulin/glucose infusions and consider prophylactic replacement or include KCl in the IV fluids.
- Continue the glucose and insulin drips through the first postsurgical meal until it is clear that the food is tolerated. Administer SC insulin as appropriate for the subsequent meal.

MANAGEMENT OF GLUCOCORTICOID-INDUCED DIABETES MELLITUS

Many patients with mild glucose intolerance may develop hyperglycemia with the initiation of glucocorticoid therapy.

Nondiabetics who experience blood glucose levels 140–200 shortly after initiation of high-dose glucocorticoids may be observed, because beta cell adaptation may correct the metabolic derangement in 1–2 wks. If normoglycemia is not obtained, then therapy is indicated. Therapy should be initiated in patients with glucose levels >200.

Poorly controlled diabetics starting glucocorticoid therapy should have anticipatory increases in diabetic therapy. Even well-controlled diabetics receiving more than the equivalent of 20 mg of prednisone daily should have a 20% increase in their insulin doses or advancement of their oral therapy.

The hyperglycemic effects of oral glucocorticoids should remit 48 hrs after cessation of therapy. IM and intraarticular glucocorticoids may have effects lasting up to 10 days.

KEY POINTS TO REMEMBER

- Physicians must anticipate that patients under significant physiologic stress or receiving glucocorticoids may have worsening hyperglycemia or increasing insulin requirements.
- Sliding scale insulin may prevent severe hyperglycemia but rarely provides good glucose control. One must anticipate insulin needs before the patient becomes hyperglycemic.
- Diabetics who are NPO need both calories and insulin to prevent ketosis and catabolism. This may be best provided by continuous glucose infusions and continuing a low-dose insulin regimen while NPO.

REFERENCES AND SUGGESTED READINGS

Alberti K. Diabetes and surgery. *Anesthesiology* 1991;74:209–211.
Hirsch IB. Role of insulin in management of surgical patients with diabetes mellitus. *Diabetes Care* 1990;13:980–991.
Hirsch IB. Inpatient management of adults with diabetes. *Diabetes Care* 1995;18(6):870–878.

Jacober SJ, Sowers JR. An update on perioperative management of diabetes. *Arch Intern Med* 1999;159:2405–2411.

Marhoffer W. Impairment of PMN function and metabolic control of diabetes. *Diabetes Care* 1992;15:256–259.

McMurry JF. Wound healing and diabetes mellitus. *Surg Clin North Am* 1984;64:769–778.

Watts NB. Perioperative management of diabetes mellitus: steady-state glucose control with bedside algorithm for insulin adjustment. *Diabetes Care* 1987;10:722–728.

40

Thyroid Diseases

Jennifer M. Quartarolo

HYPERTHYROIDISM

Hyperthyroidism is defined by increased circulating levels of T_4 and/or T_3. T_4 is a prohormone, which is peripherally monodeiodinated to the active hormone T_3. Hyperthyroidism is ten times more common in women than men.

Excess thyroid hormone has also been associated with osteoporosis, cardiac arrhythmias (especially atrial fibrillation), angina, and heart failure.

Differential Diagnosis

The etiologies of increased circulating hormone can be broken down into disorders involving increased production of T_4 (Table 40-1), increased release of preformed hormone (Table 40-2) from the thyroid gland, or exogenous sources of T_4.

Consider the possibility of **euthyroid sick syndrome** in patients with abnormal thyroid function tests and acute illness (see Euthyroid Sick Syndrome).

Presentation

History
Symptoms may include weight loss, heat intolerance, increased sweating, anxiety, insomnia, palpitations, dyspnea, diarrhea, tremor, or oligomenorrhea. Symptoms are often less pronounced in elderly patients (apathetic hyperthyroidism). Take a thorough medication history because several medications alter thyroid hormone physiology (Table 40-3).

Thyroid storm is an overwhelming presentation of thyrotoxicosis, often presenting with fever, delirium, and systemic symptoms such as nausea and vomiting. This often presents in patients with underlying hyperthyroidism in which additional T_4 release is precipitated by severe stress such as surgery, infection, stroke, diabetic ketoacidosis, parturition, iodine contrast administration, or thyroid medication withdrawal. It may also be seen in patients being treated for hyperthyroidism who are noncompliant with their medications or are on inadequate regimens.

Physical Exam
Vital signs may reveal tachycardia (sometimes with atrial fibrillation and an irregularly irregular pulse) or HTN. Fever, hypotension, or delirium suggest thyroid storm.

Common exam findings include proptosis, lid lag, smooth/warm skin, an infiltrative dermopathy (specific to Graves' disease), onycholysis, proximal muscle weakness, and tremor. A brisk uptake and release of the deep tendon reflexes are commonly found and may be best examined at the Achilles tendon.

Do a good thyroid exam to feel for nodules, enlargement, or tenderness. Also listen and feel for a bruit over the thyroid, which may occur in Graves' disease.

Lab Evaluation
Associated lab abnormalities may include an elevated alkaline phosphatase, normochromic normocytic anemia, decreased high-density lipoprotein and total cholesterol, hypercalcemia, and elevated transaminases.

TABLE 40-1. DISORDERS OF INCREASED THYROXINE PRODUCTION

Disorder	Prevalence	Mechanism	Clinical course
Graves' disease	Up to 80% of cases in United States	Antibodies to thyrotropin (TSH) receptor	Chronic, waxing and waning, some remissions
Toxic adenoma or multinodular goiter	Higher in middle-aged and elderly	Increased production of hormone independent of TSH	Chronic, unremitting
Iodine-induced	—	Secondary to iodine load or amiodarone	Self-limiting
Central/secondary	Rare (<5% of total cases)	Hypersecretion of TSH by pituitary adenoma	Chronic
Molar pregnancy or hyperemesis gravidarum	Rare	Hypersecretion of hCG	Self-limiting

The TSH is used for initial screening, followed by free T_4 (FT_4) ± free T_3 if TSH is abnormal or if there is high suspicion of hyperthyroidism. See Table 40-4 for patterns.

In thyroid storm, there may be an elevated WBC count and associated adrenal insufficiency. Consider a Cortrosyn stimulation test to test the adrenal axis (see Chap. 41, Adrenal Insufficiency).

Imaging Evaluation: Radioactive Iodine Uptake Nuclear Scan
Functioning or hyperproducing areas of thyroid are seen on the scan, whereas nonfunctioning or "cold" areas are not visualized. The patterns may suggest diffuse hyperfunction or hyperfunctioning nodules. Low uptake is seen with preformed release or exogenous sources of T_4.

Management

Pharmacologic Therapy
Beta blockers provide symptomatic relief of tachycardia and tremor. Titrate to effect starting at a low dose [e.g., propranolol (Inderal), 20 mg PO tid, or atenolol (Tenormin), 25 mg PO qd]. Consider adding digoxin (Lanoxin) for atrial fibrillation.

Antithyroid thionamide drugs [propylthiouracil (PTU; start 100 mg PO tid unless severly symptomatic, in which case 150 mg PO tid is appropriate) and methimazole (Tapazole; 15–60 mg PO per day to start depending on degree of symptomatology)] may also be provided. Follow-up should be monthly with monitoring of FT_4 until the patient is euthyroid. Thereafter, follow TSH q3–6mos.

TABLE 40-2. DISORDERS OF INCREASED PREFORMED HORMONE RELEASE

Disorder	Prevalence	Mechanism	Course
Subacute granulomatous thyroiditis (de Quervain's)	Female to male ratio: 3–6:1 Average age at onset: 30–50 yrs	Immune-mediated, likely secondary to virus	Self-limiting with full recovery after 4–6 wks
Chronic lymphocytic thyroiditis (Hashimoto's)	Highest in middle-aged and elderly	Autoimmune, associated with antithyroid antibodies	Chronic, unremitting Most progress to hypothyroidism

TABLE 40-3. DRUGS THAT AFFECT THYROID FUNCTION

Mechanism	Drugs
Decreased TSH secretion	Dopamine, glucocorticoids, octreotide
Altered thyroid hormone secretion	
Decreased secretion	**Lithium**, iodide, **amiodarone**, aminoglutethimide
Increased secretion	Iodide, amiodarone
Decreased T$_4$ absorption	Colestipol, cholestyramine, aluminum hydroxide, ferrous sulfate, sucralfate
Altered T$_4$ and T$_3$ transport in serum	
Increased serum TBG	Estrogens, tamoxifen, heroin, methadone, mitotane, fluorouracil
Decreased serum TBG	Androgens, anabolic steroids, slow-release nicotinic acid, glucocorticoids
Displacement from protein-binding sites	Furosemide, fenclofenac, mefenamic acid, salicylates
Altered T$_4$ and T$_3$ metabolism	
Increased hepatic metabolism	Phenobarbital, rifampin, phenytoin, carbamazepine
Decreased conversion of T$_4$ to T$_3$	Propylthiouracil, amiodarone, beta blockers, glucocorticoids
Associated with transient thyroiditis	Interleukin-2
Development of antiperoxidase Ab	Interferon alpha

TBG, thyroid-binding globulin.
Adapted from Surks M, Sievert R. Drugs and thyroid function. *N Engl J Med* 1995;333(25):1688–1694.

Definitive Therapy (Ablative Therapy)
Radioactive iodine ablation is the definitive therapy for Graves' disease, toxic adenomas, and multinodular toxic goiters. Recurrence rates are high, and follow-up for return of symptoms and posttherapy hypothyroidism is important.

Subtotal thyroidectomy may be performed if the previously mentioned therapies are contraindicated or there is significant mass effect from goiter.

Preoperative Management
Patients with well-controlled hyperthyroidism have no significant increased operative risk but should receive perioperative beta blockers. Patients who have uncontrolled

TABLE 40-4. PATTERNS OF THYROID FUNCTION TESTS WITH HYPERTHYROIDISM

TSH	Free T$_4$	Free T$_3$	Thyroid function
↔	↔	↔	Euthyroid
Increased	Increased	Increased	Central hyperthyroidism
Decreased	Increased	Increased	Primary hyperthyroidism
Decreased	↔	↔	Subclinical hyperthyroidism

↔, unchanged.

hyperthyroidism are at high risk for perioperative thyroid storm. Elective surgery should be delayed until they are euthyroid. If surgery cannot be delayed, then many clinicians treat preoperatively with a loading dose of antithyroid medication, stress-dose steroids, iopanoic acid, and beta blockade with the aid of an endocrinologist.

Thyroid Storm

Thyroid storm requires urgent therapy. Give liberal IV fluids and glucose, and consider therapy in an ICU setting. To decrease T_4 levels, one may provide thionamides (e.g., propylthiouracil, 200–250 mg q4h PO or per rectum) followed 2–3 hrs later by high-dose iodinated medications (e.g., iopanoic acid, 1 g q8h for 1 day, then 500 mg PO bid).

Provide stress-dose steroids, which may treat an underlying adrenal insufficiency as well as decreasing peripheral conversion of T_4 to T_3.

Beta blockers should be strongly considered (e.g., propranolol, 20 mg PO tid and titrate to effect).

HYPOTHYROIDISM

Hypothyroidism is defined as deficient secretion of T_4 by the thyroid. The majority of cases occur in women and the elderly. Deficient secretion of T_4 can result from impaired TSH stimulation of the thyroid gland or impairment of T_4 production or release. The vast majority of cases are primary in origin (Table 40-5).

Secondary or tertiary causes are rare and include pituitary macroadenoma, empty sella syndrome, pituitary infarction, radiation induced, or postsurgical.

TABLE 40-5. CAUSES OF PRIMARY HYPOTHYROIDISM

Disorder	Prevalence	Mechanism	Clinical course
Hashimoto's thyroiditis	Most common cause in iodine sufficient areas	Antithyroid antibodies (antithyroglobulin and antiperoxidase)	May have transient increase in T_4 Most progress to subclinical or overt hypothyroidism
Iatrogenic hypothyroidism	Second most common cause in United States	Destruction or removal of thyroid follicular cells after treatment for hyperthyroidism	Chronic
Iodine deficiency	Most common cause worldwide, rare in the United States	Inhibition of hormone synthesis	Chronic if iodine deficiency not corrected
Subacute (de Quervain's) thyroiditis	Exact prevalence not known	Postviral immune-mediated	Self-limiting May have transient increase in T_4 followed by decrease in T_4 Full recovery after 4–6 wks
Postpartum thyroiditis	5–9% of postpartum women	Associated with antiperoxidase Ab	Usually decrease in T_4 is transient but may be permanent in up to 25–30%

Presentation

History

Symptoms may include fatigue, weight gain, depression, cold intolerance, hoarseness (with a compressive goiter), constipation, or menorrhagia. Most signs and symptoms have an insidious onset. Inquire about anginal symptoms or coronary artery disease because therapy for hypothyroidism may worsen cardiac ischemia.

In its most severe form, it is called myxedema coma, often presenting with hypotension, heart failure, and altered mental status. A medication history is essential, because thyroid hormone physiology may be altered by several medications (Table 40-3).

Physical Exam

Findings may include slight bradycardia, goiter (painful in subacute thyroiditis), lateral eyebrow thinning, dry skin, myxedema skin changes (with severe disease), muscle weakness, pericardial or pleural effusions, and slowed relaxation of deep tendon reflexes. Hypothermia, bradypnea, depressed mental status, and ileus may all be seen with myxedema coma.

Lab Evaluation

Associated abnormalities may include hypercholesterolemia (increased low-density lipoprotein and total cholesterol, reduction in high-density lipoprotein), mild normochromic normocytic anemia, hyponatremia, and increased creatine kinase and LDH. The ECG may show T wave flattening on inversions. In severe hypothyroidism, one often sees small voltages on the ECG.

For thyroid function tests, TSH is used as the first test for initial screening, followed by FT_4 if the TSH is high or there is a suspicion of central hypothyroidism. T_3 does not have a role in diagnosis. TSH is elevated in primary hypothyroidism. A combination of low TSH and low FT_4 is seen in central hypothyroidism.

Antithyroid antibodies (antiperoxidase most specific) can confirm a diagnosis of autoimmune thyroiditis.

Consider testing the adrenal axis with a cortrosyn stimulation test.

Management

Levothyroxine (Levoxine, Levoxyl, Synthroid) is the recommended drug:

- The therapeutic dose is generally 1.6–1.7 μg/kg PO daily. Start therapy at 50–100 μg/day with the lower dose used for the elderly. In patients with coronary artery disease, a lower starting dose of 25 μg/day PO is recommended, as replacement of T_4 can precipitate cardiac ischemia. Changing formulations of levothyroxine may result in alterations in control of hypothyroidism.
- TSH should be monitored at monthly intervals until the patient is euthyroid. Dose changes should not be made at <6-wk intervals.

Perioperative Management

Patients with mild hypothyroidism do well perioperatively. Those with severe hypothyroidism should have elective surgery delayed until they are symptomatically improved. If surgery cannot be delayed, then they may be treated preoperatively with a loading dose of levothyroxine, 200–500 μg PO followed by 100 μg/day for several days. Afterwards, they may be switched to a maintenance dose. Symptoms of hypothyroidism and the magnitude of TSHs should help guide selection of the loading dose. Remember that the effects of levothyroxine last several days, and the cumulative levels will build up rapidly.

Myxedema coma requires more urgent management:

- Provide supportive measures, including ICU monitoring and IV fluids.
- Check a random cortisol to evaluate for associated adrenal insufficiency. Stress dose steroids are generally given.

- Thyroid hormone is replaced with levothyroxine, 200–500 μg PO loading dose, then 100 μg for several days before changing to maintenance dose.

EUTHYROID SICK SYNDROME

Euthyroid sick syndrome is defined as changes in thyroid function tests associated with systemic illness, surgery, or fasting. Signs and symptoms of thyroid dysfunction are absent. There is some controversy regarding this term, as whether or not these patients are truly euthyroid is unclear. This is one of the most common causes of thyroid test abnormalities in the inpatient.

Lab Evaluation

Typical changes seen with nonthyroidal illness may include the following:

- **TSH levels may be low,** although undetectable levels usually indicate primary thyroid disease. A transient increase may be seen during recovery from illness.
- **Low serum T_3** is seen in up to 70% of hospitalized patients. The serum free T_3 is usually decreased by approximately 40%.
- **Low serum T_4,** usually with a **normal free T_4.**

Management

Studies have not consistently indicated a benefit from T_4 or T_3 supplementation in this patient population (may increase mortality).

Follow-up (preferably after recovery from acute illness) to confirm abnormal values should be completed before initiating treatment.

KEY POINTS TO REMEMBER

- Symptoms of thyroid disease may be nonspecific or vague, especially in the elderly.
- Appropriate preoperative management and surveillance of hyperthyroid patients will minimize the risk of thyroid storm.
- Many patients have abnormalities in their thyroid function tests during acute illness. Resist the temptation to treat cases of probable euthyroid sick syndrome.

REFERENCES AND SUGGESTED READINGS

Baeza A. Rapid preoperative preparation in hyperthyroidism. *Clin Endocrinol* 1991;35:439–442.

Burman KD, Wartofsky L. Thyroid Function in the intensive care unit. *Crit Care Clin* 2001;17:43–57.

Chopra IJ. Euthyroid sick syndrome: Is it a misnomer? *J Clin Endocrinol Metab* 1997;82:329–333.

Ladenson PW. Complications of surgery in hypothyroid patients. *Am J Med* 1984; 77:261.

Ladenson PW, Singer PA, Ain KB, et al. American Thyroid Association guidelines for detection of thyroid dysfunction. 2000;160:1573–1575.

Lukowsky GI. Preoperative treatment of patients with thyrotoxicosis. *Am J Surg* 1982;147:766.

Ringel MD. Management of hypothyroidism and hyperthyroidism in the intensive care unit. *Crit Care Clin* 2001;17:59–74.

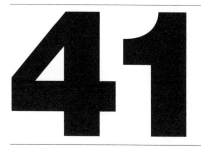

Adrenal Insufficiency

Jennifer M. Quartarolo

INTRODUCTION

Adrenal insufficiency is defined as inadequate production of cortisol ± aldosterone by the adrenal gland. Primary adrenal insufficiency refers to decreased production due to dysfunction of the adrenal gland. Secondary insufficiency occurs secondary to interruption of hypothalamic-pituitary-adrenal axis leading to decreased adrenal gland function. See Table 41-1 for differential diagnosis.

PRESENTATION

History

Acute adrenal insufficiency often presents in inpatients as a result of undiagnosed chronic insufficiency with decompensation secondary to physiologic stressors. **Obtaining a thorough medication history is essential** to rule out recent or chronic steroid use. Patients with AIDS are at high risk for adrenal failure.

Symptoms occur as a consequence of decreased levels of cortisol ± aldosterone and may include:

- Fatigue/weakness/lightheadedness
- Anorexia
- Weight loss
- Myalgias
- Nausea/vomiting
- Abdominal pain

Autoimmune adrenal insufficiency is frequently associated with other autoimmune disorders such as type I diabetes mellitus, Hashimoto's thyroiditis, vitiligo, and others. Additional symptoms in rarer cases of pituitary dysfunction or mass may include amenorrhea, cold intolerance, headache, or visual field loss.

History of recent abdominal surgery or anticoagulation should increase suspicion of adrenal hemorrhage. Overwhelming infection with *Pseudomonas*, **meningococcus,** or **pneumococcus** may result in hemorrhagic necrosis of the adrenal gland (Waterhouse-Friderichsen syndrome).

Physical Exam

Orthostatic hypotension, shock, fever, or hypothermia may be evident. Auricular cartilage calcifications may be present in chronic adrenal insufficiency. Abdominal tenderness may be present. There may be hyperpigmentation (only in primary adrenal failure secondary to increased ACTH), loss of axillary or pubic hair (especially in women), and signs of volume depletion.

Classic signs of adrenal insufficiency may be present but are nonspecific, so a high level of clinical suspicion is critical.

TABLE 41-1. CAUSES OF ADRENAL INSUFFICIENCY

Primary	Secondary
Autoimmune adrenalitis[a]	Suppression of gland secondary to chronic glucocorticoid use[a]
Adrenal hemorrhage	
Infiltrative disease (amyloidosis, malignancy)	Pituitary infection (CMV, toxoplasmosis)
Adrenal infection (tuberculosis, fungal, histoplasma, CMV)	Pituitary tumor or infarction (Sheehan's)
Medications[b]	
AIDS	

[a]Most common etiologies.
[b]Several medications may interrupt adrenal function or change cortisol metabolism, including ketoconazole (Nizoral), rifampin, phenytoin (Dilantin), opiates, and megestrol (Megace).

Lab Evaluation

Primary adrenal failure (secondary to aldosterone deficiency) may present with hyperkalemia (less common in presence of vomiting or diarrhea), urine Na >20 mEq/L, and a non–anion gap metabolic acidosis.

Primary and secondary failure (due to glucocorticoid deficiency) may present with hyponatremia, fasting hypoglycemia, normocytic anemia, hypercalcemia (mild in <10%), lymphocytosis, and/or eosinophilia.

Cortrosyn Stimulation Test
The cortrosyn stimulation test assesses the ability of the adrenal gland to respond to ACTH.

- Method: 250 μg IV or IM corticotropin given, cortisol levels measured at baseline, 30 mins, and 60 mins after injection. Some clinicians only measure at 30 mins.
- Peak cortisol levels of >20 μg/dL are normal and essentially rule out adrenal insufficiency. In the setting of severe acute illness, some use a threshold up to 34 μg /dL.

ACTH Level
An ACTH level is useful in **differentiating primary vs. secondary causes.** ACTH should be elevated in primary causes and markedly decreased in secondary causes.

Morning Cortisol Level
A morning cortisol level is useful in diagnosing insufficiency only if levels are very low (<3 μg/dL). In severe illness, levels <5 μg/dL are consistent with insufficiency. **The sensitivity of morning cortisol levels in diagnosing adrenal insufficiency is very low.** Levels are frequently elevated in acutely ill patients, although the patient still may be unable to mount an appropriate response to increased stress.

Pituitary Function Tests
Pituitary function tests are useful if there is suspicion of pituitary dysfunction. Consider serum T_4, TSH, or testosterone (in men).

Imaging Evaluation

Abdominal CT scan may be obtained to rule out adrenal hemorrhage. A head CT or MRI of the brain may be obtained if there is suspicion of pituitary mass or infarction.

MANAGEMENT

Patients with known disease or chronic steroid use should be treated empirically in situations of stress (acute illness, perioperatively, injury) with high-dose hydrocortisone. This is most important in patients receiving supraphysiologic doses (prednisone, >20 mg/day) for >1 mo in the preceding year. Stress doses should be two to three times baseline dose depending on the stressor. Some physicians give 25–50 mg hydrocortisone IV (Cortef, Hydrocortone) q8h for 1–3 days and then taper to the baseline dose.

Acute adrenal crisis is a medical emergency, and **therapy should be initiated immediately if clinical suspicion is high.** Therapy should include the following:

- Aggressive IV fluid hydration with D_5NS to support BP and correct hypoglycemia and/or hyponatremia.
- Hydrocortisone, 100 mg IV q8h, slowly tapered over several days. If the diagnosis of adrenal insufficiency is not established, then one may replace hydrocortisone with dexamethasone, which does not interfere with cortisol measurements until Cortrosyn testing has been completed.

Long-term maintenance therapy for primary adrenal sufficiency should include prednisone (2.5–5 mg PO bid) or hydrocortisone (20–25 mg IV divided bid), along with mineralocorticoid repletion with fludrocortisone (Florinef) (0.05–0.3 mg PO qd). Doses are adjusted based on correction of symptoms and electrolyte abnormalities.

Patients with established adrenal insufficiency should be provided with medical alert bracelets identifying their diagnosis.

KEY POINTS TO REMEMBER

- Symptoms may be vague and nonspecific. Maintain a high degree of suspicion and have a low threshold to test the adrenal axis. The Cortrosyn stimulation test is a good screening test.
- Provide stress-dose steroids to patients with adrenal insufficiency or who have received long-term steroids.

REFERENCES AND SUGGESTED READINGS

Cousin D. Corticosteroid supplementation for adrenal insufficiency. *JAMA* 2002;287:236–240.

Oeklers W. Adrenal insufficiency. *N Engl J Med* 1996;335:1206–1212.

Shenker Y, Skatrud JB. Adrenal insufficiency in critically ill patients. *Am J Resp Crit Care Med* 2001;163(7):1520–1523.

Zaloga GP, Marik P. Hypothalamic-pituitary-adrenal insufficiency. *Crit Care Clin* 2001;17(1):25–41.

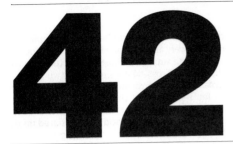

Approach to the Adrenal Incidentaloma

Christopher H. Kwoh

INTRODUCTION

Adrenal incidentalomas are found in approximately 0.5% of abdominal imaging performed for other reasons and in approximately 3% of patients at autopsy. The distribution of resultant pathologic diagnoses widely varies among studies. The medical consultant is often called to evaluate an adrenal mass found on abdominal imaging on the surgical service.

DIFFERENTIAL DIAGNOSIS

Approximately 85% of incidentalomas are nonfunctioning adenomas. Approximately 6% are secreting adenomas, with cortisol the most commonly identified and Conn's syndrome making up <1% of incidentalomas. In patients **without** known cancer, 2–3% are metastatic lesions (usually lung cancer; less commonly renal cell, breast, and melanoma). Pheochromocytoma is present in approximately 5%. Primary adrenocortical cancer is exceedingly rare, making up 1/10,000 of lesions <6 cm and perhaps 35% of lesions >6 cm.

PRESENTATION

History

Subtle signs of cortisol excess may be present in "early Cushing's syndrome" presenting as an incidentaloma without overt symptoms.

The triad of HTN, headache, and sweating makes pheochromocytoma a likely diagnosis. Its absence makes it an exceedingly unlikely diagnosis.

The presence of hypokalemia in incidentaloma gives a probability of Conn's syndrome of 6%. With HTN alone, it is 2.5%. If both are present, there is a 20% chance of Conn's syndrome.

Evidence of another primary malignancy should be sought from the history. Also look for evidence of nonclassic congenital adrenal hyperplasia, which sometimes presents as an adrenal mass in adulthood. Family history of adrenal tumors, multiple endocrine neoplasia syndromes, or other familial pheochromocytoma syndromes should be inquired about.

Lab Evaluation

Recommendations for screening evaluation by Ross and Copeland have been widely cited [1,2]. These were formulated in an era before MRI evaluation became commonplace.

All patients should have baseline electrolytes, glucose, and 24-hr urine cortisol. Depending on history, patients should have urinary catecholamines, vanillylmandelic acid, and metanephrines to evaluate for pheochromocytoma.

Pheochromocytoma should be ruled out before surgical or fine-needle manipulation of the adrenal is considered.

HTN patients should have matched aldosterone-renin levels performed (some argue that this should be done universally).

One should consider serum testosterone in women with evidence of hirsutism and estrogen levels in men with signs of feminization.

Characteristically, early Cushing's syndrome will have normal 24-hr urine and 8 A.M. serum cortisols, but without circadian rhythms. 10 P.M. cortisol may be elevated and low- and high-dose dexamethasone suppression tests will be positive. Since pituitary Cushing's disease is not a consideration, some physicians have skipped directly to the high-dose dexamethasone test.

Some recommend evaluating baseline and stimulated 17-hydroxyprogesterone levels to rule out nonclassic congenital adrenal hyperplasia.

Adrenocortical cancer is suggested by elevated 24-hr urinary 17-ketosteroids (which is also elevated in testosterone and estrogen producing tumors.) Normal urinary 17-ketosteroids and 17-hydroxycorticosteroids make a diagnosis of adrenocortical cancer highly unlikely.

Imaging Evaluation

The size of the lesion may aid in the eventual therapeutic options. Primary adrenal cancer is exceedingly rare in tumors <5 cm, and most adrenal carcinomas are >6 cm. Most benign lesions are <3 cm.

Lesions on MRI that are lipid rich are likely functioning (and therefore benign), with a reported sensitivity of nearly 100% and specificity of 81% for detecting adenomas [3]. Importantly, a significant number of lipid-poor masses will still be benign.

CT scan is less predictive of malignant vs. benign lesions, but typically benign lesions have attenuation < +10 Hounsfield and a rapid washout, whereas malignant lesions enhance at > +30 Hounsfield [4].

Metaiodobenzylguanidine scintigraphy has a high specificity for pheochromocytoma.

Tissue Evaluation

Fine-needle biopsy may be used to confirm metastatic disease. Because of the risk of seeding cancer cells if a primary adrenal malignancy is suspected, surgical exploration is indicated.

MANAGEMENT

The appropriate management of adrenal masses is not well defined.

Surgical excision should be performed for **any hormone-secreting mass or any mass that is large.** The size cutoff varies, but certainly masses >6 cm should be removed. Many clinicians would remove masses >5 cm, and some would remove masses >3 cm. Any rapidly growing tumor or complex-appearing tumor should also be removed.

Tumors of **3–6 cm** should be further characterized radiographically to determine whether they are likely malignant or benign. If the tumor is potentially malignant, most physicians would remove it. Some have recommended removal of an incidentaloma of this size in patients <50 yrs regardless of the appearance on MRI.

If a tumor is **<3 cm** and not hormone producing, then nuclear imaging or MRI should be performed to determine whether it is potentially malignant. If it is lipid rich, then no further follow-up is necessary. If it is potentially malignant, then it should be followed for change in size every 6 mos for up to 2 yrs. Any significant increase in size should lead to surgical excision. Some suggest repeating pheochromocytoma evaluation before surgical removal of an enlarging lesion.

KEY POINTS TO REMEMBER

- Adrenal tumors are very common, and the vast majority of them are benign nonfunctioning adenomas. It is the role of the medical consultant to identify tumors that are producing active hormones and those that are malignant.
- All patients with adrenal masses should have an evaluation for Cushing's syndrome. Further evaluation should be based on history, physical exam, and imaging findings.

SUGGESTED READING

Sutton MG. Prevalence of clinically unsuspected pheochromocytoma: a review of a 50 yr autopsy series. *Mayo Clin Proc* 1981;56:354–360.

REFERENCES

1. Copeland PM. The incidentally discovered adrenal mass. *Ann Intern Med* 1983;98:940–945.
2. Ross NS. Hormonal evaluation of the patient with an incidentally discovered adrenal mass. *N Engl J Med* 1990;323:1401–1405.
3. Korobkin M. Characterization of adrenal masses with chemical shift and gadolinium enhanced imaging. *Radiology* 1995;197:414–418.
4. Korobkin M. Delayed enhanced CT for differentiation of benign from malignant adrenal masses. *Radiology* 1996;200:737–742.

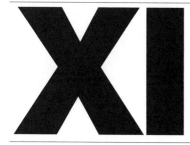

XI

Rheumatology

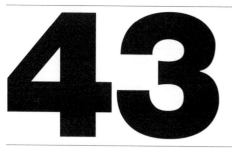

Approach to the Patient with Positive Antinuclear Antibodies

Jennifer M. Quartarolo

INTRODUCTION

ANA are autoantibodies that target nucleic acids and nucleoproteins. They are most useful in the evaluation for suspected SLE because >95% of SLE patients have a positive ANA of >1:160. **The ANA is not specific** for SLE or other rheumatologic disease; therefore, they should not be ordered unless clinical suspicion of disease exists:

- Specificity increases with rising titers (>1:160).
- One study reveals up to 30% of middle-aged patients may have positive titers of 1:40 and approximately 5% have 1:160 [1]. Thus, the majority of patients with a positive ANA ≤1:160 have no identifiable rheumatologic disorder. The incidence of a positive ANA increases with age.

The positive predictive value of ANA is highest when the titer, other specific autoantibodies, and clinical presentation are all considered.

An ANA should be ordered **after** a complete history and physical exam reveals signs and/or symptoms of rheumatologic disease.

DIFFERENTIAL DIAGNOSIS FOR POSITIVE ANTINUCLEAR ANTIBODY

- Healthy individuals (in low titers, generally <1:160)
- **Rheumatologic diseases:** See Table 43-1
- **Drug-induced lupus**
- **Infectious diseases** such as HIV
- Neoplasms

PRESENTATION

History

Try to elicit symptoms suggestive of rheumatologic disease:

- General: morning stiffness, arthritis, rash, malaise, night sweats, low-grade fevers.
- Sicca symptoms (dry eyes and dry mouth): Sjögren's syndrome.
- Proximal muscle weakness and muscle pain with skin rash: myositis and dermatomyositis.
- Raynaud's, skin changes ± dysphagia or shortness of breath: scleroderma.
- See Table 43-2 for the diagnostic criteria for SLE as established by the American College of Rheumatology. The presence of four criteria makes the diagnosis of SLE with 97% sensitivity and 98% specificity.

Other important issues to inquire about:

- A history of hydralazine or procainamide puts the patient at risk for drug-induced lupus.
- Constitutional symptoms (fever, weight loss) or localized symptoms suggesting infection or malignancy.

TABLE 43-1. ANTIBODIES ASSOCIATED WITH SPECIFIC RHEUMATOLOGIC DISEASES

Disease	Antibodies
SLE	dsDNA, Sm, nuclear ribonucleoprotein
Drug-induced lupus	Antihistone
Sjögren's syndrome	Ro(SSA), La(SSB)
Dermatomyositis	Jo-1
Scleroderma	Scl-70
CREST	Centromere
Mixed connective tissue disease	Nuclear ribonucleoprotein

CREST, syndrome of calcinosis, Raynaud's, esophageal dysmotility, sclerodactyly, and telangiectasias.

Physical Exam

- HEENT: uveitis, dry eyes or oropharynx, oral ulcers, malar rash
- Chest: crackles or pleural rub
- Cardiovascular: pericardial rub
- Musculoskeletal: joint tenderness, swelling, or effusion
- Skin: discoid rash or palpable purpura; sclerotic skin changes or Raynaud's
- Neurologic: proximal muscle weakness, psychosis without other known cause

Lab Evaluation

High titer ANA (>1:160) in an appropriate clinical situation should be followed by assays for antibodies to certain antigens (double-stranded DNA, SSA/Ro, SSB/La, ribonucleoprotein, Sm) that are more specific for SLE and other rheumatologic diseases (Table 43-1).

Studies to detect systemic involvement with SLE or scleroderma are as follows: chest x-ray, CBC, creatine, U/A, and skin biopsy, if indicated. Further evaluation should be etiology specific.

If no certain diagnosis is made, follow-up may be indicated because up to 40% of patients referred to a rheumatologist for evaluation of positive ANA who do not fulfill criteria on presentation do fulfill criteria for SLE after months to years of follow-up.

TABLE 43-2. DIAGNOSTIC CRITERIA FOR SLE

1. Malar rash	7. Renal disorder (3+ proteinuria or casts)
2. Discoid rash	8. Blood disorder (cytopenia)
3. Photosensitivity	9. Neurologic (seizures or psychosis)
4. Serositis (pericarditis, pleuritis)	10. Positive ANA
5. Arthritis in two or more peripheral joints	11. Positive Anti-dsDNA, anti-Sm, false positive VDRL, positive LE cell preparation
6. Oral ulcers	

KEY POINT TO REMEMBER

- A positive ANA of a low titer is very common, especially among the elderly. An ANA should therefore only be performed in settings in which rheumatologic disease is suspected.

SUGGESTED READING

Cabral AR, Alarcon-Segovia D. Autoantibodies in systemic lupus erythematosus. *Curr Opin Rheumatol* 1998;10(5):409–416.

Classification criteria and treatment for specific rheumatologic diseases. Available at: Web site of the American College of Rheumatology, http://www.rheumatology.org. Accessed March 2003.

Moder K. Use and interpretation of rheumatologic tests: a guide for clinicians. *Mayo Clin Proc* 1996;71(4):391–396.

Wanchu A. Antinuclear antibodies: clinical applications. *J Postgrad Med* 2000;46(2):144–148.

REFERENCE

1. Tan EM. Range of antinuclear antibodies in healthy individuals. *Arthritis Rheum* 1997;40:1601–1611.

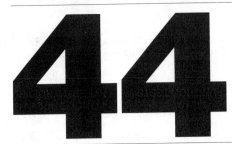

Approach to
Low Back Pain

Jennifer M. Quartarolo

INTRODUCTION

Low back pain is an exceedingly common complaint prompting medical attention in the United States, with some estimates of prevalence as high as 20%. Patients present along a wide spectrum of pain and disability, which unfortunately often does not correlate well with the seriousness of the underlying etiology. See Table 44-1 for differential diagnosis.

An effective screening technique is to develop a series of red flags that can alert the clinician to potentially serious disease (Table 44-2).

PRESENTATION

History

In assessing the possibility of malignancy-associated back pain, it is important to inquire about known primary malignancies, breast mass, smoking and family history of cancer, and systemic symptoms (weight loss, night sweats, fever, decreased appetite).

Historical clues that increase the likelihood of infection include the following:

- HIV, steroids, or other immunosuppressants.
- A history of IV drug abuse, hemodialysis, osteomyelitis/abscess, or endocarditis raises the possibility of metastatic infection.

  Mechanical injury is suggested by trauma, falls, and heavy lifting.
  Osteoporosis risk factors should be evaluated, including steroid use.
  Inquire about symptoms of inflammatory bowel disease, rheumatoid arthritis, other joint involvement, and a family history of arthritis.
  Other important questions are as follows:

- What position causes the worst pain?
  - Standing: lumbar stenosis
  - Sitting/flexion: disk herniation
- What time of day is the pain most severe?
  - Morning stiffness suggests rheumatoid arthritis or seronegative spondyloarthropathy. Pain that worsens as day progresses is typical of mechanical causes.
- Does the pain increase with walking or exercise?
  - Consider vascular insufficiency or neurogenic claudication.

Physical Exam

Look for fever and tachycardia as potential clues to infection or inflammatory arthropathy.

The back exam should focus on kyphosis, scoliosis, costovertebral angle tenderness, surgical scars, and spinal tenderness (abscess, compression fracture, lumbosacral strain).

A thorough joint exam may reveal evidence of other arthritic joints.

TABLE 44-1. DIFFERENTIAL DIAGNOSIS OF BACK PAIN

Mechanical	Infection
Lumbosacral strain	Epidural abscess
Herniated intravertebral disk	Vertebral osteomyelitis
Compression fractures	Diskitis
Lumbar spinal stenosis	**Vascular**
Spondylolysis/spondylolisthesis	Abdominal aortic aneurysm
Facet degeneration	Hematoma
Trauma	**Referred pain**
Kyphosis/scoliosis	Nephrolithiasis
Rheumatologic	Pyelonephritis
Seronegative spondyloarthropathies	Pelvic inflammatory disease
Rheumatoid arthritis	Endometriosis
Psoriatic arthritis	Cholecystitis
Arthropathy related to inflammatory bowel disease	Pancreatitis
Neoplastic	Prostatitis
Primary tumors vs. metastatic disease	

A rectal exam may reveal prostatitis. Decreased perianal sensation or rectal tone is worrisome for spinal neurologic involvement.

Provocative Tests for Sciatica

Valsalva/cough may induce pain. A straight leg raise is positive if pain is reproduced at <60 degrees with radiation down the leg.

Neurologic Exam (Sensory Motor)

- **L3-L4:** Knee extension, heel walking, patellar reflex, sensation to anterior/lateral thigh, and medial calf/ankle/foot
- **L4-L5:** Great toe dorsiflexion, sensation to posterolateral thigh, lateral calf, dorsum of foot
- **L5-S1:** toe walking, ankle plantarflexion, Achilles reflex, sensation to posterior thigh, calf, and lateral foot

TABLE 44-2. LOW BACK PAIN RED FLAGS

Symptoms >6 wks duration	Pain unresponsive to traditional analgesics
Leg weakness or numbness	Pain increasing with cough or Valsalva
Bowel or bladder retention/incontinence	Sexual dysfunction
Radiation of pain to leg or foot	Bilateral leg pain
Pain that worsens at night or when supine	Known malignancy
Perianal/saddle anesthesia	Weight loss (unexplained)
Fevers, chills, recent infections	

Lab and Imaging Evaluations

Mechanical Causes without Red Flags

It is perfectly reasonable to hold off on any imaging or lab tests for several weeks because the great majority of these conditions are both benign and self-limited.

Mechanical Causes with Red Flags

- CBC, ESR
- Consider MRI or CT
- Electromyography/nerve conduction velocity
- Plain films
- Dual-energy x-ray absorptiometry scan to evaluate for osteoporosis

Rheumatologic

- Plain films of spine and other joints involved; consider CT or MRI.
- CBC, ESR, HLA-B27, Rh factor, ANA may be considered.

Infectious

- CBC, ESR, U/A, blood cultures, chest x-ray
- MRI (or bone scan)
- Urine toxicology screen, purified protein derivative

Neoplastic

- CBC, peripheral smear, electrolytes, liver function tests, coagulations, ESR, serum protein electrophoresis/urine protein electrophoresis, Ca^+.
- Chest x-ray.
- MRI with gadolinium is crucial.

Referred Pain

- CBC, electrolytes, liver function tests, coagulations, amylase, lipase, blood cultures.
- Rest of workup is etiology specific.

MANAGEMENT

Lumbosacral Strain

- Use NSAIDs, mild muscle relaxants, hot or cold packs; and physical therapy or exercise.
- Weight loss may be helpful.
- Bed rest should not exceed 48 hrs.
- Reassurance should be provided.

Herniated Disk and Other Mechanical Causes

As per lumbosacral strain plus

- Consider steroids or low-dose narcotics for temporary relief.
- Treatment of any underlying osteoporosis.

SURGICAL INDICATIONS

Surgical indications include sciatica that correlates well with imaging or neurophysiologic findings and lasts beyond 6 wks and progressive weakness, numbness, or other neurologic deficits.

Cauda equina symptoms include bowel or bladder retention/incontinence, decreased rectal tone, and saddle anesthesia. Most etiologies of this syndrome require surgical intervention.

Decompression of abscess in the context of antibiotic failure, severe pain, or neurologic deficits is another indication, as well as tumor debulking or removal for similar scenarios.

KEY POINT TO REMEMBER

- Be aware of the red flags that identify serious pathology, including fever, neurologic symptoms, symptoms >6 wks, radiation of pain to the leg or foot, and pain that worsens with Valsalva or is unresponsive to medication.

REFERENCES AND SUGGESTED READINGS

Borenstein DG. Epidemiology, etiology, diagnostic evaluation, and treatment of low back pain. *Curr Opin Rheumatol* 2001;13:128–134.

Deyo RA, Weinstein JN. Low back pain. *N Engl J Med* 2001;26:153–159.

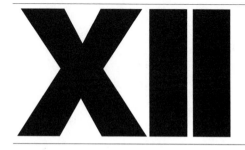

XII

Allergy and Immunology

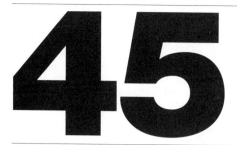

Anaphylaxis

Barbara C. Jost and
Eric F. Buch

INTRODUCTION

Anaphylaxis is a medical emergency caused by antigen-mediated release of vasoactive mediators. Anaphylactoid reactions differ from anaphylaxis in that they are not IgE dependent but are from a direct release of mediators from mast cells. The most common cause is radiocontrast medium. Clinical manifestations and management are the same as for anaphylactic reactions.

Atopy does not affect the risk of anaphylaxis but makes severe anaphylactic reactions more likely.

PRESENTATION

History and Physical Exam

Anaphylaxis is an acute, life-threatening syndrome involving multiple organ systems. Onset is typically within minutes of antigen exposure but may be delayed for hours. Median time to collapse is 30 mins for food, 15 mins for venom, and 5 mins for parenterally administered agent [1]. Delayed reactions can occur (biphasic reaction), with recurrence of symptoms 4–8 hrs after initial event.

Protracted anaphylaxis requiring hours of resuscitation occurs in up to 28% of patients. Risk factors include oral ingestion of the allergen and onset of symptoms >30 mins after exposure.

Presentation is highly variable—signs and symptoms include any of the following: flushing, hypotension, bronchospasm, tachycardia, urticaria, angioedema, laryngeal edema, abdominal or uterine cramping, diarrhea, vomiting, pruritus, or rhinorrhea/sneezing.

Lab Evaluation

If **diagnosis is uncertain,** consider measuring serum **beta-tryptase** level after patient is stabilized. Beta-tryptase peaks 15–120 mins after anaphylaxis from insect sting and has a half-life of 1.5–2.5 hrs [2].

MANAGEMENT

Regardless of severity, all anaphylactic reactions require **immediate treatment** and **careful observation;** any mild reaction can quickly become a serious one.
Epinephrine is the cornerstone of management:

- Immediately administer 0.3–0.5 mg epinephrine SC (0.3–0.5 mL of a 1:1000 solution) in the upper extremity or thigh. Consider smaller doses in the elderly (0.2 mg) and larger doses in patients on beta blockers (0.5 mg ± glucagon).
- Epinephrine may also be given via central line (3–5 mL of 1:10,000 solution) or endotracheally (3–5 mL of a 1:10,000 solution diluted in 10 mL NS) in cases of severe hypotension or respiratory failure.
- Continuous infusion of 1:10,000 epinephrine may be necessary in patients with protracted symptoms.

Airway management sometimes requires endotracheal intubation. Racemic epinephrine via metered dose inhaler may improve laryngeal edema. If laryngeal edema does not respond, consider cricothyroidotomy or tracheotomy.

Volume expansion with normal saline is indicated.

Glucocorticoids have no immediate effect but may prevent relapse of symptoms (methylprednisolone [Medrol], 125 mg IV, or hydrocortisone, 500 mg IV).

Antihistamines also have no immediate effect but may shorten symptom duration. Diphenhydramine (Benadryl) can be administered IV (25–100 mg over 5–10 mins), IM, or PO and can be given q6h for 24–48 hrs.

H_2-specific antihistamines can be added, despite lack of supporting studies (famotidine [Pepcid], 40 mg IV is a common regimen).

Close observation is advised for at least 6–8 hrs if the reaction is mild.

KEY POINT TO REMEMBER

- Anaphylaxis is a medical emergency. Therapy consists of epinephrine, corticosteroids, and antihistamines, often with an H_2-blocker.

SUGGESTED READING

Kemp SF, Lockey RF, Wolf BL, et al. Anaphylaxis: a review of 266 cases. *Arch Intern Med* 1995;155(16):1749–1754.

Practice parameters for anaphylaxis. Available at: Joint Council of Allergy, Asthma and Immunology Web site, http://www.jcaai.org/Param/Anaphylaxis. Accessed March 2003.

Ring J, Behrendt H. Anaphylaxis and anaphylactoid reactions. Classification and pathophysiology. *Clin Rev Allergy Immunol* 1999;17(4):387–389.

REFERENCES

1. Pumphrey RS. Lessons for management of anaphylaxis from a study of fatal reactions. *Clin Exp Allergy* 2000;30:1144–1150.
2. Lin RY. Histamine and tryptose levels in patients with acute allergic reactions: an emergency department-based study. *J Allergy Clin Immunol* 2000;106:65–71.

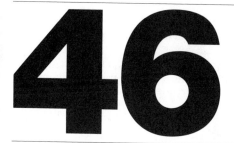

Drug Reactions and Desensitization

Barbara C. Jost and
Eric F. Buch

INTRODUCTION

Drug allergy or hypersensitivity is a form of adverse drug reaction. Up to 15% of drug administrations cause an adverse effect; the risk is doubled in the hospital setting [1].

Immunologic mechanisms of drug allergy can be stratified by Gell and Coombs' classification:

- Type I, or immediate hypersensitivity, is IgE-mediated; the premier example is anaphylaxis. Clinical manifestations include flushing, hypotension, and urticaria. Time course is usually seconds to minutes for parenteral drugs and approximately 1 hr for oral drugs.
- Type II, or antibody-dependent cytotoxic hypersensitivity, causes cell destruction via the complement system. An example is hemolytic anemia due to antibodies formed against erythrocyte-bound penicillin.
- Type III, or immune-complex-mediated hypersensitivity: serum sickness syndrome is an example.
- Type IV, or delayed-type hypersensitivity, is mediated by sensitized T cells and classically represented by contact dermatitis.

Anaphylactoid or "pseudoallergic" reactions are clinically indistinguishable from type I reactions (see Chap. 45, Anaphylaxis).

PRESENTATION

History

Hypersensitivity wanes with time. A longitudinal study of 55 patients with a history of an immediate-type reaction to penicillin and a positive skin test revealed that, after 5 yrs, only 40% of patients still had a positive skin test.

Consider all drugs taken by the patient at the time of the reaction as possible offenders, regardless of the duration of administration or a history of apparent tolerance to a drug. Remember that signs and symptoms of an illness prompting treatment with the drug in question can be mistaken for a drug reaction.

Serum sickness syndrome encompasses a broad spectrum of signs and symptoms, including fever, malaise, rash (palpable purpura and urticaria), lymphadenopathy, leukopenia, arthralgias/myalgias, and arthritis. It usually begins within 2–4 wks of drug ingestion and resolves only when the offending agent or its metabolite is completely eliminated from the body.

Drug fever may be the only evidence of hypersensitivity to a drug. Typically, it develops around days 7–10 and disappears within 36–72 hrs after the drug is stopped, although it can persist for days. Fever often reaches high levels; associated findings may include eosinophilia, leukocytosis, rash, and an elevated ESR. The mechanism is unknown.

Acute interstitial nephritis is rare but can be seen with beta-lactams, in particular methicillin, as well as rifampin, NSAIDs, sulfonamides, captopril, and allopurinol. It is associated with fever, rash, and eosinophilia. Hematuria, albuminuria, pyuria, eosinophiluria, an active urine sediment, elevated serum creatinine, and oliguria have been noted.

Physical Exam

Skin and mucous membrane alterations are the most common manifestations of drug hypersensitivity:

- **Maculopapular or morbilliform** skin eruptions are seen most often. An eruption is usually symmetric, sparing palms and soles, and consists of erythematous macules and papules. Onset is usually 4–7 days into a course of therapy, often beginning on lower extremities or over pressure points.
- **Fixed drug eruptions** occur at the same body location with each exposure to a given drug.
- **Erythema multiforme** presents with any combination of macules, papules, vesicles, bullae, and targetoid lesions. 10–20% of cases are related to drugs, especially sulfonamides, penicillin, barbiturates, salicylates, and antimalarials.
- **Stevens-Johnson syndrome, or "erythema multiforme major,"** is characterized by fever, mucus membrane involvement, and sloughing of up to 10% of the epidermis. Toxic epidermal necrolysis is the severe variant with involvement of >30% of the epidermis.

Lab Evaluation

Large-molecular-weight drugs such as insulin, toxoids, antisera, and egg-protein vaccines are complete antigens and can be used directly as skin testing reagents.

Patch testing is used to assess for type IV hypersensitivity or contact sensitivity to topical agents. A panel of antigens is applied to the skin under an occlusive dressing; results are read at 48–72 hrs.

MANAGEMENT

Immediate treatment consists of discontinuing the (most likely) offending agent and administering antihistamines and corticosteroids, if necessary.

After establishing the diagnosis of immunologic drug reaction, there are four potential approaches:

1. Administer an alternative (non–cross-reactive) drug. Review the chemical structure of the offending drug and proposed alternative.
2. Administer a potentially cross-reactive drug under close medical supervision.
   - If available and reliable, skin testing can be performed.
   - Provocative dose challenge performed by an allergy consultant in the presence of resuscitative equipment can also be used. This is contraindicated in patients with a history of Stevens-Johnson or toxic epidermal necrolysis.
3. Pretreatment protocols are available for some drugs to prevent or mitigate any reaction that might occur. Table 46-1 outlines such a protocol for radiocontrast media reactions.

TABLE 46-1. PRETREATMENT PROTOCOL FOR PATIENTS WITH A HISTORY OF RADIOCONTRAST MEDIA REACTIONS

Time before the procedure	Drug and dose		
	Prednisone[a]	Cimetidine[b]	Diphenhydramine[c]
13 hrs	50 mg PO	300 mg PO or IV	—
7 hrs	50 mg PO	300 mg PO or IV	—
1 hr[d]	50 mg PO	300 mg PO or IV	50 mg PO or IV

[a]Or methylprednisolone, 40 mg IV.
[b]Or ranitidine, 150 mg.
[c]Or chlorpheniramine, 10–12 mg.
[d]Ephedrine, 25 mg PO, may also be given 1 hr before procedure.

TABLE 46-2. CROSS-REACTIVITY AMONG BETA-LACTAMS

Beta-lactam type	Degree of cross-reactivity with penicillin
Semisynthetic penicillins	High
Cephalosporins	Low ($\leq 8\%$)
Carbapenems	High ($\sim 45\%$)
Monobactams	Trivial

4. Perform desensitization if no acceptable alternative drug exists. Desensitization does not protect against mild skin reactions such as urticaria or pruritus; treat through these. **Desensitization should only be performed under the supervision of a trained allergist** in a location outfitted with resuscitative equipment for treating anaphylaxis.

SPECIFIC DRUG ALLERGIES

PCN

PCN skin testing has been well studied and is both safe and reliable. However, it is still preferable to administer an alternative agent to a patient with a clear history of PCN hypersensitivity. Skin testing is indicated only when there is no suitable alternative. The major antigenic determinant is available commercially as benzylpenicilloyl (Pre-Pen). There is no standardized panel or radioallergosorbent assay test available for minor determinants.

The predictive value of the history of PCN allergy in combination with skin testing has been studied in two large multicenter trials [2,3]. These showed that 19% of patients with a positive history of PCN allergy (and 4–7% of those with a negative history) will have a positive skin test. See Table 46-2 for cross-reactivity of beta-lactams.

Sulfonamide Allergy

Sulfonamide antibiotics are structurally similar to thiazides, furosemide, celecoxib, and sulfonylureas.

KEY POINTS TO REMEMBER

- Skin testing may confirm sensitivity to PCN when allergy history is uncertain. Consider desensitization if history of drug allergy prevents administration of a necessary medication.
- In patients with PCN allergy, cross-sensitivity to cephalosporins is <10%, whereas sensitivity to monobactams (e.g., aztreonam) is trivial.

SUGGESTED READING

Anderson JA, Adkinson NF, Jr. Allergic reactions to drugs and biologic agents. *JAMA* 1987;258:2891–2899.

Weiss ME, Adkinson NF. Immediate hypersensitivity reactions to penicillin and related antibiotics. *Clin Allergy* 1988;18:515–540.

REFERENCES

1. Faich GA, Dreis M, Tomita D. National adverse drug reaction surveillance. 1986. *Arch Intern Med* 1988;148:785–787.

2. Sogn DD, Evans R 3rd, Shepherd GM, et al. Results of the National Institute of Allergy and Infectious Diseases Collaborative Clinical Trial to test the predictive value of skin testing with major and minor penicillin derivatives in hospitalized adults. *Arch Intern Med* 1992;152:1025–1032.

3. Green GR, Rosenblum AH, Sweet LC. Evaluation of penicillin hypersensitivity: value of clinical history and skin testing with penicilloyl-polylysine and penicillin G. A cooperative prospective study of the penicillin study group of the American Academy of Allergy. *J Allergy Clin Immunol* 1977;60:339–345.

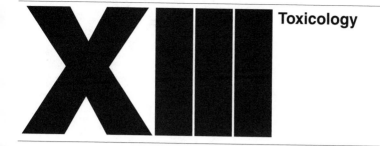

XIII Toxicology

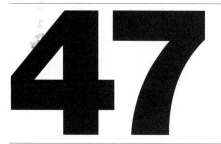

Alcohol Withdrawal

Christopher H. Kwoh

INTRODUCTION

It is estimated that 12% of patients seen by primary care physicians are alcoholics; however, most are not identified. For this reason, alcohol withdrawal is seen frequently both in the ER and on the inpatient service when patients have been abstinent for days postoperatively or because of acute illness. In this instance, a high degree of suspicion is necessary to make the diagnosis. See the Web site of the National Institute on Alcohol Abuse and Alcoholism (http://www.niaaa.nih.gov) for further details on classifying alcohol use.

PRESENTATION

History

Autonomic Hyperactivity

Autonomic hyperactivity typically begins 5–8 hrs after cessation, peaks at 2–3 days, and subsides within 7 days. There is a sensation of tremulousness with HTN, tachycardia, diaphoresis, hyperthermia, mydriasis, nausea, vomiting, and diarrhea. Insomnia, hand tremors, agitation, and anxiety can be prominent. Concurrent use of beta blockers or calcium channel blockers may mask these symptoms.

Alcohol Withdrawal Seizures

Alcohol withdrawal seizures occur in one-fourth of chronic alcohol users. A history of previous alcohol withdrawal seizures increases risk.

Most withdrawal seizures occur in the first 24 hrs, and >90% occur in the first 48 hrs. They are typically grand mal and usually single episodes. They rarely result in status epilepticus. In contrast to delirium tremens (DTs), simple withdrawal seizures do **not** alter sensorium.

Alcoholic Hallucinosis

Hallucinosis occurs in approximately 20% of hospitalized alcoholics, typically in the first 48 hrs. The hallucinations can be tactile ("formication," or the sensation of insects crawling on the skin), auditory, olfactory, or visual. The hallucinations are frequently persecutory.

Delirium Tremens

DTs usually begin at 48–96 hrs and peak at the fourth to fifth day of cessation but can persist for up to 2 wks. Altered sensorium and time of onset distinguish DTs from simple alcohol withdrawal seizures or alcoholic hallucinosis. Patients often have extreme autonomic hyperactivity, and fever is very common (35–60%). Mortality in untreated patients has been reported to be as high as 35%, but with adequate treatment the mortality is low (<5%).

Alcoholic Encephalopathy (Wernicke-Korsakoff Syndrome)

Alcoholic encephalopathy is the result of chronic thiamine deficiency, often precipitated by administration of glucose without thiamine. It is now very rare. Mortality is 10–20%.

The presentation is classically ophthalmoplegia (nystagmus, diplopia, rectus muscle weakness), ataxia (typically of the lower extremities), and altered sensorium and memory (loss of short-term memory with relative preservation of immediate and long-term memory). Confabulation can be prominent. Peripheral neuropathy is often present as well.

Affective Disturbances

Patients withdrawing from alcohol can have symptoms of depression, anxiety, insomnia, and tremor for as long as 1 yr postwithdrawal.

Physical Exam

Vital signs often reveal increased sympathetic tone and can be used to guide treatment. There may be evidence of dehydration from vomiting and polyuria. Stigmata of chronic liver disease should be sought. Neurologic exam should evaluate for evidence of focal neurologic signs, hand tremor (which can also be used to guide additional therapy), or encephalopathy.

LAB EVALUATION

Evaluation should include a complete metabolic panel, CBC, coagulation studies, UA, and chest x-ray. It is also prudent to evaluate urine toxicology given the frequency of polysubstance abuse. A bedside glucose should be considered in all patients with altered sensorium or seizures. A stool guaiac aids in identifying GI bleeding from alcoholic gastritis or portal HTN. Patients can have marked loss of magnesium and potassium from alcoholism. Other common abnormalities seen are a macrocytosis, thrombocytopenia from bone marrow suppression, elevated transaminases with AST > ALT, and hyponatremia from ingestion of extremely hypotonic alcoholic drinks.

Imaging

The need for imaging the brain in patients with alcohol withdrawal seizures is controversial. The frequency of culprit lesions in these patients as opposed to those with idiopathic epilepsy is much lower. In one series of 259 patients with alcohol withdrawal seizures, a head CT revealed clinically significant intracranial findings in 6% and altered therapy in 4% [1]. In this series, focal neurologic signs and head trauma were not predictive. Another series of 151 patients revealed potentially reversible lesions in 18% with directed surgery in 9%; however, nearly all of these patients had focal neurologic signs [2].

TREATMENT

It is prudent to administer **thiamine** (100 mg), **folate** (1 mg), and a **multivitamin** in all patients. In patients with evidence of Wernicke-Korsakoff syndrome, administration of 100 mg IV thiamine per day for several days has been used. Ophthalmoplegia can respond in hours, other symptoms may improve over the first week, but some deficits may be irreversible.

Rehydration is important in the dehydrated patient, and **glucose** should be administered in those with severe alcohol withdrawal **(never administer glucose without thiamine).** Fluid and electrolyte status should be monitored closely.

Magnesium should be replaced if hypomagnesemic; however, empiric administration in alcohol-withdrawing patients has not been shown to alter seizure frequency, DTs, or other symptoms [3].

Benzodiazepines (BZDs) have emerged as the drugs of choice in numerous controlled trials and metaanalyses in patients with moderate withdrawal symptoms. These can be administered on a fixed schedule or based on standardized symptom scales: Clinical Institute Assessment for Alcohol Scale (CIWA-Ar) is a widely used and well studied scale [4]. Symptom-based administration is as effective and often results in decreased use of BZDs and earlier discharge compared to fixed dosing [5]. Front-loaded regimens with long half-life BZDs have also shown decreased total dosages and shorter hospital stays. The BZDs can be tapered over 3–7 days in uncomplicated patients or 1–3 wks in patients with DTs.

- **Chlordiazepoxide (Librium)** is commonly used at 25–100 mg PO q2–6h prn. **Chlordiazepoxide should not be used in patients with hepatic insufficiency.** It can be used at a fixed schedule, 50 mg PO q6h × 4 doses, then 25 mg q6h × 8 doses.
- **Oxazepam (Serax),** 15–30 mg PO q6–8h prn, can be used safely in patients with liver disease.
- **Diazepam (Valium)** can be front loaded with titration until asymptomatic and calm (10–20 mg PO q1–2h or 3–5 mg IV q10mins) and then dosed additionally as needed [6]. With a half-life of 30–50 hrs, most patients do not require significant redosing.
- **Lorazepam (Ativan),** 1–2 mg q6–8h can be used in the elderly, those with altered drug metabolism, or those at risk for oversedation, because it has a short half-life.

Beta blockers are effective in controlling autonomic symptoms but have not been shown to reduce the risk for DTs or seizures. Therefore, they should not be used as monotherapy for severe withdrawal. **Atenolol (Tenormin),** 50–100 mg PO per day, is a frequently used regimen as an adjunct to BZDs.

Clonidine (Catapres), 0.1–0.2 mg PO tid or in patch form, may also control autonomic symptoms but, like beta blockers, should not be used as monotherapy.

Neuroleptics have been suspected to lead to an increase in withdrawal seizures and are not recommended. Low-dose **haloperidol** (Haldol) can be used as an adjunct to BZDs for alcoholic hallucinosis in patients who are not seizure prone, given its limited effect on seizure threshold.

Phenobarbital (Solfoton) is probably safe and may be useful in those who do not respond to high doses of BZDs because of extreme down-regulation of receptors.

Phenytoin (Dilantin) has not been shown to be more effective than placebo in double-blind controlled trials in alcohol withdrawal seizures in nonepileptics [7,8]. However, BZDs are the drugs of choice for withdrawal seizures.

Persistent memory difficulties from Korsakoff's syndrome may be marginally improved with clonidine or fluvoxamine (Luvox) [9,10].

Hospitalization is a good opportunity to arrange referral to substance abuse counseling or Alcoholics Anonymous.

KEY POINTS TO REMEMBER

- Delirium from alcohol withdrawal may begin as long as 10 days after cessation. Maintain a high degree of suspicion for alcohol withdrawal even a week or more into hospitalization.
- The cornerstone of therapy for alcohol withdrawal is long-acting benzodiazepines. Also provide multivitamins, thiamine, and folate. Look for associated nutritional deficiency or end-organ damage to the liver, bone marrow, or nervous system.

SUGGESTED READING

Mayo-Smith MF. Pharmacologic management of alcohol withdrawal: a meta-analysis and evidence-based practice guideline. *JAMA* 1997;278(2):144–151.

REFERENCES

1. Earnest MP. Intracranial lesions shown by CT scans in 259 cases of first alcohol-related seizures. *Neurology* 1988;38:1561–1565.
2. Feussner JR. Computed tomography brain scanning in alcohol withdrawal seizures. *Ann Intern Med* 1981;94:519–522.
3. Wilson A. A double-blind, placebo-controlled trial of magnesium sulfate in the ethanol withdrawal syndrome. *Alcohol Clin Exp Res* 1984;8:542–545.
4. Sullivan JT. Assessment of alcohol withdrawal: the revised clinical institute withdrawal assessment for alcohol scale. *Br J Addict* 1989;84:1353–1357.
5. Saitz R. Individualized treatment for alcohol withdrawal: a randomized double blind controlled trial. *JAMA* 1994;272(7):519–523.

6. Sellers EM. Diazepam loading: simplified treatment of alcohol withdrawal. *Clin Pharmacol Ther* 1983;34(6):822–826.
7. Alldredge BK. Placebo-controlled trial of intravenous diphenylhaydantoin for short term treatment of alcohol withdrawal seizures. *Am J Med* 1989;87:645–648.
8. Chance JF. Emergency department treatment of alcohol withdrawal seizures with phenytoin. *Ann Emerg Med* 1991;20(5):520–522.
9. McEntee WJ. Memory enhancement in Korsakoff's psychosis by clonidine. *Ann Neurol* 1980;7(5):466–470.
10. Martin PR. Effective pharmacotherapy of alcoholic amnestic disorder with fluvoxamine. *Arch Gen Psychiatry* 1989;46:617–621.

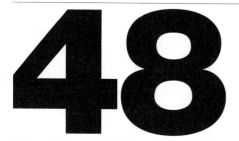

Opioid Intoxication and Withdrawal

Christopher H. Kwoh

OPIOID INTOXICATION

Presentation

History

Symptoms of opioid intoxication include altered sensorium, respiratory depression, severe constipation, nausea, and vomiting. Rare complications in massive overdose include pulmonary edema and seizures.

Physical Exam

Vital signs may reveal hypopnea, bradycardia, and, in extreme cases, hypotension. Patients classically have **constricted pupils.**

Lab Evaluation

Evaluation should include basic serum electrolytes, glucose, and urine and serum toxicology. Many opioid-intoxicated patients may be intoxicated with multiple substances.

Management

Naloxone (Narcan) can rapidly reverse the effects of opioids. Initially, 0.8 mg can be given IV (or sublingual if no IV is obtainable) and an additional dose given at double the previous dose q15mins until there is a response.

- Nearly all true opioid overdoses should have some response to the 6.4-mg dose. Some opioids are thought to be more resistant to naloxone (e.g., buprenorphine, propoxyphene, codeine, fentanyl) and may require higher doses (10–20 mg).
- Naloxone is very short acting and may need to be given by IV drip (effective dose administered per hour converted into an hourly drip, or estimated as two-thirds the initial effective bolus dose per hour).

   Gastric lavage with activated charcoal should be attempted if the ingestion is recent (within 60 mins).
   Consider **endotracheal intubation** if the patient is obtunded.

OPIOID WITHDRAWAL

Presentation

History

Opioid withdrawal may be seen in patients who are abusers of opioids and are admitted to the hospital. Also look for symptoms in the patient who has been on long-standing high-dose opioids for pain who is made NPO.

   Patients have flu-like symptoms with rhinorrhea, nausea, vomiting, myalgias, diaphoresis, insomnia, diarrhea, and anxiety. Lacrimation, hot and cold flashes, and intense drug craving are also seen. Symptoms are more common and more extreme when withdrawing from shorter-acting opioids.

   Opioid withdrawal is extremely unpleasant but not life threatening in otherwise healthy adults.

Physical Exam

Classically, one sees dilated pupils, piloerection ("chicken skin" or "going cold turkey"), tachycardia, and HTN.

Management

Methadone (Dolophine, Methadose) can be used for **objective signs** of opioid withdrawal. A common regimen includes 10 mg initially and repeat doses of 5–10 mg q4–6h. Continue the second day (in divided doses if desired) with a dose equivalent to the first day total dose and taper by 5 mg/day. Taper methadone addicts off more slowly.

Clonidine (Catapres) can be given at 0.1–0.2 mg PO q3h prn to a maximum of 1.2 mg/day and tapered over 2 wks.

Patients addicted to pentazocine (Talwin) should be detoxified on pentazocine, given its differing biochemical activities (partial agonist/antagonist).

Consider referral of substance abusers to drug rehabilitation and Narcotics Anonymous programs.

KEY POINTS TO REMEMBER

- Opioid overdoses may require reversal with naloxone, which may require delivery by IV drip owing to its short half-life.
- Opioid withdrawal may be seen in patients on opioids for chronic pain in addition to those addicted to heroin or other opioids. Methadone, with its long half-life, is useful for controlling symptoms.

REFERENCES AND SUGGESTED READINGS

Carnwath T. Randomised double blind comparison of lofexidine and clonidine in the outpatient treatment of opiate withdrawal. *Drug Alcohol Depend* 1998;50:251–254.

Farrell M. Opiate withdrawal. *Addiction* 1994;89:1471–1475.

Fishbain DA. Opiate detoxification protocols: a clinical manual. *Ann Clin Psychiatry* 1993;5:53–65.

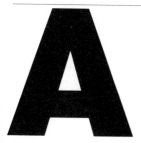

Review of Selected Clinical Trials

4S (SCANDINAVIAN SIMVASTATIN SURVIVAL STUDY)

Multiple Citations

Randomised trial of cholesterol lowering in 4444 patients with coronary heart disease: the Scandinavian Simvastatin Survival Study (4S). *Lancet* 1994;344:1383–1389. (Initial results.)

Kjekshus J. Reducing the risk of coronary events: evidence from the Scandinavian Simvastatin Survival Study (4S). *Am J Cardiol* 1995;76:64C–68C. (Reduced coronary events.)

Pederson TR. Lipoprotein changes and reduction in the incidence of major coronary heart disease events in the Scandinavian Simvastatin Survival Study (4S). *Circulation* 1998;97:1453–1460. (Reduced cholesterol and coronary events.)

Clinical Question

Does treatment with simvastatin in patients with coronary disease affect morbidity, mortality, and serum cholesterol?

Design

Randomized, double-blind, placebo-controlled trial.

Inclusion Criteria

Patients aged 35–70 yrs with a history of coronary disease and total serum cholesterol 213–290 mg/dL.

Exclusion Criteria

Patients with MI in prior 6 mos, congestive heart failure, anticipated coronary artery bypass graft/percutaneous transluminal coronary angioplasty, premenopausal women, secondary hypercholesterolemia, or triglycerides >2.5 mmol/L.

Patients and Follow-Up

4444 patients were followed up for a median of 5.4 yrs.

Intervention

Simvastatin (or matching placebo), 20 mg PO per day, titrated to 10 mg or 40 mg to target range of total cholesterol 116–201 mg/dL.

Results

Patients in the simvastatin group achieved greater improvement in serum cholesterol levels [total decrease, 25%; low-density lipoprotein (LDL) decrease, 34%; high-density lipoprotein increase, 8%; TG decrease, 10%, vs. no clinically significant change for placebo], had decreased mortality [8% vs. 12%; relative risk reduction (RRR), 30%; p <.001] owing to coronary mortality (5.0% vs. 8.5%; RRR, 42%), and reduced major coronary events (19% vs. 28%; RRR, 34%). Patients on simvastatin also experienced fewer cerebrovascular events (RRR, 28%), less frequent new or worsening angina (25.6% vs. 32.6%; RRR, 26%), and claudication (2.3% vs. 3.6%; RRR, 38%).

Conclusions

In patients with hypercholesterolemia and coronary disease, simvastatin leads to decreased total cholesterol, triglycerides, and low-density lipoprotein; increased high-density lipoprotein; decreased coronary events and mortality; decreased cerebrovascular accidents, and limits progression of claudication and anginal symptoms.

ACAS (ASYMPTOMATIC CAROTID ATHEROSCLEROSIS STUDY)

ACAS Investigators. Endarterectomy for asymptomatic carotid artery stenosis. *JAMA* 1995;274:1421–1428.

Clinical Question

Is there a benefit of carotid endarterectomy (CEA) vs. medical therapy in patients with asymptomatic carotid artery stenosis?

Design

Randomized controlled trial.

Inclusion Criteria

Patients aged 40–79 yrs with unilateral or bilateral asymptomatic carotid stenosis >60%.

Exclusion Criteria

Symptoms referable to either the stenosis or contralateral cerebral hemispheric symptoms within the previous 45 days, contraindication to aspirin, and an expected life span of <5 yrs.

Patients and Follow-Up

1662 patients with >99% follow-up at median of 2.7 yrs.

Intervention

825 patients underwent CEA with medical therapy. 834 patients underwent medical therapy alone, consisting of ASA and risk factor management.

Results

At 5 yrs, the risk of ipsilateral stroke or any perioperative stroke or death was 5.1% with CEA and 11% with medical management alone ($p = .004$). Perioperative complications included a 2.3% rate of death or stroke (5 of 19 due to arteriography).

Conclusions

Selected asymptomatic patients with carotid artery stenosis >60% may benefit from CEA in addition to medical management.

ACUTE (ASSESSMENT OF CARDIOVERSION USING TRANSESOPHAGEAL ECHOCARDIOGRAPHY)

Klein AL, Grimm RA, Murray RD, et al. Use of transesophageal echocardiography to guide cardioversion in patients with atrial fibrillation. *N Engl J Med* 2001;344(19):1411–1420.

Clinical Question

For atrial fibrillation, can transesophageal echocardiography (TEE) safely be used to shorten the period of anticoagulation before cardioversion?

Design

Multicenter, randomized, nonblinded trial.

Inclusion Criteria

Age >18 yrs, atrial fibrillation duration >2 days, atrial flutter if documented history also of atrial fibrillation.

Exclusion Criteria

Hemodynamic instability, contraindication to anticoagulation or TEE, or already on warfarin for >7 days.

Patients and Follow-Up

1222 patients with median duration of arrhythmia 13 days, followed for 8 wks.

Intervention

Patients were randomly assigned to conventional treatment, consisting of 3 wks therapeutic warfarin followed by cardioversion or TEE-guided treatment, consisting of immediate cardioversion if no thrombus detected on TEE. All patients in both groups were anticoagulated for a minimum of 4 wks after cardioversion.

Results

70% of patients in the TEE-guided group underwent early cardioversion with fewer hemorrhagic events and no significant increase in embolic events or mortality. At the end of 8 weeks, the proportion of patients in sinus rhythm was virtually identical in the two groups.

Conclusions

TEE-guided cardioversion can be considered a safe and effective alternative to the conventional strategy of 3 wks warfarin therapy before cardioversion; it shortens the time to restoration of sinus rhythm and prevents bleeding events.

AFFIRM (ATRIAL FIBRILLATION FOLLOW-UP INVESTIGATION OF RHYTHM MANAGEMENT) INVESTIGATORS

AFFIRM Investigators. A comparison of rate control and rhythm control in patients with atrial fibrillation. *N Engl J Med* 2002;347:1825–1833.

Clinical Question

Is there any difference between treating patients with atrial fibrillation with rate control and anticoagulation vs. rhythm control in terms of stroke, cardiovascular events, or death?

Design

Randomized, controlled trial.

Inclusion Criteria

Patients with atrial fibrillation who did not have "lone atrial fibrillation" and were considered to require long-term medical management for atrial fibrillation.

Exclusion Criteria

Patients with lone atrial fibrillation (aged <65 yrs and no stroke risk factors) or contraindications to anticoagulation.

Patients and Follow-Up

2027 patients in the rate control group and 2033 patients in the rhythm control group, with mean age of 70 yrs, were followed for 5 yrs.

Intervention

The rate control patients received medications to keep resting heart rate <80 bpm and exercise heart rate (HR) <110 bpm, as well as warfarin anticoagulation with a goal INR of 2–3 (an average of 85% were on warfarin over the course of the trial). The rhythm control group was given approved antiarrhythmic therapy and required to receive anticoagulation unless sinus rhythm was maintained for at least 4 wks (an average of 70% of the rhythm control group were on warfarin over the course of the trial).

Results

Sinus rhythm was regained in 35% of the rate control group and 63% of the rhythm control group at 5 yrs. Crossover was high, with 15% crossing from rate control to rhythm control and 38% crossing from rhythm control to rate control by 5 yrs. The risk of ischemic stroke was similar in the two groups (5.5% in rate control vs. 7.1% in rhythm control; $p = .79$). Most ischemic strokes occurred after discontinuation of warfarin or with subtherapeutic INRs. There was a trend toward lower mortality in the rate control group (25.9% vs. 26.7%; $p = .08$).

Conclusions

There is no clear difference between rate control and anticoagulation and rhythm control in terms of mortality or ischemic stroke. Patients on rhythm control may still benefit from full anticoagulation.

PERIOPERATIVE BETA BLOCKADE WITH ATENOLOL

Mangano DT, Layug EL, Wallace A, et al. Effect of atenolol on mortality and cardiovascular morbidity after noncardiac surgery. *N Engl J Med* 1996;335:1713–1720.

Clinical Question

Does atenolol decrease the rate of perioperative mortality or cardiovascular morbidity?

Design

Randomized, double-blind, placebo-controlled trial.

Inclusion Criteria

Patients with coronary artery disease (prior MI, typical angina, or atypical angina with a positive stress test) or risk factors (aged >65 yrs, HTN, diabetes, total cholesterol >240 mg/dL, or current smoker).

Exclusion Criteria

Patients with asthma, heart failure, third-degree heart block, HR <55 bpm, or SBP <100 mm Hg.

Patients and Follow-Up

99 patients in the atenolol group and 101 patients in the placebo group with 96% follow-up at 2 yrs.

Intervention

Patients received atenolol, 50 mg PO or 5 mg IV, starting 30 mins before surgery and continuing daily through the postoperative period as long as HR >55 bpm and SBP >100 mm Hg. The dose was doubled as tolerated for HR >65 bpm and SBP >100 mm Hg. The control group received matching placebo.

Results

Mortality at 6 mos was 0% in the atenolol group and 8% in the placebo group ($p < .001$). Mortality benefit of atenolol continued at 2 yrs (10% vs. 21%; $p = .014$).

Conclusions

Atenolol decreased the risk of perioperative mortality in patients with high cardiac risk. However, the placebo group did have more risk factors than the atenolol group.

BARI (BYPASS ANGIOPLASTY REVASCULARIZATION INVESTIGATION)

Comparison of coronary bypass surgery with angioplasty in patients with multivessel disease. The Bypass Angioplasty Revascularization Investigation (BARI) investigators. *N Engl J Med* 1996;335:217–225.

Outcomes of noncardiac surgery after coronary bypass surgery or coronary angioplasty in BARI. *Am J Med* 2001;110:260–266.

Clinical Question

In patients with multivessel coronary artery disease, is coronary artery bypass graft (CABG) or percutaneous transluminal coronary angioplasty (PTCA) more effective in reducing mortality and preventing subsequent MI?

Design

Randomized, nonblinded trial.

Inclusion Criteria

Patients with angiographically proven multivessel coronary artery disease suitable for both CABG and PTCA.

Patients and Follow-Up

1829 patients (mean age, 62 yrs; 73% men) with 5.4-yr mean follow-up.

Intervention

Patients were randomized to CABG or PTCA, and 98% had the assigned treatment.

Results

In-hospital death and stroke were not significantly different between the groups. Patients in the PTCA group were less likely to have an in-hospital MI (2.1% vs. 4.6%). There was no difference in 5-yr survival, but patients in the CABG group were less likely to require repeat revascularization [8% vs. 54%; number needed to treat (NNT), 2.2]. Diabetics assigned to CABG had significantly higher 5-yr survival (65.5% vs. 80.6%; NNT, 6.6).

In addition, 501 patients in the BARI trial had noncardiac surgery in the 8 yrs after enrollment. Perioperative cardiac mortality was similarly low in both groups (0.9% in CABG group, 1.2% in angioplasty group) as were perioperative nonfatal MIs (0.4% in each group).

Conclusions

Unselected patients with multivessel coronary artery disease have similar survival whether treated with CABG or PTCA. However, those assigned to CABG required less revascularization, and diabetics treated with CABG have higher 5-yr survival. The rates of perioperative cardiac mortality and MI were low when performed within 5 yrs of coronary intervention.

PERIOPERATIVE BETA BLOCKADE WITH BISOPROLOL

Poldermans D, Boersma E, Bax JJ, et al. The effect of bisoprolol on perioperative mortality and myocardial infarction in high-risk patients undergoing vascular surgery. *N Engl J Med* 1999;341:1789–1794.

Clinical Question

Does bisoprolol reduce perioperative mortality and MI in high-risk patients undergoing vascular surgery?

Design

Randomized, placebo-controlled trial.

Inclusion Criteria

Patients with at least one cardiac risk factor (history of congestive heart failure, prior MI, pathologic Q waves on ECG, diabetes, angina pectoris, aged >70 yrs, therapy for ventricular arrhythmias, or limited exercise capability) **and** evidence of inducible myocardial ischemia on dobutamine echocardiography.

Exclusion Criteria

Patients with extensive regional wall-motion abnormalities or strong evidence of left-main or severe three-vessel disease, patients already taking beta blockers, and those with asthma.

Patients and Follow-Up

Of 1351 screened, 112 qualified for the trial with 100% follow-up.

Intervention

Bisoprolol, 5 mg PO qd, was started 7 days preoperatively and continued for 30 days postoperatively. The dose was increased to 10 mg after 7 days, as tolerated, to keep HR >60. Other patients received standard medical therapy.

Results

Bisoprolol was associated with a cardiac mortality reduction of 80% (3.4% vs. 17%; $p = .02$) and a reduction of nonfatal MI (0% vs. 17%; $p < .001$).

Conclusions

Bisoprolol appears to reduce the risk of perioperative cardiac death and MI in high-risk patients undergoing vascular surgery. Because of the selection criteria used in this trial, the efficacy of bisoprolol in the group at highest risk could not be determined. This highest-risk group included those patients in whom coronary revascularization was considered or for whom the surgical procedure might ultimately be canceled. However, the rate of events in the standard care group (34%) suggests that patients at significant risk were enrolled in the trial.

CARE (CHOLESTEROL AND RECURRENT EVENTS)

Sacks FM, Pfeffer MA, Moye LA, et al. The effect of pravastatin on coronary events after myocardial infarction in patients with average cholesterol levels. Cholesterol and Recurrent Events Trial investigators. *N Engl J Med* 1996;335:1001–1009.

Clinical Question

In patients with previous MI and average blood lipid levels, does pravastatin prevent coronary events and stroke?

Design

Randomized, double-blinded, placebo-controlled trial.

Inclusion Criteria

Acute MI within previous 3–20 mos; total cholesterol <240 mg/dL; LDL, 115–174 mg/dL.

Exclusion Criteria

Age <50 yrs or >80 yrs, diastolic BP >115 mm Hg.

Patients and Follow-Up

1283 patients (mean age, 69 yrs; 82% men) with 5-yr median follow-up.

Intervention

Patients were assigned to pravastatin, 40 mg PO per day, or placebo. All patients also received dietary counseling according to National Cholesterol Education Program (NCEP) step 1 guidelines.

Results

Pravastatin significantly reduced the rate of major coronary events (RRR, 24%; NNT, 33), stroke (RRR, 31%; NNT, 34), coronary artery bypass graft (RRR, 26%; NNT, 40), and percutaneous transluminal coronary angioplasty (RRR, 23%; NNT, 45). Benefits were greater for women and those with higher pretreatment LDL. There was no significant difference in overall mortality or cardiovascular mortality.

Conclusions

There was clear benefit from pravastatin in reducing major coronary events and strokes among those with coronary disease and average cholesterol levels (LDL, 115–174). NCEP guidelines recommend target LDL of ≤ 100 mg/dL in those with known coronary artery disease or equivalent.

COPERNICUS (CARVEDILOL PROSPECTIVE RANDOMIZED CUMULATIVE SURVIVAL)

Packer M, Fowler MB, Roecker EB, et al. Effect of carvedilol on the morbidity of patients with severe chronic heart failure: results of the carvedilol prospective randomized cumulative survival (COPERNICUS) study. *Circulation* 2002;106(17):2194–2199.

Clinical Question

Does the beta blocker carvedilol reduce morbidity and mortality in stable patients with severe congestive heart failure?

Design

Randomized, double-blinded, placebo-controlled trial.

Inclusion Criteria

New York Heart Association (NYHA) class III or IV heart failure for >2 mos; LV ejection fraction <25%; minimal peripheral edema with no ascites or rales; no recent intravenous vasodilators or inotropes.

Exclusion Criteria

Recent coronary intervention, acute MI, stroke, or ventricular arrhythmia; SBP <85 mm Hg, HR <68 bpm, or creatinine >2.8; uncorrected primary valvular disease or presumed reversible cardiomyopathy.

Patients and Follow-Up

2289 patients with mean age of 63 yrs, followed for average of 10.4 mos with 100% follow-up.

Intervention

Placebo vs. carvedilol, started at 3.125 mg bid for 2 wks, then titrated to maximum of 25 mg bid as tolerated. The majority of patients in both groups were also on ACE inhibitors and diuretics.

Results

The group treated with carvedilol had a highly significant reduction in mortality at 1 yr (RRR, 35%; NNT, 15). The combined end point of death or hospitalization was also reduced (RRR, 24%; NNT, 10).

Conclusions

Although beta blockers had been previously proven effective in mild heart failure, many clinicians were still reluctant to use them in severe heart failure. COPERNICUS showed that carvedilol can be used safely in patients with class III and IV heart failure and provides even greater absolute mortality benefit. All patients in this study were compensated and euvolemic before starting beta blocker therapy.

CURE (CLOPIDOGREL IN UNSTABLE ANGINA TO PREVENT RECURRENT EVENTS)

Clopidogrel in unstable angina to prevent recurrent events. *N Engl J Med* 2001; 345(7):494–502.

Clinical Question

Does clopidogrel decrease mortality and myocardial infarction in patients with unstable angina or non–Q-wave MI?

Design

Randomized, double-blinded, placebo-controlled trial.

Inclusion Criteria

Patients hospitalized within 24 hrs with unstable angina and ECG changes or elevated cardiac enzymes.

Exclusion Criteria

Patients with ST elevation on ECG, contraindications to antithrombotic or antiplatelet therapy, severe heart failure, taking oral anticoagulants, PTCA or CABG in prior 3 mos, or glycoprotein IIb/IIIa receptor inhibitors in the prior 3 days.

Patients and Follow-Up

12,562 patients (6259 in clopidogrel, 6303 in placebo).

Intervention

Clopidogrel was administered with a 300-mg load followed by 75 mg PO qd or matching placebo for 3–12 mos (mean 9 mos). ASA, 75–325 mg/day, was also given.

Results

The clopidogrel group had a lower rate of combined death from cardiovascular causes, MI, and stroke (9.3% vs. 11.4%; $p < .001$). Major bleeding events occurred in 3.7% in the clopidogrel group vs. 2.7% in the placebo group ($p = .001$).

Conclusions

Clopidogrel decreases the rates of cardiovascular death, MI, or cerebrovascular accident in selected patients with unstable coronary syndromes but increases bleeding events.

ELITE II

Pitt B, Poole-Wilson PA, Segal R, et al. Effect of losartan compared with captopril on mortality in patients with symptomatic heart failure: randomised trial—the Losartan Heart Failure Survival Study ELITE II. *Lancet* 2000;355:1582–1587.

Clinical Question

In patients with symptomatic heart failure, is losartan more effective or better tolerated than captopril?

Design

Randomized, double-blinded trial.

Inclusion Criteria

Age ≥ 60 yrs, NYHA class II–IV heart failure, LV ejection fraction <40%.

Exclusion Criteria

Treated with ACE inhibitor in previous 3 mos, intolerant to ACE inhibitors, SBP <90 mm Hg or DBP >95 mm Hg, recent cardiac or cerebral event, or renal insufficiency.

Patients and Follow-Up

3152 patients (mean age, 71 yrs; 69% men) with median 1.5-yr follow-up. 99.9% follow-up.

Intervention

Patients were assigned to losartan, 12.5 mg PO daily, titrated to 50 mg PO daily, or captopril, 12.5 mg PO three times daily, titrated to 50 mg PO three times daily.

Results

There was no significant difference in mortality, sudden death or cardiac arrest, all-cause hospital admission, or heart failure–related hospital admission. Fewer patients discontinued losartan because of adverse effects (RRR, 34%; NNT, 20) and cough (RRR, 89%; NNT, 42).

Conclusions

Losartan did not prove more effective than captopril in treating symptomatic heart failure but was better tolerated. Until further studies document the efficacy of angiotensin receptor antagonists, ACE inhibitors remain the first-line treatment.

EPIC (EVALUATION OF PLATELET IIB/IIIA INHIBITION FOR THE PREVENTION OF ISCHEMIC COMPLICATIONS)

Multiple Citations

Topol EJ. Randomised trial of coronary intervention with antibody against platelet IIb/IIIa integrin for reduction of clinical restenosis: results at six months. The EPIC Investigators. *Lancet* 1994;343:881–886. (6-mo results.)

Use of a monoclonal antibody directed against the platelet glycoprotein IIb/IIIa receptor in high-risk coronary angioplasty. The EPIC Investigation. *N Engl J Med* 1994;330:956–961.

Topol EJ. Long-term protection from myocardial ischemic events in a randomized trial of brief integrin beta3 blockade with percutaneous coronary intervention. EPIC Investigator Group. Evaluation of Platelet IIb/IIIa Inhibition for Prevention of Ischemic Complication. *JAMA* 1997;278:479–484. (3-yr outcome.)

Clinical Question

Does IIb/IIIa inhibition with abciximab improve long-term results of restenosis and survival?

Design

Randomized, double-blinded, placebo-controlled trial.

Inclusion Criteria

Patients aged <80 yrs having angioplasty or atherectomy for coronary artery disease.

Patients and Follow-Up

2099 patients with 3-yr follow-up.

Intervention

Patients were randomized to placebo or abciximab, 0.25 mg/kg, bolus 10 min before procedure. Those receiving abciximab were randomized to 10 μg/min infusion $\times$ 12 hrs or matching placebo. All patients received ASA and heparin.

Results

At 30 days, patients receiving bolus and infusion of abciximab had decreased combined end point of death, MI, or need for revascularization (8.3% vs. 12.8%; $p = .008$). This benefit was still seen at 3 yrs (41.1% vs. 47.2%; $p = .009$) with no difference between placebo and bolus without infusion.

Conclusions

Bolus and infusion therapy of a IIb/IIIa platelet inhibitor decreases the combined end point of death, infarction, and need for revascularization for up to 3 yrs in patients undergoing coronary interventions.

ESSENCE (EFFICACY AND SAFETY OF SUBCUTANEOUS ENOXAPARIN VS. INTRAVENOUS UNFRACTIONATED HEPARIN, IN NON–Q-WAVE CORONARY EVENTS)

Cohen M, Demers C, Gurfinkel EP, et al. Low-molecular-weight heparins in non-ST-segment elevation ischemia: the ESSENCE trial. Efficacy and Safety of Subcutaneous Enoxaparin versus intravenous unfractionated heparin, in non-Q-wave Coronary Events. *Am J Cardiol* 1998;82(5B):19L–24L.

Clinical Question

Is the low-molecular-weight heparin enoxaparin comparable to unfractionated heparin in the treatment of unstable angina and non–Q-wave myocardial infarction?

Design

Randomized, double-blinded, placebo-controlled trial.

Inclusion Criteria

Angina at rest for >10 mins within 24 hrs of randomization along with objective evidence of underlying ischemic heart disease (new ST depression, documented history of myocardial infarction, revascularization, or myocardial ischemia).

Exclusion Criteria

Persistent ST elevation, left bundle branch block or paced rhythm, contraindication to anticoagulation, established precipitating cause for angina, creatinine clearance <30 mL/min.

Patients and Follow-Up

3171 patients followed for 30 days.

Intervention

In addition to standard therapy for unstable angina, patients received enoxaparin, 1 mg/kg SC every 12 hrs, or unfractionated heparin with PTT target of 55–85 secs.

Results

The triple end point of death, myocardial infarction, or recurrent angina was significantly lower in the enoxaparin group (RRR, 18%; NNT, 29) and there was no significant difference in major bleeding events.

Conclusions

Enoxaparin was shown to be a safe and effective alternative to unfractionated heparin in unstable angina, is easier to administer and monitor, and may provide more predictable anticoagulation.

FRISC II (FAST REVASCULARISATION DURING INSTABILITY IN CORONARY ARTERY DISEASE)

Wallentin L, Lagerqvist B, Husted S, et al. Outcome at 1 year after an invasive compared with a non-invasive strategy in unstable coronary-artery disease: the FRISC II invasive randomised trial. FRISC II Investigators. Fast Revascularisation during Instability in Coronary artery disease. *Lancet* 2000;356:9–16.

Clinical Question

In patients with unstable angina, is an invasive or noninvasive strategy better for reducing mortality, later cardiac procedures, MI, and hospital readmission?

Design

Randomized trial with 1-yr follow-up.

Inclusion Criteria

Patients with unstable coronary ischemia (increasing, at rest, suggestive of MI) and abnormal ECG or myocardial enzymes.

Exclusion Criteria

Need for thrombolysis in previous 24 hrs, bleeding or anemia, recent percutaneous transluminal coronary angioplasty, age >75 yrs, serious noncardiac illness.

Patients and Follow-Up

257 patients (70% men; mean age, 66 yrs) with 1-yr follow-up >99%.

Intervention

Invasive strategy was immediate angiography and revascularization, if necessary. Noninvasive strategy was angiography only if persistent symptoms, severe angina, or abnormal exercise test before discharge and revascularization only if incapacitating symptoms, recurrent unstable angina, or MI.

Results

Patients randomized to invasive strategy had significantly lower rates of MI (RRR, 25%; NNT, 35), death (RRR, 43%; NNT, 60), readmissions at 1 yr (RRR, 35%; NNT, 5), and cardiac procedures after discharge (RRR, 76%; NNT, 5).

Conclusions

Patients with unstable coronary artery disease benefited from an early invasive strategy, with lower rates of death, MI, readmission, and further invasive procedures.

Commentary

The results of FRISC II showed clear benefit to an early invasive strategy, in contrast to TIMI IIIB and VANQWISH trials. This may have been due to aggressive revascularization with coronary stents and abciximab in FRISC II.

GUSTO IIB (GLOBAL USE OF STRATEGIES TO OPEN OCCLUDED CORONARY ARTERIES IN ACUTE CORONARY SYNDROMES)

A clinical trial comparing primary coronary angioplasty with tissue plasminogen activator for acute myocardial infarction. The Global Use of Strategies to Open Occluded Coronary Arteries in Acute Coronary Syndromes (GUSTO IIb) Angioplasty Substudy Investigators. *N Engl J Med* 1997;336:1621–1628.

Clinical Question

In patients with acute ST-elevation MI, is primary angioplasty better than tissue plasminogen activator in preventing death, reinfarction, and stroke?

Design

Randomized, nonblinded trial.

Inclusion Criteria

Patients with ST-segment elevation on ECG who presented to the hospital within 12 hrs of onset of symptoms of acute MI.

Exclusion Criteria

Current warfarin treatment, bleeding, prior stroke, contraindication to heparin, renal insufficiency, BP >200/110, possible pregnancy.

Patients and Follow-Up

1138 patients (77% men) with 6-mo follow-up.

Intervention

Patients were assigned to primary angioplasty or accelerated tissue plasminogen activator (100 mg total).

Results

The primary composite end point of death, nonfatal reinfarction, and nonfatal stroke within 30 days occurred in significantly fewer patients in the angioplasty group (RRR, 30%; NNT, 25). At 6 mos, there was no significant difference in the primary end point.

Conclusions

Primary angioplasty showed a modest benefit over thrombolysis in patients with ST-elevation MI within 12 hrs. This benefit was apparent at 30 days, but not at 6 mos. In hospitals in which immediate angioplasty is available, it is a viable alternative to thrombolysis with similar long-term outcomes.

HOT (HYPERTENSION OPTIMAL TREATMENT)

Hansson L, Zanchetti A, Carruthers SG, et al. Effects of intensive blood-pressure lowering and low-dose aspirin in patients with hypertension: principal results of the Hypertension Optimal Treatment (HOT) randomised trial. HOT Study Group. *Lancet* 1998;351:1755–1762.

Clinical Question

In patients with HTN, does low-dose ASA prevent cardiovascular events and reduce cardiovascular mortality?

Design

Randomized, double-blinded, placebo-controlled trial.

Inclusion Criteria

Adults with HTN.

Exclusion Criteria

Age <50 yrs or >80 yrs, diastolic BP <100 mm Hg or >115 mm Hg.

Patients and Follow-Up

19,193 patients (mean age, 62 yrs; 53% men) with 3.8-yr mean follow-up (97%).

Intervention

Patients were assigned to ASA, 75 mg PO per day, or placebo. All patients were also treated for HTN with target diastolic BP of 90, 85, or 80 mm Hg.

Results

ASA significantly reduced the rate of major cardiovascular events (RRR, 15%; NNT, 176) and MI (RRR, 36%; NNT, 208). There was no significant increased risk of bleeding or intracranial hemorrhage.

Conclusions

Adults with treated HTN showed a modest absolute benefit from daily low-dose ASA.

MADIT (MULTICENTER AUTOMATIC DEFIBRILLATOR IMPLANTATION TRIAL)

Moss AJ. Improved survival with an implanted defibrillator in patients with coronary disease at high risk for ventricular arrhythmia. Multicenter Automatic Defibrillator Implantation Trial Investigators. *N Engl J Med* 1996;335:1933–1940.

Clinical Question

Does placement of an automatic implantable cardioverter-defibrillator (AICD) decrease mortality in patients with coronary disease at high risk for ventricular arrhythmia?

Design

Randomized, nonblinded trial.

Inclusion Criteria

Patients aged 25–80 yrs with known coronary artery disease (prior MI), LV ejection fraction <35%, documented asymptomatic nonsustained ventricular tachycardia who had inducible ventricular arrhythmia on electrophysiology study that was **not** suppressed by procainamide.

Exclusion Criteria

Patients with NYHA class IV heart failure, nonischemic cardiac disease, need for revascularization, MI in the last 3 wks, prior cardiac arrest/VT causing syncope or hypotension, diminished life expectancy from noncardiac disease, advanced cerebrovascular disease, recent coronary artery bypass (within 2 mos) or PTCA (within 3 mos), and women of childbearing age not on oral contraceptives.

Patients and Follow-Up

196 patients with mean follow-up of 27 mos.

Intervention

Patients were randomized to placement of a transthoracic or transvenous defibrillator or medical therapy determined by the patient's physician.

Results

Patients in the AICD group had decreased mortality (15/95 vs. 39/101; RRR, 54%; $p =$ .009). Six patients in the medical therapy group died of unknown causes.

Conclusions

Patients with ischemic cardiomyopathy with systolic dysfunction and inducible, nonsuppressible ventricular arrhythmia at EP study have decreased mortality by placement of an AICD.

MOCHA (MULTICENTER ORAL CARVEDILOL HEART FAILURE STUDY)

Bristow MR. Carvedilol produces dose-related improvements in left ventricular function and survival in subjects with chronic heart failure. MOCHA Investigators. *Circulation* 1996;94:2807–2816.

Clinical Question

Is there benefit from increasing doses of carvedilol in patients with stable, symptomatic heart failure?

Design

Randomized, double-blinded, placebo-controlled trial.

Inclusion Criteria

Age 18–85 yrs with symptomatic dilated cardiomyopathy and EF <35% for at least 6 mos and on stable doses of ACE inhibitors and diuretics.

Exclusion Criteria

Resting HR <68 bpm, sitting SBP >160 or <85 mm Hg, uncorrected valvular disease, hypertrophic or postpartum cardiomyopathy, uncontrolled sustained or symptomatic ventricular tachycardia, MI in the last 3 mos, anticipated PTCA/CABG/heart transplant within 6 mos, sick sinus syndrome, second- or third-degree AV block, COPD requiring therapy, cerebrovascular accident in the previous 3 mos, creatinine >2.5 mg/dL, transaminases >3× upper limits of normal, untreated endocrine disorder, alcohol intake >100 g/day, pregnant or lactating women, platelets <10 K, WBC <3 K, use of antiarrhythmics, monoamine oxidase inhibitors, calcium channel blockers, or amiodarone in the last 3 mos.

Patients and Follow-Up

345 patients followed for 6 mos.

Intervention

Patients were randomized to placebo or carvedilol at 6.25 mg PO bid (low dose), 12.5 mg PO bid (medium dose), or 25 mg PO bid (high dose).

Results

Patients on carvedilol had improved mortality at 6 mos compared to placebo (1.1% vs. 6.7% vs. 6.0% vs. 15.5% in high dose, medium dose, low dose, and placebo, respectively; p <.001), fewer hospitalizations (0.13, 0.15, 0.14 vs. 0.36 hospitalizations per patient, respectively; p = .01), and an improvement of radionuclide-calculated LV ejection fraction which was dose dependent.

Conclusions

Carvedilol may result in dose-related decrease in mortality and hospitalization, as well as improvement in LV function.

NASCET (NORTH AMERICAN SYMPTOMATIC CAROTID ENDARTERECTOMY TRIAL)

Barnett HJ. Benefit of carotid endarterectomy in patients with symptomatic moderate or severe stenosis. North American Symptomatic Carotid Endarterectomy Trial Collaborators. *N Engl J Med* 1998;339(20):1415–1425. (<70% stenosis.)

NASCET collaborators. Beneficial effect of carotid endarterectomy in symptomatic patients with high-grade carotid stenosis. North American Symptomatic Carotid Endarterectomy Trial Collaborators. *N Engl J Med* 1991;325:445–453. (>70% stenosis.)

Clinical Question

In patients with symptomatic carotid artery stenosis, is endarterectomy better than medical management?

Design

Randomized, nonblinded trial.

Inclusion Criteria

Carotid artery stenosis confirmed by angiography and symptoms of transient ischemic attack or nondisabling stroke.

Exclusion Criteria

Intracranial stenosis more significant than the carotid lesion, life expectancy <5 yrs, cardiac lesions likely to cause cardioembolism, nonatherosclerotic carotid disease, and severe ipsilateral cerebral infarction in the at-risk territory.

Patients and Follow-Up

2226 patients with average follow-up of 5 yrs and data on 99.7% in 1987–1996.

Intervention

Carotid endarterectomy vs. medical management (antiplatelet therapy; attempted smoking cessation; and control of diabetes, lipids, and HTN).

Results

In patients with >70% stenosis, the trial was stopped early with a 17% absolute risk reduction (ARR) of ipsilateral stroke at 2 yrs for surgery. In patients with 50–69% stenosis, the rates of stroke at 5 yrs were 15.7% for surgery and 22.2% for medical therapy (RRR, 29%; ARR, 6.5%; NNT, 15; $p = .045$). Greatest benefit was seen in men, recent stroke, and hemispheric symptoms (vs. retinal symptoms). In patients with <50% stenosis, there was no benefit from endarterectomy.

Conclusions

Endarterectomy is beneficial for patients with symptomatic carotid artery stenosis >70%. With stenosis 50–69%, benefit depends on rate of surgical complications and other risk of stroke. With stenosis <50%, endarterectomy is rarely indicated.

PRISM-PLUS (PLATELET RECEPTOR INHIBITION IN ISCHEMIC SYNDROME MANAGEMENT IN PATIENTS LIMITED BY UNSTABLE SIGNS AND SYMPTOMS)

Inhibition of the platelet glycoprotein IIb/IIIa receptor with tirofiban in unstable angina and non-Q-wave myocardial infarction. Platelet Receptor Inhibition in Ischemic Syndrome Management in Patients Limited by Unstable Signs and Symptoms (PRISM-PLUS) Study Investigators. *N Engl J Med* 1998;338(21):1488–1497.

Clinical Question

Does tirofiban, a glycoprotein IIb/IIIa inhibitor, decrease the rates of death and MI in patients with unstable angina or non–Q-wave MI?

Design

Randomized, double-blinded, placebo-controlled trial.

Inclusion Criteria

Patients with symptoms of unstable angina with new T ischemic changes on ECG (ST-segment changes of 0.1 mV or more, T-wave inversion of 0.3 mV or more in >2 limb leads or >3 precordial leads excluding V_1, or pseudonormalization of 0.1 mV or more) or an elevation of serum myocardial enzymes (CK-MB).

Exclusion Criteria

ST-segment elevation >20 mins, thrombolysis in the previous 48 hrs, PTCA <6 mos prior, CABG <1 mo prior, history of a platelet disorder, platelets <150 K, active bleeding or a high risk of bleeding, and creatinine >2.5 mg/dL.

Patients

1915 patients (347 in tirofiban only, 797 in heparin only, 773 in tirofiban + heparin).

Intervention

Three regimens were assigned: IV tirofiban + IV placebo heparin, tirofiban (0.4 μg/kg/min for 30 mins, then 0.1 μg/kg/min) + heparin titrated to 2× control value of PTT, or adjusted-dose heparin + placebo tirofiban. Study infusions were given for at least 48 hrs. No mechanical interventions were performed in this period unless there was refractory ischemia or new MI. All patients received ASA, 325 mg/day.

Results

Patients receiving tirofiban alone had an increased 7-day mortality (4.6% vs. 1.1%), and the tirofiban-only arm was stopped prematurely. The composite primary end points (death, MI, refractory ischemia) were lower among the tirofiban + heparin vs. heparin only (12.9% vs. 17.9%, $p = .004$ at 7 days; 27.7% vs. 32.1%, $p = .02$ at 6 mos), as were the frequency of death or MI (4.9% vs. 8.3%, $p = .006$ at 7 days; 8.7% vs. 11.9%, $p = .03$ at 30 days). Major bleeding occurred in 4% of the tirofiban + heparin group and 3% of the heparin-only group.

Conclusions

Tirofiban + heparin and ASA decreased the rate of death or MI up to 30 days in patients presenting with unstable angina or non–Q-wave MI.

RALES (RANDOMIZED ALDACTONE EVALUATION STUDY)

Pitt B. The effect of spironolactone on morbidity and mortality in patients with severe heart failure. Randomized Aldactone Evaluation Study Investigators. *N Engl J Med* 1999;341:709–717.

Clinical Question

Does the addition of spironolactone (Aldactone) to standard medical management for patients with a history of NYHA class IV heart failure improve morbidity or mortality?

Design

Randomized, double-blind, placebo-controlled trial.

Inclusion Criteria

Must have had NYHA class IV heart failure within 6 mos before enrollment and class III or IV at time of enrollment, ejection fraction of <35%, and treated medically with an ACE inhibitor and loop diuretic.

Exclusion Criteria

Treatment with K^+-sparing diuretic, serum K^+ >5.0, creatinine >2.5 mg/dL, post–heart transplant or on the transplant list, primary operable valvular disease, active cancer, unstable angina, congenital heart disease, primary hepatic failure, or other life-threatening conditions.

Patients and Follow-Up

1663 patients with mean follow-up of 24 mos.

Intervention

Spironolactone, 25 mg PO qd, or matching placebo. Dose was increased to 50 mg PO qd if progressive congestive heart failure and no hyperkalemia. Dose was decreased to 25 mg PO qod if hyperkalemia developed.

Results

At mean follow-up of 24 mos, patients randomized to spironolactone had decreased mortality (35% vs. 46%; p <.001), fewer hospitalizations for congestive heart failure (515 hospitalizations for 822 patients in intervention group vs. 753 for 841 patients in placebo group; RRR, 35%; p <.001), and greater improvement in NYHA classification (p <.001). Benefit was seen as early as 2–3 mos.

Conclusions

Spironolactone, when added to standard medical therapy, decreases mortality, hospitalizations, and improves symptoms in patients with class IV heart failure.

SAVE (SURVIVAL AND VENTRICULAR ENLARGEMENT TRIAL)

Pfeffer MA, Braunwald E, Moye LA, et al. Effect of captopril on mortality and morbidity in patients with left ventricular dysfunction after myocardial infarction. Results of the survival and ventricular enlargement trial. The SAVE Investigators. *N Engl J Med* 1992;327:669–677.

Clinical Question

Among those with asymptomatic LV dysfunction, does captopril, given 3–16 days after MI, reduce morbidity and mortality?

Design

Randomized, double-blinded, placebo-controlled trial.

Inclusion Criteria

Acute MI within previous 3–16 days, LV ejection fraction ≤ 40%, age 21–80 yrs.

Exclusion Criteria

Unstable clinical course, overt heart failure, symptoms of continuing ischemia, compelling indication or contraindication for captopril, or renal failure.

Patients and Follow-Up

2231 patients (mean age, 59 yrs; 82% men) with 42-mo mean follow-up. Follow-up was 99.7%.

Intervention

Patients were assigned to placebo or captopril, initially 12.5 mg PO tid, then increased to 50 mg PO tid if no side effects.

Results

Captopril significantly reduced 42-mo mortality (RRR, 17%; NNT, 24), cardiovascular deaths (RRR, 20%; NNT, 24), incidence of serious heart failure (RRR, 34%; NNT, 56), hospitalization for heart failure (RRR, 14%; NNT, 29), and MI (RRR, 22%; NNT, 30).

Conclusions

Captopril started 3–16 days after MI reduced long-term mortality and cardiovascular morbidity among those with LV dysfunction but not overt heart failure.

SOLVD (STUDIES OF LEFT VENTRICULAR DYSFUNCTION)

Effect of enalapril on mortality and the development of heart failure in asymptomatic patients with reduced left ventricular ejection fractions. The SOLVD Investigators. *N Engl J Med* 1992;327:685–691.

Clinical Question

In patients with asymptomatic LV dysfunction, does enalapril reduce mortality, progression to symptomatic heart failure, and hospitalization?

Design

Randomized, double-blinded, placebo-controlled trial.

Inclusion Criteria

Patients with LV ejection fraction <35% but not taking digoxin, diuretics, or vasodilators for heart failure. Patients could be taking these medications for other indications.

Exclusion Criteria

Symptomatic heart failure during 3-wk run-in period.

Patients and Follow-Up

4228 patients (mean age, 59 yrs; 89% men) with 37-mo mean follow-up.

Intervention

Patients were assigned to treatment with enalapril (2.5 mg PO twice daily then 10 mg PO twice daily if no side effects) or placebo.

Results

Patients in the treatment group were significantly less likely to develop symptomatic heart failure (RRR, 31%; NNT, 11), be hospitalized for heart failure (RRR, 32%; NNT, 14), and be hospitalized for other cardiovascular reasons (RRR, 9%; NNT, 24). There was no significant mortality difference.

Conclusions

Enalapril reduced the development of heart failure and hospitalizations in patients with asymptomatic ventricular dysfunction.

Commentary

The SOLVD study showed that, in addition to their established role in overt heart failure, ACE inhibitors can slow progression in patients with asymptomatic LV dysfunction.

SPAF (STROKE PREVENTION IN ATRIAL FIBRILLATION)

SPAF Investigators. Preliminary report of the Stroke Prevention in Atrial Fibrillation Study. *N Engl J Med* 1990;322:863–868. (Preliminary results.)
SPAF Investigators. Stroke Prevention in Atrial Fibrillation Study. Final results. *Circulation* 1991;84:527–539. (Final results.)

Clinical Question

Are ASA and warfarin effective in reducing rates of stroke and systemic embolism in patients with nonrheumatic atrial fibrillation?

Design

Randomized, double-blinded, and placebo-controlled (to ASA); open label to warfarin.

Inclusion Criteria

Patients with atrial fibrillation (chronic or paroxysmal).

Exclusion Criteria

Congestive heart failure, prosthetic valves, or rheumatic heart disease.

Patients and Follow-Up

There were four study cohorts. 627 patients in group 1 were randomized to warfarin and then randomized and blinded to ASA or placebo. 703 patients in group 2 were randomized to no warfarin and then to blinded ASA or placebo. The trial was halted early at 1.1 yrs and the placebo arm discontinued. Total follow-up was 1.3 yrs.

Intervention

Warfarin with INR target of 2–4.5 and ASA vs. placebo.

Results

Warfarin with ASA or placebo reduced ischemic stroke or embolism (2.3% vs. 7.4%; RRR, 67%; $p = .01$) as did ASA with or without warfarin (3.6% vs. 6.3%; RRR, 42%; $p = .02$). The risk of significant bleeding was not increased by warfarin or ASA (1.5% vs. 1.4%, respectively, vs. 1.6% for placebo).

Conclusions

Warfarin and aspirin are effective in decreasing the rate of ischemic and embolic strokes in patients with nonrheumatic atrial fibrillation.

SPAF III (STROKE PREVENTION IN ATRIAL FIBRILLATION)

SPAF Investigators. Adjusted-dose warfarin versus low-intensity, fixed-dose warfarin plus aspirin for high-risk patients with atrial fibrillation: Stroke Prevention in Atrial Fibrillation III randomised clinical trial. *Lancet* 1996;348:633–638.

Clinical Question

Is adjusted-dose warfarin or ASA + fixed-dose warfarin a superior anticoagulation strategy for preventing stroke in patients with atrial fibrillation at high risk for stroke?

Design

Randomized, nonblinded trial.

Inclusion Criteria

Patients with atrial fibrillation and at least one risk factor (as identified in SPAF II): congestive heart failure or LV dysfunction, SBP >160 mm Hg, prior cerebrovascular accident or thromboembolism, or woman >75 yrs old.

Exclusion Criteria

Patients with prosthetic valves, hemodynamically significant mitral stenosis, recent pulmonary embolism, or frequent NSAID use were excluded.

Patients and Follow-Up

1044 patients with a mean follow-up of 1.1 yrs with early termination.

Intervention

Patients were randomized to (a) warfarin with an INR goal of 2–3 or (b) ASA, 325 mg PO qd + fixed-dose warfarin (0.5–3 mg PO per day titrated to achieve INR 1.2–1.5 on consecutive measurements).

Results

Combined events of ischemic stroke and embolism were decreased in the adjusted-dose warfarin group (1.9% vs. 7.9%; p <.0001) as were disabling or fatal stroke (1.7% vs. 5.6%; p = .0007). Major bleeding episodes were comparable for adjusted-dose warfarin and ASA/fixed-dose warfarin (2.1% vs. 2.4%).

Conclusion

Patients with atrial fibrillation and at least one other risk factor (congestive heart failure, prior embolism, prior cerebrovascular accident/transient ischemic attack, SBP >160 mm Hg, or woman aged >75 yrs) benefit from adjusted-dose warfarin instead of ASA + low-intensity fixed-dose warfarin.

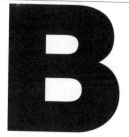

Preoperative Antibiotic Prophylaxis

Nature of operation	Likely pathogens	Recommended preoperative antibiotic (one dose on call to OR unless otherwise specified)
Cardiac		
Prosthetic valve, coronary artery bypass, other open heart surgery, implantation of pacemaker or defibrillator	*Staphylococcus epidermidis*, *Staphylococcus aureus*, *Corynebacterium*, enteric gram-negative bacilli	Cefazolin, 1–2 g IV Or cefuroxime, 1–2 g IV Or vancomycin, 1 g IV
GI		
Esophageal	Enteric gram-negative bacilli	High risk only: cefazolin, 1–2 g IV
Gastroduodenal	Enteric gram-negative bacilli	High risk only: cefazolin, 1–2 g IV
Biliary tract	Enteric gram-negative bacilli, enterococci, clostridia	High risk only: cefazolin, 1–2 g IV
Colorectal	Enteric gram-negative bacilli, anaerobes, enterococci	PO: neomycin + erythromycin base Parenteral: cefoxitin, 1–2 g IV Or cefotetan, 1–2 g IV Or cefazolin, 1–2 g IV + metronidazole, 500 mg IV
Appendectomy (non-perforated)	Enteric gram-negative bacilli, anaerobes, enterococci	Cefoxitin, 1–2 g IV Or cefotetan, 1–2 g IV
Genitourinary	Enteric gram-negative bacilli, enterococci	High risk only: ciprofloxacin, 500 mg PO or 400 mg IV
Gynecologic or obstetric		
Vaginal or abdominal hysterectomy	Enteric gram-negatives, anaerobes, group B streptococci, enterococci	Cefazolin, 1–2 g IV Or cefotetan, 1–2 g IV Or cefoxitin, 1 g IV

(continued)

Nature of operation	Likely pathogens	Recommended preoperative antibiotic (one dose on call to OR unless otherwise specified)
Cesarean section	Enteric gram-negatives, anaerobes, group B streptococci, entero-cocci	High risk only: cefazolin, 1 g IV after cord clamping
Abortion	Enteric gram-negatives, anaerobes, group B streptococci, entero-cocci	First trimester, high risk: aqueous penicillin G, 2 MU IV Or doxycycline, 300 mg PO
Head and neck surgery		
Incisions through PO or pharyngeal mucosa	Anaerobes, enteric gram-negative bacilli, S. aureus	Clindamycin, 600–900 mg IV Or gentamicin, 1.5 mg/kg IV
Neurosurgery		
Craniotomy	S. aureus, S. epidermidis	Cefazolin, 1–2 g IV Or vancomycin, 1 g IV
Ophthalmic	S. aureus, S. epidermidis, streptococci, enteric gram-negative bacilli, Pseudomonas	Gentamicin, tobramycin, ciprofloxacin, ofloxacin Or neomycin-gramicidin-polymyxin B; multiple drops topically over 2–24 hrs
Orthopedic		
Total joint replacement, internal fixation of fractures	S. aureus, S. epidermidis	Cefazolin, 1–2 g IV Or vancomycin, 1 g IV
Thoracic (noncardiac)	S. aureus, S. epidermidis, streptococci, enteric gram-negative bacilli	Cefazolin, 1–2 g IV Or vancomycin, 1 g IV
Vascular		
Arterial surgery involving prosthesis, abdominal aorta, or groin incision	S. aureus, S. epidermidis, enteric gram-negative bacilli	Cefazolin, 1–2 g IV Or vancomycin, 1 g IV
Lower-extremity amputation for ischemia	S. aureus, S. epidermidis, enteric gram-negative bacilli, clostridia	Cefazolin, 1–2 g IV Or vancomycin, 1 g IV
Contaminated surgery		
Ruptured viscus	Enteric gram-negative bacilli, anaerobes, enterococci	Cefoxitin, 1–2 g IV q6h Or cefotetan, 1–2 g IV q12h ± Gentamicin, 1.5 mg/kg IV q8h
Traumatic wound	S. aureus, group A streptococci, Clostridia	Cefazolin, 1–2 g IV q8h

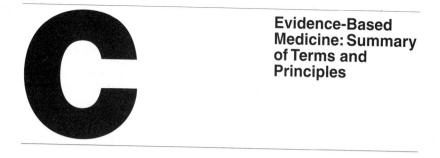

Evidence-Based
Medicine: Summary
of Terms and
Principles

Below is a description of some of the terms most commonly used in evidence-based medicine and used throughout this manual.

The **p value** is used throughout clinical trials and represents the likelihood that the results of a trial may be due to chance alone. For instance, a p value of .01 means that there is a 1% chance that the results of the trial are due to chance alone; a p value of .2 means that there is a 20% chance that the results are due to chance. In medicine, a p value of $<.05$ is taken to be statistically significant. The 95% confidence interval is the range of values that within which we can be 95% certain that the true result lies.

TERMS USED IN DIAGNOSTIC STUDIES

Many of the terms are based on calculations using the following table:

	Has the tested disorder	Doesn't have the tested disorder
Test positive	**a** (True-positive)	**b** (False-positive)
Test negative	**c** (False-negative)	**d** (True-negative)

Sensitivity: The proportion of those who have the disorder who test positive = $(a/[a + c])$.
Specificity: The proportion of those who do not have the disorder who test negative = $(d/[b + d])$.

Tests with high sensitivity have few false negatives, and a negative result is then useful in ruling out a disorder.

Tests with high specificity have few false positives, and a positive result is useful in ruling in a disorder.

Likelihood ratios (LRs) represent the ratio of the probability of the test result (positive or negative) among those who **have** the tested disorder to the probability of the test result among those who **do not have** the tested disorder.

The LR for a positive test = sensitivity / (1-specificity) = a/(a + c)/b/(b + d)

The LR for a negative test = (1-sensitivity) / specificity = c/(a + c)/d/(b + d)

The usefulness of the likelihood ratio is that it allows the clinician to extrapolate the results of the test to different populations where the disease prevalence differs. The clinician may estimate the likelihood of the patient having the disease (pretest odds) based on the available information (disease prevalence based on epidemiology, historical factors, exam, other data). The influence of the test result may then be expressed simply as follows:

Posttest odds = Pretest odds × LR.

TERMS USED IN THERAPEUTIC TRIALS

The **experimental event rate** (EER) is the rate (percentage of patients experiencing the event) of events in the group receiving the intervention. The **control event rate** (CER) is the rate of events among those not receiving the intervention.

Absolute risk reduction (ARR) represents the difference in adverse events between the experimental and control groups = EER − CER. Absolute risk increase (ARI) is used if more adverse events occur in the experimental group.

Relative risk reduction (RRR) represents the proportion of the reduction in event rates from the tested intervention = (EER − CER) / CER. Relative risk increase (RRI) is the correlate used to quantify harm.

The **number needed to treat** (NNT) is the number of patients that need to receive the intervention to prevent one event = 1/ARR. If the experimental group has more adverse events, then number needed to harm (NNH) is used.

Index

Note: Page numbers followed by *f* refer to figures; page numbers followed by *t* refer to tables.

Notes